The Quest to Know the Human Heart

The Disruptors Who Created Modern Cardiology and Cardiac Surgery

by Stephen B Guss, M.D.

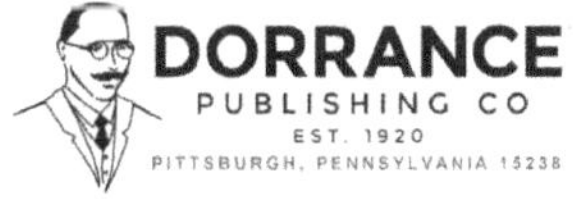

DORRANCE PUBLISHING CO

EST. 1920

PITTSBURGH, PENNSYLVANIA 15238

Dorrance Publishing Co
585 Alpha Drive
Suite 103
Pittsburgh, PA 15238
Visit our website at *www.dorrancebookstore.com*

ISBN: 979-8-89211-914-6
eISBN: 979-8-89211-842-2

The Quest to Know the Human Heart

The Disruptors Who Created Modern Cardiology and Cardiac Surgery

I want to thank my wife, Toni, for her love, patience, support, encouragement, and editorial advice during the year-and-one-half writing process of this book.

I am especially grateful to scientists who graciously and patiently gave me time, editorial critiques, and advice for my book, including:

Dr. Eugene Braunwald
Dr. Gary Roubin
Dr. K. Peter Rentrop
Dr. Richard Schatz
Dr. Alden Harken
Dr. Bruce Fye
Dr. Audrey Von Poelnitz
Dr. Mark Goldman
Dr. Igor Palacios
Dr. Robert Kipperman

Dr O.H Frazier

And to those who graciously gave permission to use their personal photos:

Dr. James Shelburne
Dr. Ronald Scherlag
Dr. Joseph Alpert
Dr. Yong-jian Geng
Dr. Moses Menendez
Dr. Goran Hansson
Dr. Gary Roubin
Dr. Richard Schatz
Dr. Peter Rentrop
Dr. Mark Goldman
Dr. Alden Harken
ARTIST JAMES CROWLEY
Dr. Gerald Pohost
Dr. Igor Palacios
Dr. Matthew Budoff

And to David Gavasheli and Dr. Roy Nuzzo, whose artistic talents in portraiture I relied upon.

And to Dr. Jennifer Guss for her editing and ideas.

Special thanks to Paul Gibilisco for his understanding and hours of computer technical support.

CONTENTS

FOREWORD

THE DISRUPTORS – THE SCIENTISTS WHO GAVE US TODAY'S CARDIOLOGY AND CARDIAC SURGERY

I have written this book hoping that learning about the past will help the reader better understand our present knowledge, diagnostic techniques, and treatments of today's cardiology and maybe even anticipate what may come in the future. I am also hopeful that this knowledge will allow patients who already have heart disease to better understand what their disease is and why their treatment program has been chosen by their internist or cardiologist. This book is about over five hundred years of "Disruptors," scientists who broke the mold, implemented something entirely new, and changed the course of cardiology and cardiac surgery.

Why study the history of cardiology at all? As Maya Angelou said, "You can't really know where you are going until you know where you have been" (Jan. 9, 2021).

This book also demonstrates over and over again during cardiac scientific discovery the principle espoused by that wise philosopher, my own personal favorite philosopher, Yogi Berra: "You've got to be very careful if you don't know where you are going, because you might not get there" and "If you don't know where you are going, you might wind up someplace else."

The reader also will see how progress was sometimes impeded by other scientists due to pride, arrogance, professional jealousy, desire for failure of others (schadenfreude), or failure to follow the scientific principles of inquiry and questioning. Sometimes researchers abandoned cardiology pursuits because cardiac disease was not considered very important in the scheme of other medical diseases at the time.

And sometimes scientists were seduced by other new discoveries being discussed in scientific circles, such as the new field of bacteriology, rather than concentrating or studying the heart.

It would be wise for all of us to remember the words of the great Sir William Osler, often considered the Father of Modern Medicine: "How eminent so ever a man may become in science, he is apt to carry with him errors which were in vogue when he was young—errors that darken his understanding, and make him incapable of accepting even the most obvious of truths."

During the 47½ years that I have practiced cardiology, my patients have been the beneficiaries of great advances, discoveries, revolutionary medications and new medical inventions and devices. I also enjoyed as a practitioner the amazing changes in technology not available when I first entered the field that have excited me almost daily and continued to evolve or even totally change with time. I have been living through the "Golden Era of Cardiology." Cardiology was the main medical beneficiary of space-age technology and even more than many medical specialties continued to look for even newer technologies and adapt them for better patient care. For example, it was important to monitor remotely the vital signs of astronauts in space, and this became the basis of today's cardiac monitoring. But it wasn't always this way.

Before the seventeenth century, very little was known about the heart and how it worked except for anatomic descriptions from autopsies, which were often wrongly described or the findings misinterpreted. Before the 1600s, the common wisdom about how the heart functioned and its purpose was totally in error. This ignorance was largely due to the fact that cardiac knowledge was static for nearly fourteen hundred years and limited to anatomic information without live physio-logical experiments to explain the abnormalities found at autopsies. The autopsy abnormalities found rarely could be related to live people. Galen of Pergamon (Greek physician, a.k.a. Galen, 129 A.D.-216 A.D., born Pergamon, Turkey, and died Rome, Roman Empire) ascended to the pinnacle of medicine. He claimed knowledge in most fields and amazingly was challenged by none. He was even known for verbally bullying others into accepting his premises. During this medically dark 1400-year period, new theories were not even proposed, and Galen's teachings were blindly accepted by other physicians. In the 1600s European doctors started experimenting and challenging the old teachings of the great guru of medical thought, Galen, who was often wrong. In the mid-1600s some thoughtful physicians for the first time began performing physiologic experiments and correlating their findings on living hearts of animals and blood vessels of living humans. These studies revealed not only how a normal heart worked but also explained some clinical disease states allowing for the first-time diagnoses to be made while patients were still alive rather than postmortem.

Dr. James Herrick in his book (*A SHORT HISTORY OF CARDIOLOGY,* 1942) wrote that Galen "muddied rather than clarified the conception of heart disease for so long a time… in some respects he materially retarded the advance of medical science."

I have organized this book by what I consider important topics into seventeen chapters with discussion of specific physicians in each chapter who brought cardiology into the modern era and out of the Dark Age of beliefs. Finally, I have tried to put most of the scientists discussed in the historical context of his or her time in the world and country in which they lived to give the reader an idea of what was happening around the scientists when they made their contribution. Although not a comprehensive survey, in my judgment it includes some of the most important advances, the main scientists and cardiologists of each era and topic discussed, and the most important topics in cardiology that we care about today. Each chapter will also have a personal anecdote from my own 47-plus years of clinical experience that is related to that chapter, some of which I hope the reader will find as amusing as I did at the time as cardiology is not always serious.

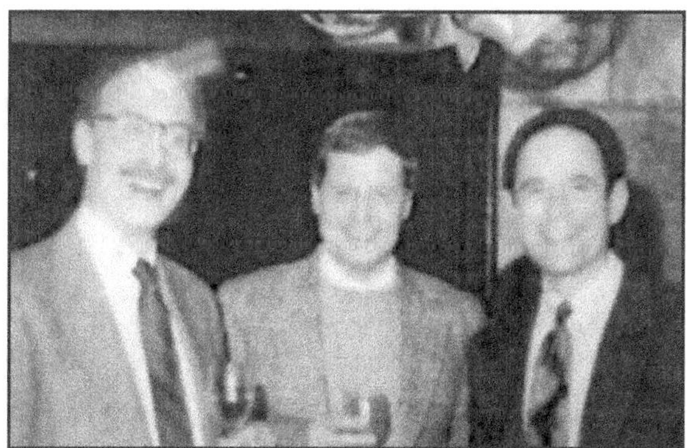

Author,Dr Lawrence Lubow, Dr Arthurs Fisch original Morristown
Cardiology Associates doctors
author's personal collection

I have had an unique opportunity, as I have practiced cardiology until age eighty and began my cardiology training way back in 1972, fifty years before. I have lived through the most rapid improvements in technology and cardiac knowledge in history. Furthermore, I have even known many of the people discussed in this book personally or met many of the 20th- and 21st-century leaders and cardiology pioneers casually at meetings and lectures. When I started as an internal medical intern, coronary care units (CCUs) were just being opened. The only in-hospital monitoring technologically available then required a three-to-four-foot cord tethered to the patient from the monitor with no remote "Bluetooth" monitoring we take for granted today. Few hospitals were performing heart catheterization, and angioplasty and stenting were not even imagined by any of us in the field. Stress testing was just changing over from a primitive and less sensitive two-step Master's test with two electrocardiograms (EKG) taken (before and after walking up and down two steps for a period of time) to electric treadmills for exercising a patient with continuous electrocardiographic monitoring of the entire 12-lead EKG while walking. Nuclear stress tests were not as yet invented; pacemakers were in their infancy and quite primitive compared to those of today; echocardiography was simple and of limited utility diagnostically. The reader will be introduced to how the cardiology profession came to perform coronary artery stenting, echocardiography, complicated and multifunctional pacemakers, and various modern cardiac surgeries. Today, cardiology is an entirely different specialty than even fifty years ago. At the mid-20th century, most cardiologists also practiced general internal medicine. The true specialty of practicing only cardiology did not emerge until the mid-1960s, when I entered the specialty. Because of the explosion of medical knowledge, today cardiology is so subspecialized that many cardiologists no longer practice anything but their sub or even sub-sub specialty within cardiology. These recent areas of specialization include interventional cardiology (cardiac catheterization and coronary artery stenting), structural cardiology (fixing and replacing heart valves without surgery), electrophysiology (the abnormal rhythms of the heart and pacemakers), imaging (echocardiography, nuclear cardiology, cardiac MRI and cardiac PET scanning), pediatric cardiology, and heart failure specialists performing preop evaluation and post-surgical care. There are even cardiac oncologists who deal with the side-effects of cancer drugs on the heart. I am certain that within a decade, other subspecialties of cardiology will also emerge.

I have at the end of each chapter defined in a glossary of terms some of the words that we cardiologists use but are not commonly used by non-physicians. So let's start our story.

CHAPTER 1
THE DEVELOPMENT OF CARDIAC PHYSICAL DIAGNOSIS

I followed her course for at least ten years. Sally was mildly short of breath when I first saw her, and she had a systolic murmur (a noise made by turbulent blood flow in the pumping phase of the heart) heard where the heart impulse is felt in the chest (called the apex). I categorized her heart murmur as grade II/VI. The echocardiogram (ultrasound of the heart) only showed mild mitral regurgitation or leakage of the valve separating the left atrium and left ventricle on the left side, as some of the blood went in the wrong direction out of the left ventricle back to the left atrium instead of out to the body. She did well for the next ten years and continued to exercise but a year ago developed increasing shortness of breath once again, and her heart murmur was now longer in the cycle and grade IV/VI in loudness. I was certain that her mitral regurgitation had worsened and ordered a follow-up echocardiogram, which confirmed what I heard with my stethoscope. After undergoing surgical repair of her mitral valve, she was exercising normally again. Sometimes all you need is a stethoscope and properly listening ears to make a diagnosis. My Harvard Medical School physical diagnosis instructor Dr. Howard Corning used to say, "It's not what's between the tubes but what's between the ears that counts." He also criticized us Harvard Medical students for always thinking that when hearing hoofbeats, zebras were coming rather than horses.

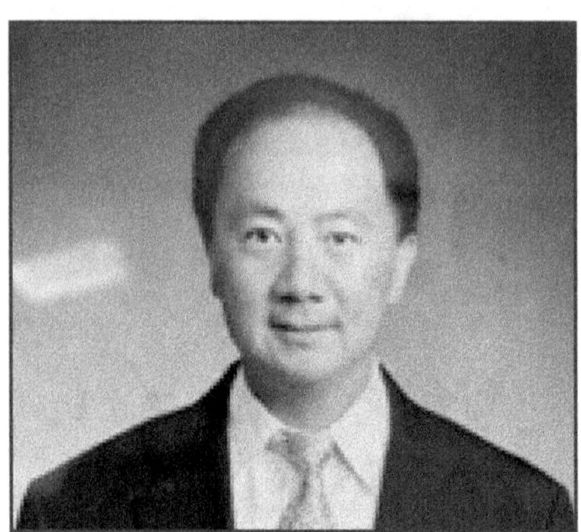

Dr Alan Hsieh, director of echocardiogrphy, Morristown Cardiology Assoc
author's personal collection

Until the 1800s most cardiac diagnoses were made after a patient died, usually by autopsy, until physical diagnosis came into being. This required new approaches to examining a patient, percussing (tapping) the chest and a new unique instrument, the stethoscope, which allowed physicians to make many diagnoses while patients were still alive by listening for certain noises (called heart murmurs) only made by abnormally diseased hearts. By and large, until this era, the physical diagnosis of the heart was confined to feeling the pulse at the wrist, watching the breathing pattern, and looking at the patient's skin color for signs of pallor or blueness known as cyanosis. We can thank much of early cardiac progress to the Disruptors who changed the way we examined patients and the information that could be gleaned from physical diagnosis that remains important even today despite our high-tech sophisticated equipment.

The first of the diagnosticians went a step further than his contemporaries and used his fingers to percuss (i.e. tap) the chest. Leopold Auenbrugger (1722-1809, born Graz, Austria, and died Vienna, Austria) lived at the time when the United States was still a British colony fighting for the English against the French in the French and Indian War (1754-1763) on the American continent. After two years into the war, England declared war on France (the Seven Years' War). This war ended in France, ceding Canada and its land along the Mississippi to England. Auenbrugger lived in the Habsburg Empire in Austria, then ruled by Maria Theresa from 1740-1780, the only female to have the title of Holy Roman Empress. Although primarily a German-speaking aristocracy, the empire also included Hungary and Italian-speaking Lombardy and Venetia, as well as what later became Czechoslovakia, the Balkan Peninsula and parts of Romania and Poland. In 1804 the Habsburgs changed the name to the Austrian Empire, and later split into the Austro-Hungarian Empire in 1867.

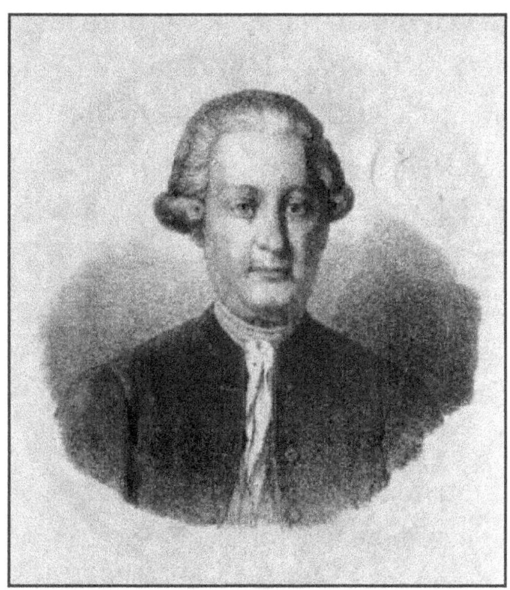

LEOPOLD AUENBRUGGER
National Library of Medicine, public domain

Due to his experiences with percussing his family's wine barrels in their wine business to assess the level of wine inside, Auenbrugger adopted this technique to evaluate the lung and was able to make conclusions about lung disease from tapping on the chest. He published in 1754 his observations on his new physical diagnostic technique, noting normal chest percussion findings and abnormalities. His findings took some time to be adopted by other doctors, but to this day his percussive methods are used by skilled physical diagnosticians along the lines described by Auenbrugger.

The real breakthrough for the Era of Cardiac Physical Diagnosis, that is, examining the heart from the outside of the body, was due to Theophile Hyacinthe Rene Laennec (1781-1826, born Quimper, France, and died Ploare, France). Laennec is the inventor of the first stethoscope and is rightly referred to as the Father of Physical Diagnosis. He was carving his new invention, the stethoscope, at the time of the signing of the Treaty of Paris in 1815, when Napoleon was defeated for a second time after his escape from Elba in the Battle of Waterloo. Laennec, who already knew how to carve wooden flutes, made his new invention from carved wood in 1816 and published his findings in 1819.

He first had the inspiration for his idea after observing two children sending signals from one piece of wood to another connected by scratching a needle on the wood. Looking much different than those of today, his stethoscope was a straight, hollowed-out short wooden tube (one end to the doctor's ear and the other against the patient's chest). By putting distance between patient's bare chest and the doctor's ear, his invention's design was Laennec's attempt to preserve modesty for young female patients. His ability to carve wooden flutes helped him invent the stethoscope especially after noticing that a cylindrical piece of paper placed on the chest at one end and to one's ear at the other increased sound transmission. Subsequently, others made variations in the shape of the earpiece. The stethoscope continued to undergo further improvements with time and is still used today, much improved and even continuing to improve, being now binaural rather than monaural and sometimes even electrical. Laennec's instrument paved the way for diagnostic cardiology to determine the cause, type and severity of heart disease before a postmortem was performed, simply by listening to the heart sounds through the chest wall. He was the first physician to describe the sound made by blood coursing through fused and thickened mitral valve leaflets (the two normally thin pieces of tissue that open and close with each heartbeat to allow blood to flow synchronously from the upper-left atrium to the left ventricle below). This thickening of the mitral valve is known as mitral stenosis and is usually caused by rheumatic fever, although its cause was not understood back in 1816. When the leaflets are fused tightly in the semi-closed position, blood backs up into the lungs, causing severe shortness of breath followed by leg swelling. Thus, his invention and some of his auditory observations ushered in a new era of physical diagnosis for heart disease diagnosis and treatment. He was primarily interested in lung disease despite his cardiac contributions, probably because his mother died when he was age five of tuberculosis.

Laennec lived in France at the time of the French Revolution, although he was a small child when it occurred. In 1802 General LeClerc led troops to suppress the uprising of the black population in Haiti. In 1803 the Louisiana Purchase occurred when France sold Louisiana to the U.S. during Jefferson's presidency. Napoleon crowned himself emperor in 1804, and his first major battle victory occurred in 1805 at the Battle of Austerlitz against Austria, Russia, England, and Sweden. In 1814 Napoleon surrendered, abdicated, and was exiled on the island of Elba, allowing the Bourbon Monarchy with Louis XVIII to return to the French throne. One year before Laennec's invention, Napoleon in 1815 escaped from Elba but lost in his famous Battle of Waterloo against an opposition coalition army and died in 1821. In 1830 another revolution occurred in France, overthrowing the Bourbon king and replacing him with Louis-Philippe as King of France. A failed attempted assassination occurred in 1832. French troops withdrew from Mexico in 1839, and the February Revolution occurred in 1848. At the end of that year, Louis Napoleon Bonaparte started his term as the first president of the French Republic. He was the son of Louis Bonaparte, King of Holland, the younger brother of Napoleon.

By 1855 the first binaural stethoscope was invented. Remember that Laennec's was for only one ear. The new changes were made by Golding Bird (1814-1854, born Downham, Norfolk, UK, and died London, UK), who first described a stethoscope with flexible tubes but only a single earpiece. In 1851 Arthur Leared (1822-1879, born Wexford, Ireland, and died London, UK) invented a binaural stethoscope for the first time with flexible tubes similar to today's instruments with a tube going into each ear. Maurice Rappaport, an electrical engineer, and Howard B. Sprague, a cardiologist (1895-1970, born Swampscott, Mass., and died Boston, Mass., U.S.), changed the stethoscope to two heads in the 1940s, one with a bell shape and one with a flat diaphragm to better hear either low- or higher-pitched murmurs and sounds. David Littman (1906-1981, born Chelsea, Mass., U.S., and died Boston, Mass., U.S.) in 1960 developed the first of his lighter stethoscopes all with improved acoustics, which have become the standard for doctors of today.

Subsequently electronic stethoscopes to enhance sound amplification have been marketed but provide little value unless amplification is required by a physician with reduced hearing. These electronic stethoscopes often capture too much background noise. Besides its value over the years diagnostically, the stethoscope has become the iconic symbol of the medical profession and medical care.

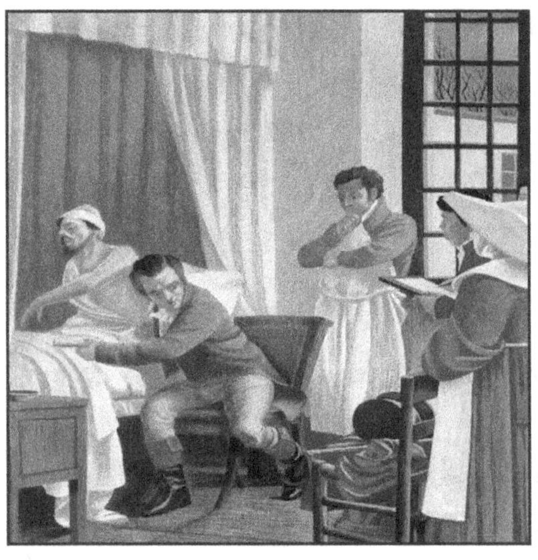

Courtesy of the Wellcome Collection
Painting by T. Chartran of Laennec
Examining a patient and license by Alamy

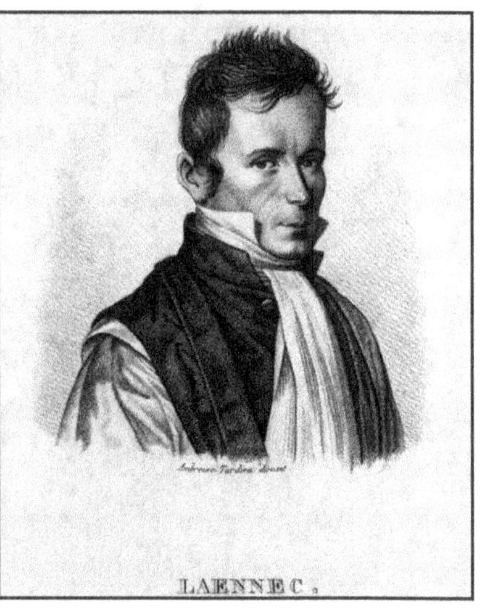

RENE LAENNEC,
licensed by Alamy

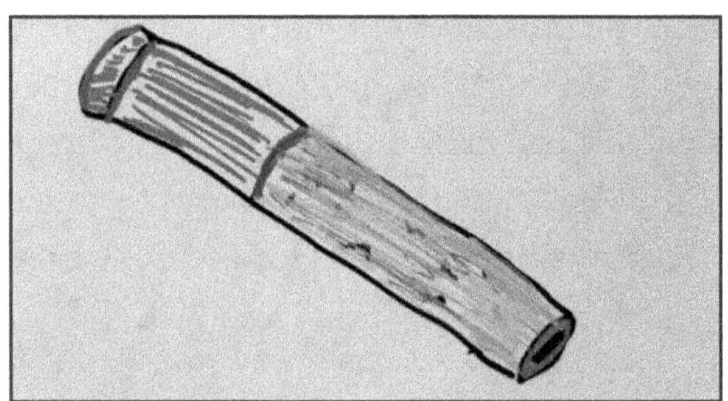

Laennec's first stethoscope; drawing by author

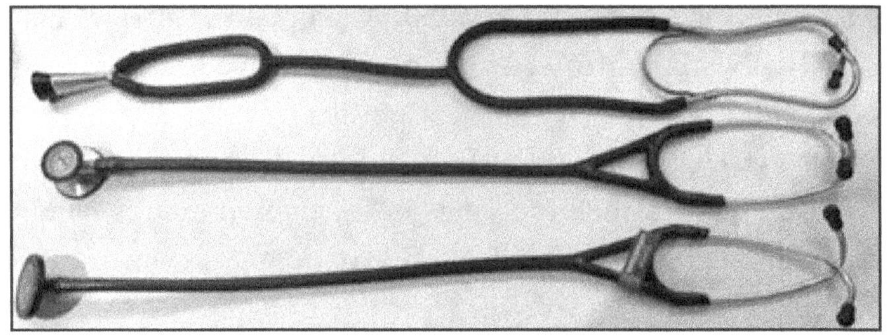

Stethoscopes owned by author above: Single-head used by author's surgeon
father-in-law, Dr. Otto Weiss, in the 1950s
Middle: Double-headed Littman, owned by author
Below: Single-headed Littman, owned by author

JOSEF SKODA (1805-1881, born Pilsen, Bohemia, Czech Republic, and died Vienna, Austria) was the scientific inheritor of Laennec. In 1867 Austria was joined with Hungary after its defeat in the Austro-Prussian War of 1866. He lived much of his life in Vienna at the time when the opera house was built. The world exposition was held in Vienna in 1873. By the time of his death, Vienna had a population over one million while the Austrian Empire became the third most populous country in Europe after Russia and the United Kingdom. With Emperor Franz Joseph I (1830-1916) ruling as a constitutional monarch (1848-1916), Vienna became the cultural capital of Europe.

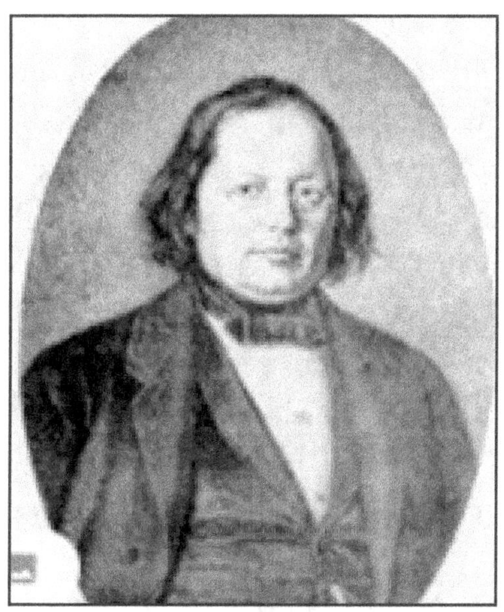

JOSEF SKODA
National Library of Medicine, public domain

Whereas Laennec was primarily interested in the lung, using his stethoscope to diagnose pulmonary disease, Skoda advocated and taught not only the auscultation of Laennec but also the percussion of Auenbrugger, and he correlated for the first time physical findings with necropsy findings. He heralded the new era in MODERN PHYSICAL DIAGNOSIS. Skoda published his findings in 1839. He showed that lung auscultatory sounds corresponded to whether the tissue below the chest wall was either healthy or diseased, but these findings were not specific of a particular diagnosis. He recognized that the characteristics, loudness and timber of heart murmurs were the result of anatomic abnormalities with physiologic consequences. He correlated these findings with the underlying heart disease on auscultation. Skoda was first to make the distinction between heart sounds (noise made by opening and closing of heart valves) and heart murmurs (whirring or swishing noise created usually by abnormal heart valves, causing blood flow turbulence to create this noise) heard with the stethoscope. He showed that the diagnosis was aided by knowing the position of the heart murmur in the chest and where it was transmitted. Skoda's teachings quickly spread to Germany and beyond. In 1846 he was made head of internal medicine in Vienna. Some consider him the Father of Cardiology as a specialty. Interestingly, he also was a dermatologist.

The third of the great early physical diagnosticians was Ludwig Traube (1818-1876, born in Ratibor, Poland, and died in Berlin, Germany). Traube lived in Germany when it became unified as one country in 1871. Prussia, the dominant state militarily and economically, was ruled by William I (Kaiser Wilhelm I), and the unity of Germany was brought about due to the efforts of the Chancellor of Prussia, Otto von Bismarck (Chancellor from 1870-1890), who created the modern German state out of many principalities after the defeat of France in the Franco-Prussian War of 1870.

Traube studied under Skoda and taught physical diagnosis using the stethoscope (known as auscultation) and percussion (tapping on the chest). He also performed experiments showing the scientific basis for digitalis treatment. The famous pathologist and medical leader Virchow ranked Traube third after Laennec and Skoda as furthering the field of physical diagnosis. His major scientific contribution to cardiology was the recognition of the connection of the kidney to heart disease, and he correctly wrote that heart disease would lead to kidney congestion and dysfunction. After being held back from promotion for years because of his religious beliefs, he was finally appointed as Professor of Medicine at the Medical School of the University of Berlin in 1872.

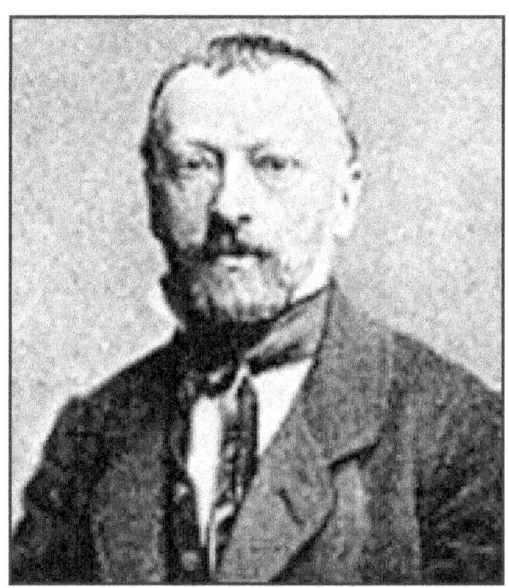

LUDWIG TRAUBE
National Library of Medicine, public domain

The skills of physical diagnosis could not be contained to Europe and eventually spread across the Atlantic Ocean, where JACOB MENDES DACOSTA (1833-1900, born St. Thomas, U.S. Virgin Islands (then a Danish colony), and died Villanova, PA, U.S.) inherited the mantle from Skoda for proselytizing physicians in the U.S. to use physical diagnostic techniques.

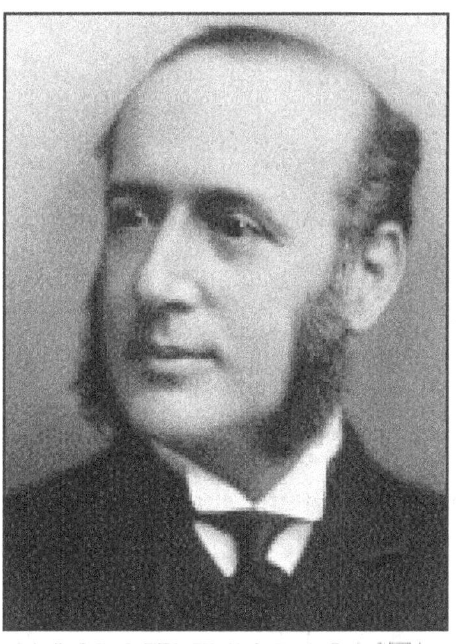

JACOB MENDES DACOSTA
National Library of Medicine, public domain

He taught at what became Jefferson Medical College. He described the syndrome of "Soldier's Heart" associated with symptoms of sweating, palpitations, and shortness of breath. Originally the symptoms were thought to be cardiac in origin but subsequently were determined to be psychological (probably Post-Traumatic Stress Disorder). DaCosta was the first to describe and study this problem in four hundred patients during the U.S. Civil War, where he served as a physician for the Union Army. The syndrome became known as DaCosta Syndrome, named after him in 1871.

At the time of DaCosta, Harriet Beecher Stowe wrote *Uncle Tom's Cabin* in 1852. In 1856 Senator Charles Sumner of the Republican Party denounced slavery on the U.S. Senate floor, and two days later the South Carolina proslavery Senator Preston Brooks beat Sumner nearly to death with his cane on the Senate floor. In 1860 South Carolina seceded from the U.S., and in 1861 the South formed the Confederate States and captured Fort Sumter in Charleston, South Carolina, starting the U.S. Civil War. In 1863 the U.S. slaves were emancipated. President Lincoln was assassinated in 1865. The Thirteenth Amendment to the U.S. Constitution to abolish slavery was ratified in 1865, and President Andrew Johnson began his Reconstruction plan for the South. Everyone born in the U.S., including slaves, was granted citizenship in the U.S. in 1868, after the passage of the Fourteenth Amendment.

Although not known for his specific cardiology contributions, Sir William Osler (1849-1919, born Bond Head (forty miles from Toronto, Canada) and died Oxford, England) made such a mark on American and later British medicine that his influence must be acknowledged. He was a great teacher, and his major contribution was making the third-year medical students an experience of bedside examining and talking to the patient on the ward and not just learning from textbooks or watching others perform the examination from a distance. This was a major change in medical education. He pioneered making rounds with just a small number of students for better teaching, a tradition of American medical schools today. His philosophy was that medical students learned by doing, and he is said to have stated that he hoped for no more than that his tombstone would say "I taught medical students in the wards, as I regard this as by far the most useful and important work I have been called upon to do." In short, he took medical teaching out of the classroom and into the medical wards for medical students to gain clinical experience. He changed U.S. medical education forever. He was at first chairman of the Department of Medicine at the University of Pennsylvania. He was one of the four founding fathers of Johns Hopkins Medical School and later moved on to a professorship at Oxford University in England. He is well known for his description of "Osler Nodes," which are raised painful small nodules (bumps) on the fingers as a sign of infectious endocarditis, i.e. infection of a heart valve. He is named for the finding of extremely high blood pressure due to stiff arteries (Osler's sign) and for Osler-Weber-Rendu disease, which are enlargements of very small arteries, sometimes with bleeding (including in the lung). Most importantly, he recognized the third component of blood, platelets (they are much smaller than red and white blood cells and clump to form white clots that can cause heart attacks and strokes), and documented that they were important in clotting (thrombosis). His revolutionary teaching led people to call him the Father of Modern Medicine. His views on race and the indigenous New World populations are unacceptable by today's standards, and doubtless, if he were living today, he would no longer hold these views. In his address to Albany medical students, he advised, "Care more particularly for the individual patient than for the especial features of the disease." He is quoted as advising, "Use your five senses. We miss more by not seeing than we do by not knowing.... See, then reason and compare and control. But see first. No two eyes see the same thing." His most memorable quotation is "Listen to your patient; he is telling you the diagnosis," meaning that listening to your patient's symptoms and concerns is so important to being a successful diagnostic physician. But he also taught some general principles for good science. He warned that "The greater the ignorance, the greater the dogma." He was wary of scientists who presumed to hold the truth without acknowledging that our knowledge is limited or that more than one way of treating a patient usually existed.

And he warned in an oblique but fairly explicit way that even the most esteemed scientists are not immune from their formed biases when he said in his William Harvey lecture in 1906 (delivered at the Harveian Oration at the Royal College of Physicians, London), "How eminent so ever a man may become in science, he is apt to carry with him errors which were in vogue when he was young—errors that darken his understanding, and make him incapable of accepting the most obvious truths." To his personal sadness, he lost a son at birth and another son in battle during WWI at the Battle of Ypres in Belgium. Tragically, the medical world lost Osler to the Spanish Flu in 1919.

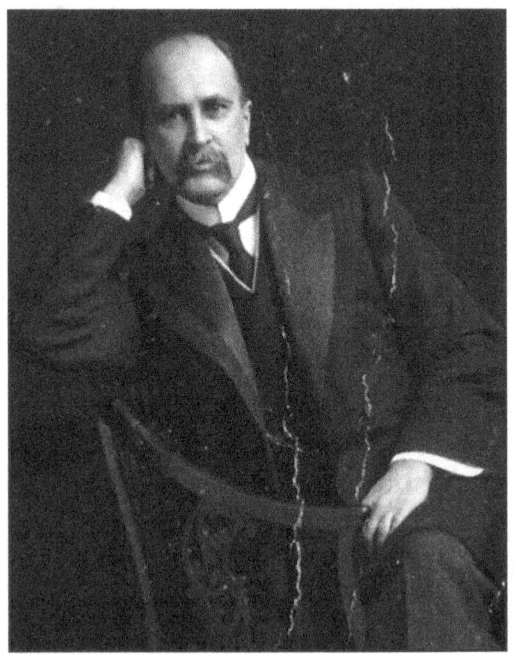

SIR WILLIAM OSLER
National Library of Medicine, public domain

Joseph Perloff (1924-2014, born New Orleans, Louisiana, U.S., and died Los Angeles, California, U.S.) was my chief when I was a cardiology resident. He was leaving Georgetown Medical School to become the Chief of Cardiology at the Hospital of the University of Pennsylvania, and I was lucky enough to meet him just after he finished giving a lecture in 1972 at the National Institutes of Health, where I was serving from 1970-1972. I told him that I was leaving dermatology and asked if he needed any more cardiology residents at Penn. To my lasting good fortune, he said he had one spot left and hired me "on the spot." I joined him in Philadelphia in the summer of

1972 for my two-year residency in cardiology. This was near the end of the Vietnam War, when the U.S. was going through great turmoil, including the impeachment of President Nixon in 1973. In 1978 there was hope of peace between the Israelis and Palestinians with the Camp David accords. In 1979 the yearlong Iranian hostage crisis of the U.S. personnel kept prisoner within the U.S. Embassy in Iran occurred. In 1986 the space shuttle *Challenger* exploded.

Joseph Perloff had been the disciple of the chief of cardiology at Georgetown Medical School, Proctor Harvey (1918-2007, born Lynchburg, Virginia, U.S.A., and died in Richmond, Virginia). Both men clearly carried on the tradition of those early cardiac diagnosticians and inherited the responsibility as the premier teachers of cardiac physical diagnosis in the U.S. Dr. Harvey was famous for dividing first-year medical students sitting in an amphitheater into groups, which he designated as horns, violins, woodwinds, etc., although no one actually held an instrument. At first it seemed weird to these medical students until he began playing a symphonic recording and asked each "section" to stand when they heard their instrument. If you were in the room, you witnessed a group of students standing and sitting, bobbing up and down, as their instrument could be heard playing by the real orchestra. This taught medical students to listen better for heart murmurs with their stethoscopes as they learned to hear their designated instrument playing. The exercise taught the students an unforgettable lesson, that one needs to hear the trees and not the forest in listening to the heart (i.e. eliminate all extraneous noise) in order to differentiate where the murmur was best heard on the chest wall and in what part of the cardiac cycle it occurred, i.e. listening for the trees rather than the forest to make a diagnosis with a stethoscope.

Dr. Joseph Perloff, as chief of cardiology at the Hospital of the University of Pennsylvania, spent hours teaching us to properly examine the heart and would say that all he needed to make a cardiac diagnosis were four pieces of information: the symptoms, the physical examination findings, the chest x-ray and the ECG. During a presentation by one of the residents, as each piece of information was revealed he would give a differential diagnosis (possibilities) of the problem until the fourth piece (and

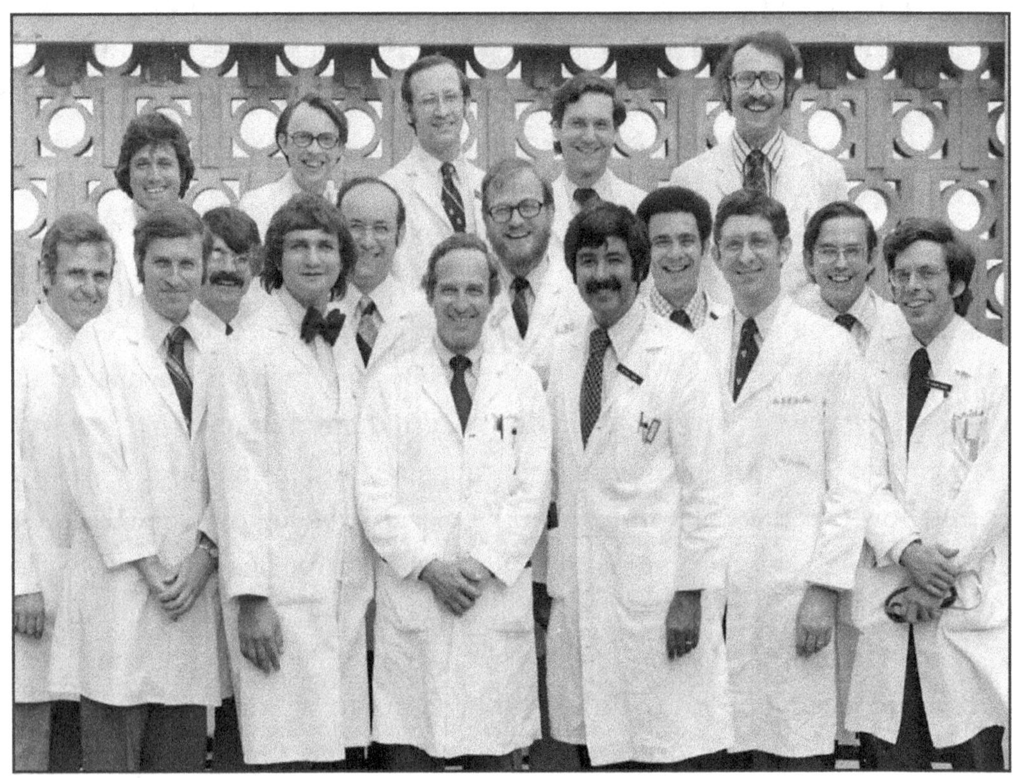

JUNE 1974, Hospital of the University of Pennsylvania Cardiology Fellows and Staff
Dr. Mark Josephson (see EPS chapter), top left; Dr. Joseph Perloff, first row center; the author, Stephen Guss, top right with more and darker hair than currently
Dr. James Shelburne, second row middle with Dr. Arthur Fisch, my practice partner of 47½ years, to the right with very thick curly hair, the style of the 1970s
The author's personal collection

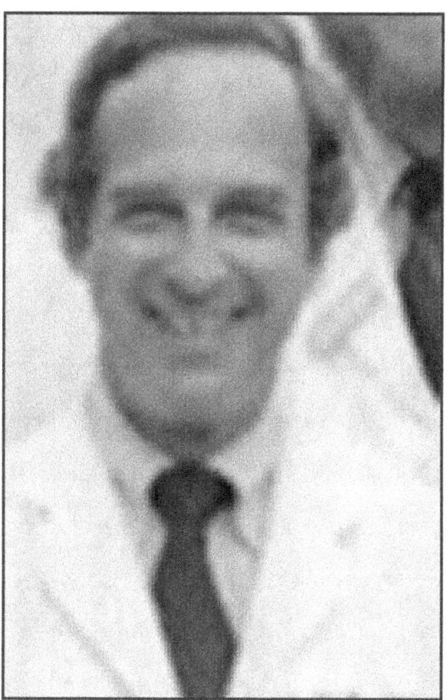

JOSEPH PERLOFF, author's personal collection

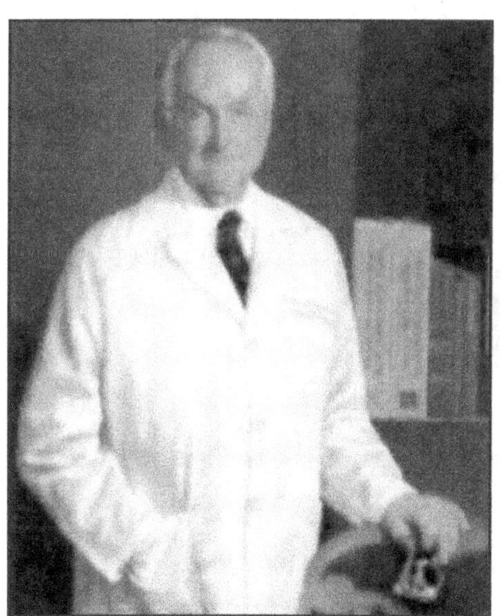

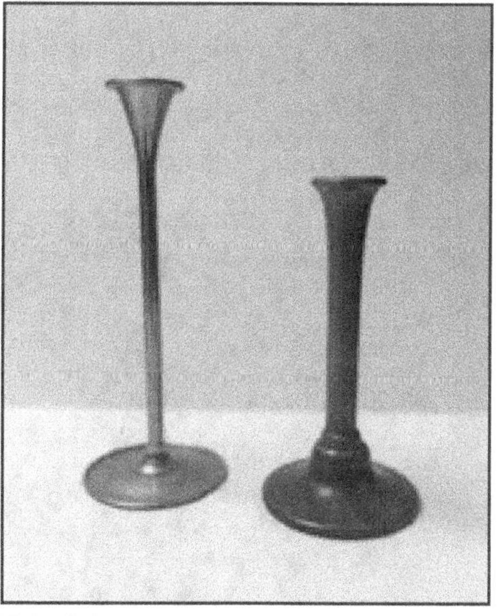

W. PROCTOR HARVEY, M.D.
by James Crowley, Collection of Georgetown School of Medicine
Image courtesy of the artist
Monaural stethoscopes used until 1960s for obstetrical use by Dr. Anna
Weiss, who brought them to the U.S. from Vienna in 1938 To viewer's left a
metal stethoscope, and to viewer's right a wooden monaural scope

The monoaural stethoscope, much to my surprise, did not go entirely out of use for some physicians well into the 20th century. Above are two used by my mother-in-law, Dr. Anna Weiss, who used them as a GP for obstetrical purposes in Mattoon, Illinois, from 1953-1968. She brought them with her from Vienna, Austria, where she grew up and studied medicine, but fled with my future father-in-law, Dr. Otto Weiss, from the Nazis in 1938.

Dr. James Shelburne at the Hospital of the University of Pennsylvania and director of the Cardiac Catheterization Laboratory was also a wonderful teacher. While "making rounds" to discuss the cardiac patients on our service, we would usually stand in a small circle. Dr. S. would ask someone in the group, often to his right side, a question. If they were wrong or did not know the answer, unlike many medical school and residency teachers he would not make you feel small or stupid but in his most Southern drawl possible (he was from Alabama originally) would turn to one of the residents on his other side and say, "I'll engage him in conversation. You call security and tell them there is someone here masquerading as a physician." Although we knew we answered incorrectly, his demeaner was never to belittle us but to help us remember next time. It is unusual to laugh (even at yourself) when you are wrong and in a group of peers, but Dr. S. accomplished this for us without tearing us down our deflating our self-esteem.

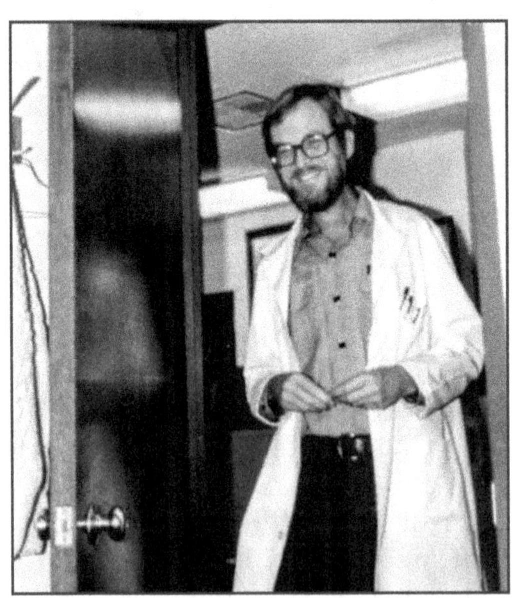

JAMES SHELBURNE,
Dr. Shelburne's personal collection by permission of Dr. Shelburne

GLOSSARY CHAPTER 1

Heart murmur – noise made by the heart and heard with a stethoscope usually due to turbulence from abnormal heart valves

Regurgitation – referring to leaking of blood in the wrong direction through one of the four heart valves

Percussion – tapping with the fingers, usually on the chest or at the liver in the abdomen

Auscultation – listening, usually with a stethoscope

Mitral stenosis – thickening of the bi-leaflet valve on the left side of the heart separating and controlling blood flow between the upper-left atrium and lower-left ventricle. Usually caused by previously remote rheumatic fever inflammation.

Nodules – bumps above or below the skin that one can feel

Endocarditis – infection of one of the four heart valves

Thrombosis – clotting

Differential diagnosis – considering the multiple possible causes of a patient's disease or symptoms until it is narrowed down

CHAPTER 2

THE LINK BETWEEN CORONARY ARTERY NARROWING AND ANGINA AND HEART ATTACKS – WHY DID IT TAKE 400 YEARS TO FIGURE IT OUT?

Mike was a personal friend, prominent lawyer in the area, and a patient of mine for years. He was traveling in the South of France with his wife when he ended up in a very, very small medical facility with a physician who did not know how to treat his heart attack and who spoke only French. It was 3:30 in the morning in NJ when my phone rang (I wasn't even on call that night), and it was Mike telling me his story. Fortunately, Mike was fluent in French and translated my recommendations into French to the French doctor and the doctor's response back to me from French to English. The three of us managed to get treatment started and get Mike transferred to a larger facility, where an emergency coronary angioplasty and stenting procedure was successfully performed. For years afterwards Mike and I laughed at the picture in our minds of the sick patient acting as the translator between two physicians, an ocean apart, who could not speak each other's language. We could laugh because the outcome was so favorable.

The general public has a basic understanding that blocked or clotted coronary arteries lead to heart attacks. Yet what is common knowledge even to many high school students today concerning how the heart works and its function in the body was a mystery to physicians of the 16th-19th centuries. Some of this ignorance was a result of very primitive or even no instrumentation. Some was due to the failure to take one more step in the scientific process of discovery, often because the next logical question was not asked. Part of this failure was due to bias handed down over the ages or even failing to see what was right in front of their eyes. To finally sort out the mystery of the heart and its function took four hundred years. And it took an additional thirty years after confirming the cause (medical term "etiology") of heart attacks to convince the medical profession that the disease that we now call "coronary artery atherosclerosis" was an important disease for their patients. Why was this? The answer is the finale of a medical mystery, which not only took a long time to solve but was pieced together like a jigsaw puzzle, one piece at a time, in fits and starts. The road to discovery was not linear.

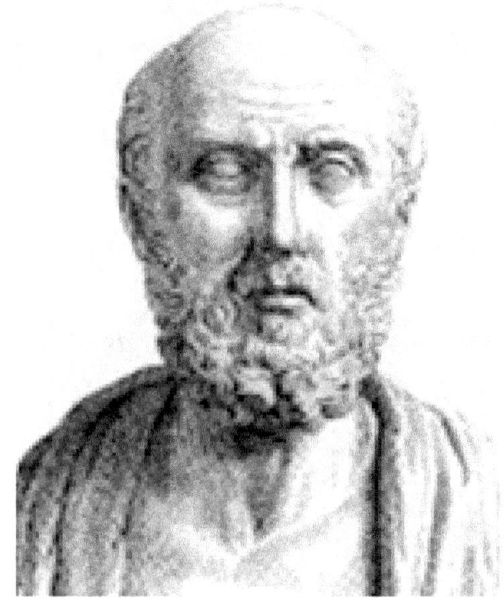

HIPPOCRATES, public domain

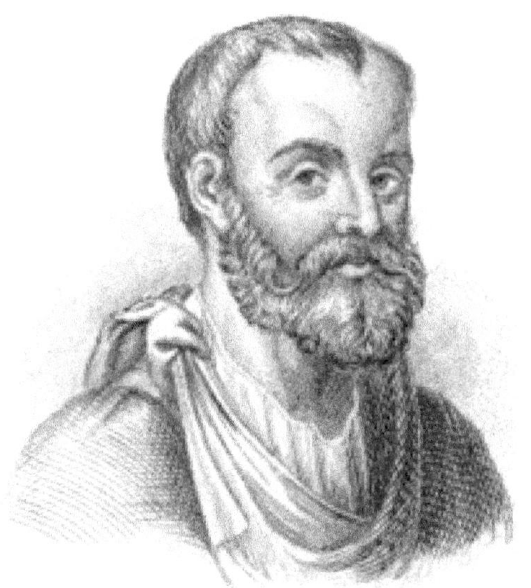

GALEN, courtesy Wellcome Collection, public domain

One might wonder if Hippocrates (460-370 B.C., born Kos, Greece, and died Larissa, Greece) found any clues to the coronary artery disease link. As it turned out, he was the Father of Medicine but not of cardiology and gave us little knowledge of the heart during the time he lived. Although Hippocrates had some theories on the heart, he never systematically studied the heart. He did use an extract of the bark of the willow bark tree (a derivative of modern aspirin) but not for cardiac purposes but to relieve the pain of childbirth.

One might ask if the great Galan provided any answer about the coronary artery dilemma. Galen of Pergamon (129-216 A.D., born Pergamon, Turkey, and died Rome, Italy) was a Greek who lived in Rome but had to leave since he was performing autopsies prohibited by the Roman authorities and Roman law. He had been the physician to five Roman emperors. It appears from history that although brilliant, his personality was vain, and Galen often bullied his opponents with his loud voice into submission and acceptance of what he said, often obscuring inaccuracies as the truth. He was the guru of medicine for 1400 years and almost singlehandedly prevented original thought or questioning since he was accepted almost blindly as the genius of medicine by the medical profession. Unfortunately for mankind, most of his conclusions about the heart were inaccurate. He wrongly thought that air went through the skin directly into the arteries and that the arteries and veins were not connected by capillaries. He taught that tiny pores (i.e. mini-holes) in the interventricular septum, the muscle that divides the right from the left ventricle, allowed dark blood to become bright red blood for the body. In short, he was not a help but a hindrance to our question. Presumably Galen's impeding of medical knowledge and progress was unintentional for these 1400 years and, to a large degree, was the fault of the students who came after his death who failed to ask questions or challenge the current wisdom of the time.

It turns out that there was one genius who understood the heart and how coronary arteries affect health. He was Leonardo DaVinci, but unfortunately he never published his investigations, and his paper became lost for 265 years. But I am getting ahead of the story.

By way of introduction, the heart has three coronary arteries, tubes that supply different segments of the heart with oxygen-rich blood primarily to the left ventricle (oxygen is the fuel for heart muscle to pump). One of the three arteries is known as the 1) Left Anterior Descending Coronary Artery, which supplies the front wall of the heart (LAD in common parlance and sometimes known as the "widow maker" since the LAD supplies the largest segment of heart muscle, accounting for 40%-45%). The other two coronary arteries are the 2) Circumflex Coronary Artery, which runs to the left-outer side and back of the heart in most patients and accounts for about 30-35% of the heart territorial supply; and 3) the Right Coronary Artery, which in 85% of patients is the underside of the heart muscle (15-20% of total heart muscle) blood supply and lies on the diaphragmatic muscle separating the chest from the abdominal contents of the body. Interestingly, everyone's coronary artery anatomy is unique to them, although everyone has three basic arteries. It is the side branches and where they start or run that make the coronary artery tree unique to a patient like fingerprints. The segmental distribution is fortunate since a heart attack (medical term: myocardial infarction) causes death to some of the heart muscle but may leave enough alive muscle behind to allow life to continue and, for many patients, even a normal daily life.

THE CAUSE OF A HEART ATTACK

Heart attacks occur when a yellow lipid-filled plaque tears or splits (we in cardiology say "rupture") and a reaction occurs in the artery to fill the void by causing a blood clot to form, basically to fill the hole. Sometimes the amount of clotting is overzealous and leads to a total block of the artery channel (occlusion) so no blood can travel beyond the blockage. The heart muscle supplied beyond this block dies if the blood is not restored within a few hours, just as your lawn will not be watered if someone steps on or squeezes off a segment of your perforated garden hose. The amount of damage is dependent upon how much muscle is affected, which in turn is related to whether the blockage occurs upstream or very downstream. This concept is what took scientists four hundred years to figure out.

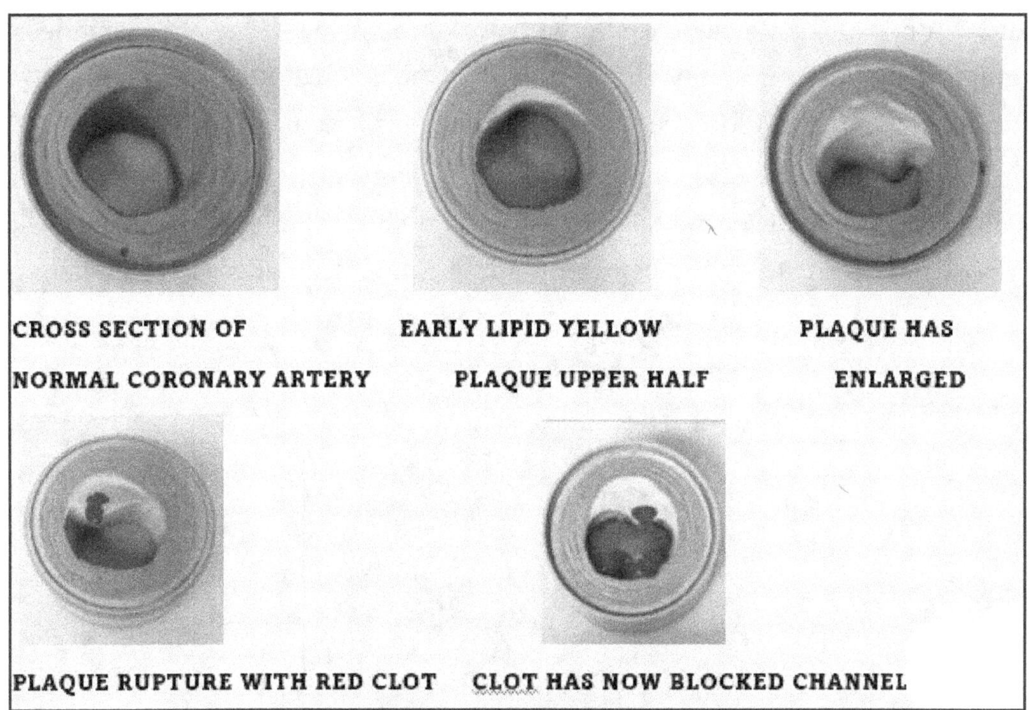

Author's personal collection

Today most high school students are taught that the venous and arterial circulations are connected by small blood vessels called capillaries. Most know that oxygen from the air passes into the lung sacs and then diffuses into small capillaries. The capillaries then connect to the pulmonary veins, bringing oxygenated blood from the lungs, then to the left side of the heart to pump to the body organs. The veins of the body then bring the deoxygenated blood back to the right side of the heart and pump the blood via the pulmonary artery into the lungs for a resupply of oxygen.

There was one person who had curiosity and insight and had the function of the heart figured out. It took a well-known artist to be the first to understand the workings of the heart. It was Leonardo DaVinci (1452-1519, born Anciano, Italy, and died Amboise, France). He was a singular genius and accurately described the anatomy of the heart in his drawings. He is often thought of as the first person to really study the heart, and it is amazing how much he understood back in the early 1500s. Leonardo spent much of his productive life in Florence, which was ruled by the Medici family and Lorenzo "the Magnificent." The Medici family attracted to Florence the best and the brightest and the most creative minds of the Renaissance in the fields of mathematics, science, engineering, art, and literature, including Leonardo DaVinci, who lived some his most productive years in Florence. Leonardo began his famous painting, *Mona Lisa*, in 1503 in Florence. Also coming to Florence were such geniuses as Botticelli, Michelangelo, Raphael and the politician and noted writer Niccolo Machiavelli, whose name became the adjective for a politically calculating and evil person.

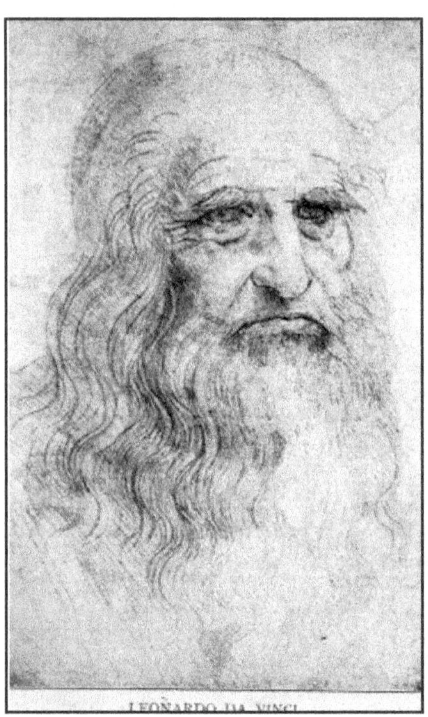

LEONARDO DAVINCI, public domain

Leonardo suggested that coronary artery atherosclerosis (another word is plaque) was a buildup of material, which we today now know includes cholesterol, other fats, cells, and material, to hold it all together called ground substance to compose the plaque. He most importantly understood that this plaque (not his term) caused heart damage when he wrote in 1512-1513 that "vessels in the elderly restrict the transit of blood through thickening of the tunic." However, few people were aware of his findings, and his ideas and papers remained unknown and unpublished for over two hundred and fifty years after his death. Ironically, if you look closely at the inner corner of the left side of the nose at the eye, one will see a small vertical elliptical area, which probably is a xanthelasma, or small collection of cholesterol under the skin.

In 1764, over 250 years after DaVinci recorded his findings and theories, William Hunter (1718-1783, born East Kilbride, Scotland, and died London, England) came in possession of DaVinci's papers and tried to call attention to them to the medical profession, but his call fell on deaf ears. Because of his lost papers, DaVinci lost his opportunity to become a Disruptor in Cardiology. Hunter lived before and during the American Revolution in the United Kingdom when it was ruled by George III. He was alive in the time of Samuel Johnson and James Boswell, the famous battle of Culloden when Bonnie Prince Charles failed in his attempt to free Scotland from the English, golf became formalized at St. Andrews in Scotland, Charles MacIntosh invented waterproof clothing, and John McAdam invented the macadam road surface first in America but then brought his talents back to Scotland. Had doctors listened to William Hunter, who tried to spread the substance of the writings of DaVinci, the medical profession might have awakened from its slumber in the dark ages of medicine much earlier, but they did not seem to care or notice. Hunter's discovery did little to attract the medical profession's attention to the link between coronary artery disease and heart attacks. It required another four hundred years after DaVinci to solve this mystery and about 120 years after Hunter. The question is, why did it take so long?

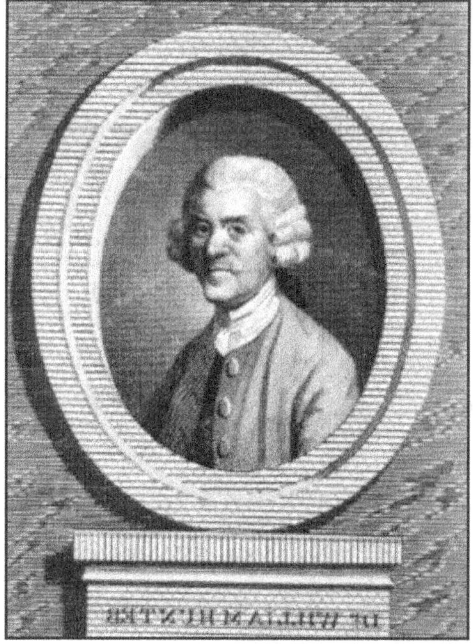

WILLIAM HUNTER
National Library of Medicine, public domain

Someone was required to advance the field of heart study given the hundreds of years of darkness. Living at the time of Leonardo was ANDREAS VESALIUS (1514-1564, born Brussels, Belgium, and died Zakynthos, Greece), who assumed the mantle of scientific discovery.

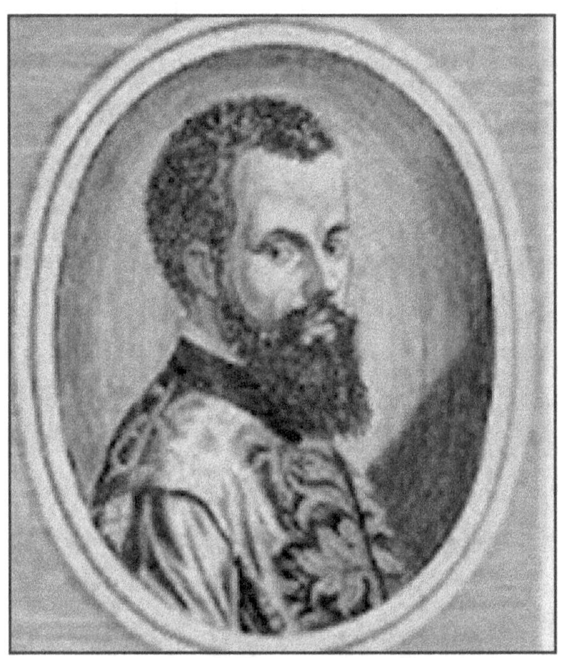

ANDREAS VESALIUS
Courtesy National Library of Medicine, public domain

As the founder of descriptive anatomy, Vesalius became the most influential figure in medicine after Galen and is given credit for stimulating the field of histology (studying tissue under a microscope) and cellular pathology (individual cells which are abnormal) before the microscope was even invented. He was a forerunner of the 17th-century breakthroughs. Educated in the famous Padua School of Medicine in Italy, which was the leading medical center of learning at the time, his grand work was *DE HUMANI CORPORIS FABRICA* (1543). He recognized that there were valves in veins to prevent backflow (reflux) of blood. Most importantly, he became an early discoverer in the field of the circulation. Anatomic study was the first of the modern cardiological studies and eventually gave birth to cardiac physiology (performing experiments on how the heart works) and pathological anatomy (anatomy of sick patients) as physicians became more and more curious and were able to cast off the yoke of the arbitrary and incorrect knowledge handed down for centuries in exchange for the new scientific inquiry. Vesalius opened the door a crack into the modern era, but only a crack.

It would take four hundred years to solve the problem and an additional thirty years to gain acceptance of this link among coronary artery disease, angina, and heart attacks by the medical community once proof was available.

To find the answer about how coronary atherosclerosis (i.e. fatty cholesterol inside the coronary arteries that supplies the heart muscle with oxygenated blood) to the symptom of angina pectoris (chest discomfort with effort from narrowed coronary arteries) and the catastrophe of a heart attack (myocardial infarction due to total blockage of a coronary artery resulting in heart muscle death so the heart segment no longer pumps), five answers were required:

1. How the normal heart works
2. What normal and abnormal heart muscle looks like and what its function was normally
3. What diseased coronary arteries both on the surface and inside the hollow channel look like
4. What the symptoms of coronary artery disease, e.g. angina pectoris, heart attacks, and how doctors could recognize them
5. Proving a connection among #2, #3, and #4

STEP ONE: THE NORMAL HEART AND HOW IT WORKS

WHO CAME AFTER LEONARDO DAVINCI?
Something changed in the seventeenth century, which was to become THE AGE OF NEW DISCOVERY and The BEGINNING OF CARDIAC EXPERIMENTATION.

Cardiology was not yet a specialty, although knowledge was advanced even in the 1500s by such people as MICHAEL SERVETUS (1511?-1553, born Villanueva de Signina, Spain, and died Geneva, Switzerland). He had a theory of the pulmonary circulation receiving air and then transporting this air back to the left side of the heart and not passing, as Galen thought, into the arterial blood through pores in the muscle separating the right and left ventricles. Although his conclusions turned out to be correct, they were only unproven theories, not supported by any experimental observations for proof. This required the entrance of William Harvey onto the scene, the first major Disruptor of the status quo.

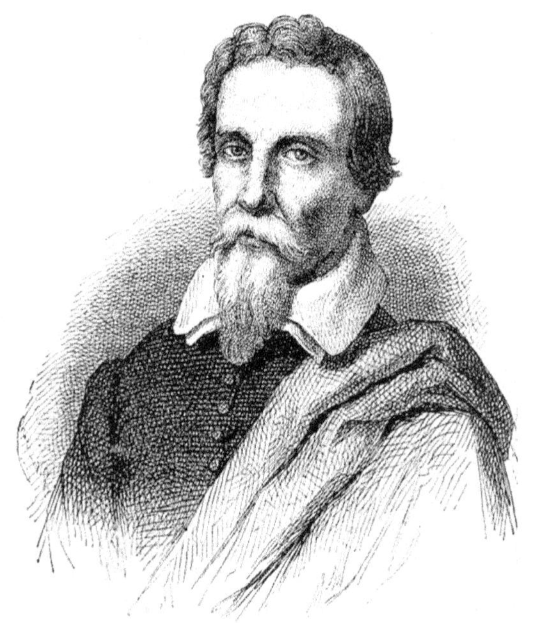

MICHAEL SERVETUS
Collection Abecasis/Science Photo Library License

The person who was at the vanguard of this new age of discovery and experimentation and the first Disruptor was WILLIAM HARVEY (1578-1657, born Folkestone, England, and died London, England). Harvey was the first scientist to use physiologic experiments on animals and humans rather than rely upon static autopsy (also known as necropsy) results.

During his time, King James II of England asserted the Union of the Crowns (1603) joining England and Scotland to create Great Britain, although it took another one hundred years to bring this about in a practical manner. England and Scotland remained separately governed during his time until 1707. The English civil war began in 1642.

Harvey's findings lay the groundwork for proving the link between coronary disease with angina pectoris and heart attacks. Harvey lay down only the first of many pieces of the jigsaw puzzle that were required to solve this question.

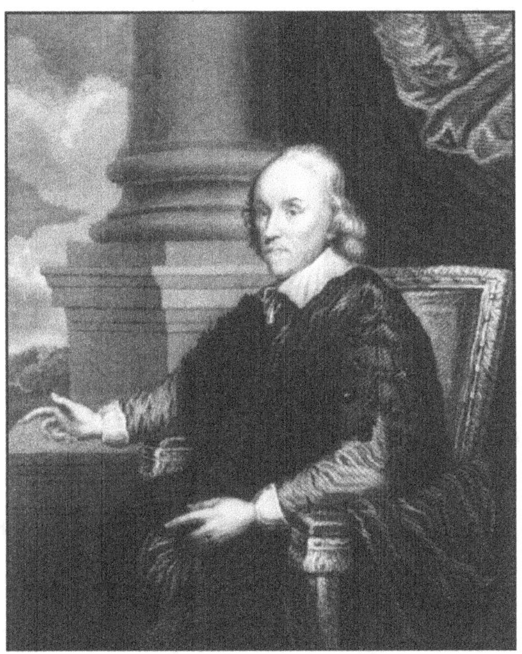

WILLIAM HARVEY,
courtesy National Library of Medicine, public domain

Harvey was the first to perform scientifically based physiologic research on the heart, whereas predecessors only advanced theories about the heart without experimentation to prove their theories. His monumental work, *DE MOTU CORDIS ET SANGUINIS* ("Movement of the Heart and Blood"), was published in 1628 (often referred to as *MOTU CORDIS*), the same year that the "Petition of Right" passed as an English document setting out specific individual protections against the state, which many consider as important as the Magna Carta. With experiments and direct observations, Harvey found proof of how the circulation of the heart functioned, often disagreeing with the dicta of the ages from such greats as Galen. Like many of the great doctors of the 17th century, he also studied medicine in Padua. Some of his Italian contemporaries hinted that Italians had previously demonstrated many of his scientific conclusions, and some of Harvey's contemporary Italian historians contended that Harvey merely plagiarized from others such as Columbo, Fabricius and Desalpino. But modern historical experts dispute the Italian historians' assertions and are convinced that Harvey's ideas and research were original. Expert historians of the twentieth century accept the originality of Harvey and the uniqueness of his proof. Some historians have actually written that if Italian critics had read Harvey's book, there would be no such conflicting claims.

Anatomically Harvey proved that the heart pumped blood in two separate but linked circulations (arterial and venous) and that the heart did not manufacture blood as many previously thought (the bone marrow does). He proved that air did not come directly through the skin into the arteries (which Galen wrongly thought) but via the lungs and into the pulmonary venous circulation. He described the pulmonary circulation of arteries going to the lungs to accept air (oxygen) and then bringing the oxygenated blood back to the left side of the heart to be pumped to the body. He realized that the circulation received air (later determined that oxygen was the critical component of air) that was breathed in. He hypothesized and in his mind was certain that very small blood vessels, later to be known as capillaries, connected the unoxygenated pulmonary arteries to the oxygenated pulmonary veins and that air did not pass directly through the skin. He was certain that small pulmonary arteries emptied into these very small blood vessels before continuing as pulmonary veins to the left side of the heart. However, without a microscope (not perfected for another forty years), he could not prove his theory of capillaries using the magnifying glasses available at the time with their limited magnification. The observation of capillaries awaited the later findings of Malpigi (see below) using a microscope invented by others.

Harvey observed that the left ventricle pumped in systole, the phase of heart muscle contraction and enlarged by filling with blood but without pumping in diastole, the relaxation phase. He performed experiments to prove that arteries became smaller when relaxing in diastole when the heart relaxed but enlarged when the heart pumped blood into them in systole. They were able to enlarge due to arterial wall elasticity. He demonstrated that blood propelled forward in systole due to the force of the left ventricle contraction. He proved with experiments that when an isolated arm artery was placed under water or oil, the artery continued to enlarge in systole, which would be impossible if air diffused through the artery wall directly from the ambient air as Galen proclaimed as the arterial wall would be compressed by the heavier oil and would not enlarge. Harvey, through direct observations, also described how blood first entered the right atrium and then into the right ventricle and then into the left atrium followed by the left ventricle with each circulatory cycle. Although his studies were crude, given the equipment available, they were revolutionary, brilliant, and ground-breaking. He correctly discovered that blood did not pass through small pores from the right ventricle into the left ventricle but traveled from the right ventricle through the lung circulation to regain entrance into the left side of the heart, first through the left atrium and then into the left ventricle. Harvey observed that the heart chambers became smaller after pumping (systole) and that the heart muscle thickened as it pumped in systole, causing the pulse to be felt, for instance at the wrist or at the apex of the heart palpated through the chest wall. Harvey also determined by experiments that the heart relaxed in diastole.

In his masterpiece *DE MOTU CORDIS*, he concluded, "The heart, consequently, is the beginning of life…for it is the heart by whose virtue and pulse the blood is moved." James Herrick, who later convinced the medical community in 1918 about the link between coronary atherosclerosis and heart attacks, wrote, "It is plain that he (i.e. William Harvey) created cardiology." Harvey was the first scientist to look at the living heart rather than the anatomic heart at autopsy and the first scientist to perform experiments connecting anatomy with physiology. Whereas he performed physiologic experiments on the heart, others before only theorized from anatomic findings on necropsy specimens. His monumental work was *DE MOTO CORDIS ET SANGUINIS* ("Movement of the Heart and Blood"). With direct experiments and observations he based his conclusions, often disagreeing with the dicta of the times and the ages.

However, it took MARCELLO MALPIGHI (1628-1694, born Crevalcore near Bologna, Italy, and died Rome, Italy) to prove Harvey's capillary hypothesis. Malpighi lived in Italy at a time of scientific exchange and the establishment of Italian scientific academies. But it was also a time of transition when old families were replaced by a new nobility of wealth with a new disparity between the wealthy and impoverished.

Famine at the end of the 16th century and new waves of plague in the 1630s and 1650s caused a population loss of 20-25%, throwing Italy into economic despair made worse by the war in 1623-39 between the Turkish Ottomans and the Iranians, causing a disruption of Italian trade. Agriculture and urban industrialization went into a tailspin at this time. Thus, Italy collapsed except for the province of Lombardy, where Milan with oil, wine, and silk retained a buoyant economy. Despite the decline of Italy, Malpighi was able to make one of the major cardiac discoveries of that time, to prove the existence of capillaries, which were only theorized by Harvey so Malpighi was the second great Disruptor of old thought.

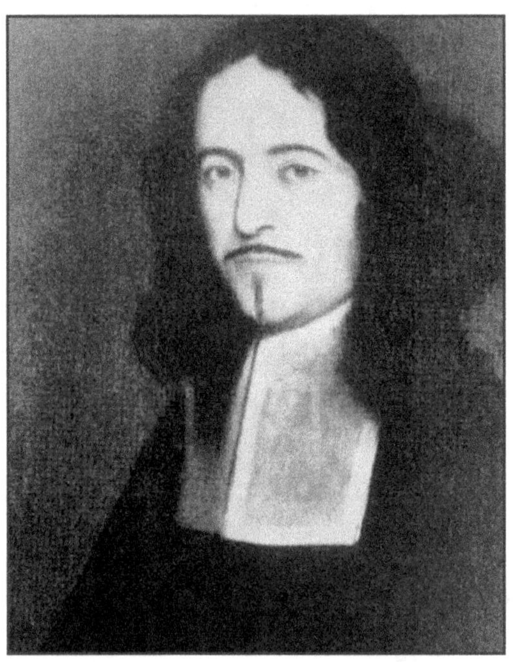

MARCELLO MALPIGHI
Science Photo Library License

Marcello Malpighi was the first modern histologist (study of tissue under a microscope). Owing to the invention of the microscope and its improvements by Van Leeuwenhoek, he was able to prove what Harvey could only theorize, i.e. tiny blood vessels later called capillaries connected the small pulmonary arteries to the pulmonary veins and were the active site of air uptake (i.e. later determined to be oxygen) from the small lung sacs known as alveoli. Of course, this was true of all blood delivered by arteries and returned to the heart by veins from all the body's organs and tissue as capillaries are found in all organs between arteries and veins. Malpighi also described red blood and white blood cells.

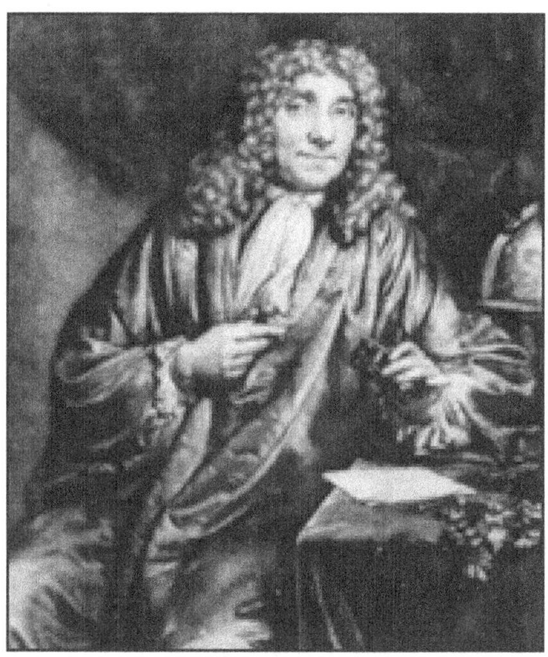

Most people were taught in school that Van Leeuwenhoek invented the microscope, which was the tool that opened many of the new frontiers of scientific research. Actually the first microscope was invented around 1590 (twenty-two years before he was born) by the Dutch lens maker father-and-son team of Hans (dates unknown) and Zacharias Janssen (1585-1638, born the Hague, Netherlands, and died Amsterdam, Netherlands). Unfortunately their microscope did not provide sharp enough detail to reveal very small life forms or fine vascular structure. Van Leeuwenhoek's contribution was making improvements to the existing microscopes so that the magnification was three hundred times greater than before and with far clearer detail than from existing microscopes. This allowed the viewing of tiny life forms such as bacteria and protozoa. But even if someone else had technically improved the microscope instead of Van Leeuwenhoek, his contribution of scientific description was equally important if not more so, making him a great Disruptor. In 1677 he published his famous paper describing what he called protozoa, but in fact he was also describing bacteria that he obtained from the human mouth (he kept his teeth very clean after his observation and had healthy teeth much longer than most people of the time). He also examined animal and human sperm under his microscope. Van Leeuwenhoek is considered the Father of Microbiology (the study of very small creatures like bacteria and protozoa). He also confirmed Malpighi's observations of capillaries.

Van Leeuwenhoek wrote: "I never looked upon the heart as a maker of blood (as many predecessors did) but as the engine that caused the blood to circulate, driving it forcibly into the arteries and by its opening, giving way for the blood to come in and out of the veins." He subsequently bequeathed twenty-six microscopes to the Royal Society at his death.

The second pioneering experimental cardiac physiologic scientist came a century after William Harvey. This physiologic research scientist was Stephen Hales (1677-1761, born Bekesbourne, UK, and died Teddington, UK). Stephen Hales lived in the time when England and Scotland formed one kingdom (1707, Acts of Union). England was still poor but with a growing population. The century was a period of change with new ideas and scientific progress. It was the Age of the Enlightenment but also of political upheaval. After fighting wars with the Netherlands and France, England became the main political force in the colonial new world and a major European power.

Hales arrived slightly over one hundred years after Harvey. Although he was a protestant minister by day and scientist by night, he spent much of his free time experimenting in science. He attended Cambridge University in what is now Corpus Christi College, where he took an interest in science but became a fulltime minister in Teddington the rest of his life. His first physiology of the heart book was not published until he was 55 years old, a late start some might say. But he already was a plant biologist and is considered the founder of plant physiology (how plants function) and for a century was considered the world's expert in this field. In addition he became quite versed with the machines of the age and devised a machine to show the motion of the planets, all the while still preaching from his church pulpit. He was the second cardiac physiologist in history to enter the field after Harvey and the first scientist to make quantitative physiologic measurements. He was the first person to measure blood pressure (which he termed "force") and was a pioneer in the study of blood pressure. His experiments on what we now call blood pressure started in 1712. Ironically, he really wanted to measure the force in vegetables, but we are eternally grateful that he found the horse for his experiments and not a radish. He used a vertical hollow glass rod inserted into a hollow brass pipe as a monometer, which he then placed into a horse's crural artery (the artery just beyond and downstream from the horse's knee). In 1733 Hales published his findings in his book, *HAEMASTATICKS*. He noted that the blood column would rise and fall with each pulse (he correctly concluded it was systole and diastole) and he determined that the resting heart rate was 36 beats a minute for most horses, he assessed. When the horse exhibited pain, he observed the pulse rose from sixty to one hundred beats a minute and the "force" increased (i.e. the column of blood rose in the glass tube). He found the column height of blood decreased as he bled the horse (i.e. the blood pressure was falling as he phlebotomized (removed blood) the horse) and the blood pressure fell as more and more blood was removed. He called his finding "force," not "blood pressure," although it was blood pressure he was measuring. His description is the first of hypovolemic shock (extremely low blood pressure due to blood loss) and the physiology of blood pressure change with animal motion as he determined that blood pressure rose with movement or struggle. But more practical ways of measuring blood pressure awaited to be invented.

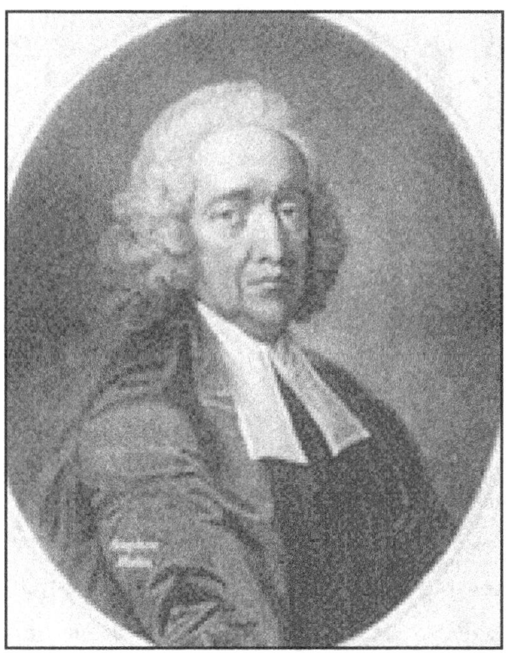

Stephen Hales, National Library of Medicine, public domain

Step one was now solved, how the heart worked. But there was more to learn.

STEP TWO: THE HEART MUSCLE (MYOCARDIUM) IN HEALTH AND DISEASE

1600s and 1700s

Still no one understood how the heart muscle was composed, organized, or functioned until three other pioneers came along. The first was NIELS STENSEN (1638-1686, born Copenhagen, Denmark, and died

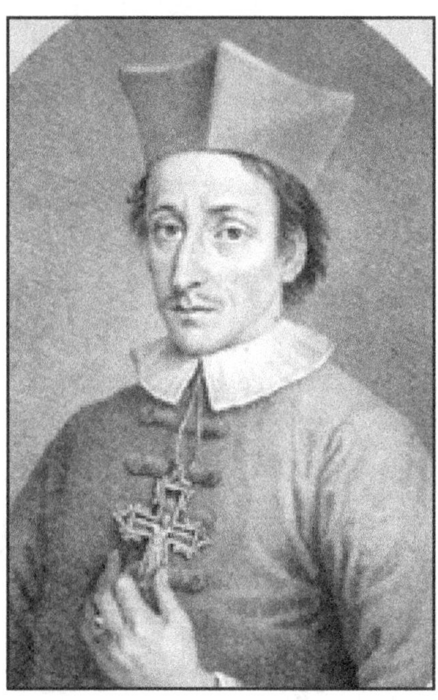

NIELS STENSEN,
public domain

Schwerin, Germany). Denmark during the time of Stensen was at almost continuous war with its Nordic neighbor Sweden and ceded provinces to Sweden in 1658, which now compose the southern part of Sweden.

Stensen (also known as Steno) discovered the muscular fiber composition of the heart, "nothing except arteries, veins, nerves, fibers and membranes…I omit fat and bone because all hearts do not have this, and no muscle has it…truly the heart merits the name of muscle because it has tendons and flesh and nerves."

Stensen also wrote, "The heart can not generate certain substances as heat (fire), innate warmth, the seat of the soul, nor can it produce certain humors as blood, certain spirits or vitality.....thus from the fibers proceeds all movement of the heart, occurring as a phenomenon of its own" (4, Willius). In 1664 he published that the heart met the criteria of muscle with flesh, tendon, and nerves.

Next came RICHARD LOWER (1631-1691, born Bodmin, UK, and died London, UK).

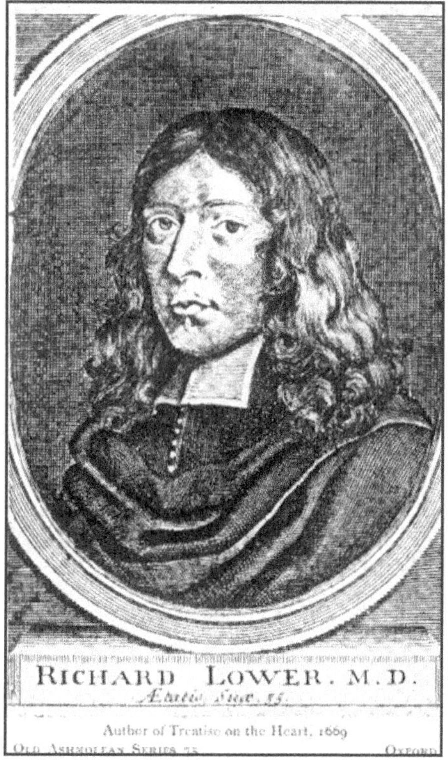

RICHARD LOWER
National Library of Medicine, public domain

England during the time of Richard Lower was nearly at continuous war from 1639-1644. In 1642 England began its civil war. In 1652 tea first was brought back to England from China. The Great Fire of London occurred in 1666, and in 1688 the Glorious Revolution occurred, replacing James II, the last Catholic monarch of England, with Willian III, a protestant also known as William the Orange. In 1689 a Bill of Rights was enacted by both parliaments of England and Scotland.

Lower described the spiral helical nature of cardiac muscle (Tractus de Corde, 1691). Ironically, his important observation was largely ignored until the early 2000s but now has become an important subject of echocardiographic studies of cardiac function. In addition electrical physiologic studies now often depend on his observations with new applications on how the heart really contracts. The new findings affect open heart surgery and ventricular surgical tailoring procedures of today to remove dead heart muscle while avoiding contracting muscle. Lower also studied blood flow and noted the change in color of the blood in the veins versus the arteries as air was inspired. He injected a fluid into the coronary arteries and observed for the first time that some arteries connected with others coronary arteries in other areas, known as making an anastomosis. These vessels are also known collateral vessels, but he did not understand their significance, providing an alternative source of blood to areas of the heart where arterial flow is insufficient due to narrowing (stenoses).

Nearly a century later appeared JEAN NICOLAS CORVISART (1755-1821, born Dricourt, France, and died Dricourt, France). Corvisart was the physician to Napoleon Bonaparte and lived during the French Revolution and the Napoleonic Wars that followed. He was the first to distinguish that the heart could enlarge by thickening of the heart muscle (hypertrophy), enlargement of the chambers (dilation AKA dilatation), or both. His findings were published in the late 1700s and became crucial subsequently in diagnosing the severity of many types of valvular heart disease and weakened hearts with congestive heart failure of many causes, including from heart attacks.

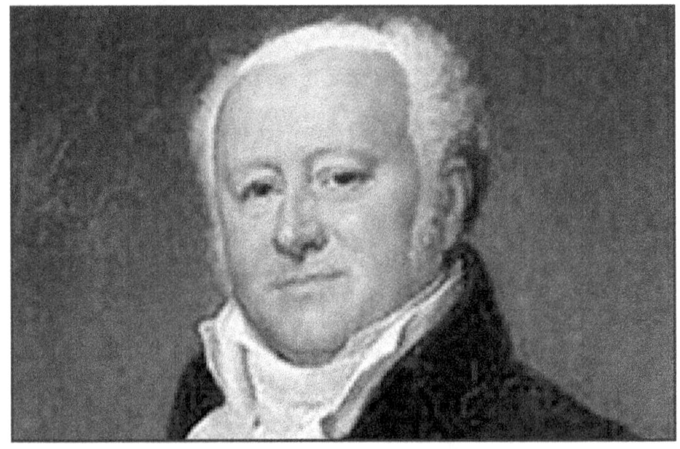

JEAN NICOLAS CORVISART
National Library of Medicine, public domain

Many physicians described the thinning or scarring of the heart muscle in the 1700s, now called a "ventricular aneurysm." Although blocked or narrowed coronary arteries were most likely the cause of these findings, the connection remained obscure to the medical profession for another two hundred years.

STEP THREE: DESCRIPTION OF CARDIAC SYMPTOMS OF ANGINA PECTORIS

Even the symptom that we now know as common in coronary artery disease, angina pectoris, was not understood or well described until 1768, when WILLIAM HEBERDEN (1710-1801, born London, UK, and died London, UK) described the symptoms now known caused by narrowed coronary arteries, angina pectoris. Heberden was born in the year of food shortages in England from a harsh winter with riots occurring in March of 1710. Queen Anne was the English monarch and Louis XIV was king of France. By midsummer of 1710, the Habsburgs of Austria and England defeated Spain in the War of Spanish Succession. By mid-century, John Canton had created a new method of making artificial magnets. Of course, by the end of the century the American colonies won their independence in a hard-fought war with England.

Heberden described symptoms in patients who exerted themselves physically and associated with a pressure in the middle of the chest, often going to the left arm or neck and receding when the patient again rested. He termed this "Angina Pectoris," the term we use to this day to describe the chest discomfort occurring when the demand for oxygenated blood by the heart outstrips the supply brought to it by narrowed coronary arteries (the balance of supply-and-demand is upset) due to a narrowing in the channel with a fatty substance known as an atherosclerotic plaque.

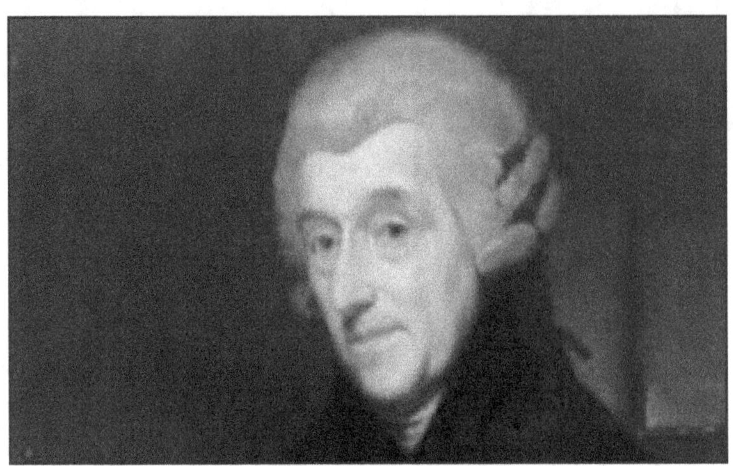

WILLIAM HEBERDEN
National Library of Medicine, public domain

Although first describing angina pectoris in 1768, Heberden did not publish his results on his first one hundred patients with this symptom until 1802, probably because it took 34 years to collect even this size sample in a disease that was not common. Interestingly, the average cardiologist today will see this number of patients with angina pectoris in a single year. This difference may help explain why it took four hundred years to figure out the link between coronary artery disease and the problems it can cause, such as angina pectoris and heart attacks. Even Heberden did not describe the symptoms of an acute heart attack, let alone its link to blocked coronary arteries or that blocked coronary arteries caused his classically described symptom. But more to come. Heberden found that some patients often lived for many years with angina pectoris and some seemed "cured" while other patient died suddenly. Although his description was accurate, Heberden did not understand the anatomic origin (heart and coronary arteries), physiology (i.e. a change in supply-and-demand in a narrowed coronary artery), or even the variable prognosis, much less that his description was even a cardiac originated symptom. It took later cardiologists to understood that when the demand by the heart muscle for blood outstrips the supply in a narrowed coronary artery such as during exertion, a discomfort often occurs in the center of the chest but not actually within the heart itself (this is known as referred pain). In his book published in 1802, *Commentaries on the History and Cure of Disease*, (Willius) Heberden discussed one hundred patients he had seen in his practice with this symptom. He correctly concluded that it could lead to sudden death or, as he wrote, "falling down dead." He had no explanation for the cause or even the origin from the coronary arteries, much less the heart itself, and only could suggest opium as a treatment.

STEP FOUR: BEGINNING STEPS ASSESSING THE OUTSIDE AND INSIDE OF CORONARY ARTERIES AND EARLY ATTEMPTS TO LINK DISEASED CORONARY ARTERIES TO CARDIAC MUSCLE PATHOLOGY

GIOVANNI LANCISI (1654-1720, born Rome, Italy, and died Rome, Italy). Interested in epidemiology (how disease is spread), he recognized that malaria came from mosquito-laden swamps and proposed draining them. He also published papers on vegetations on heart valves (now called endocarditis) and findings in the heart due to syphilis. He challenged the Hippocratic notion that the heart could not be affected by disease. Lancisi's work published posthumously in 1728 in his *De Motu Cordis et Aneurysmatibus* ("Motion of the Heart and on Aneurysms") describes the ossification of coronary arteries. He observed that often portions of the arteries were as hard as bone (with calcium). He even discussed that they might be the cause of cardiac enlargement and aneurysms, yet never linked this to heart attacks or even cardiac damage, although he came close but only mentioned the possibility in passing without going into detail.

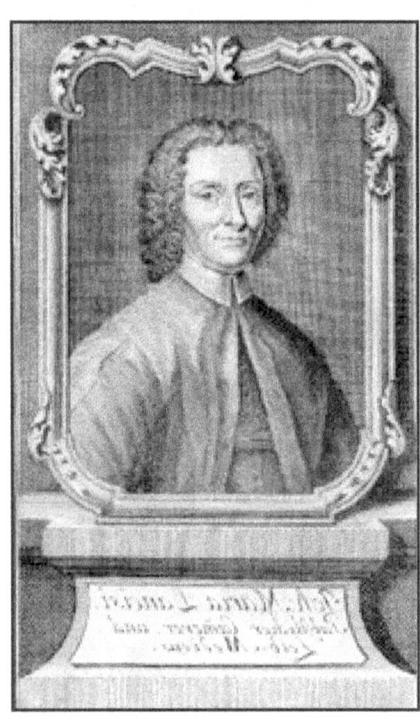

GIOVANNI LANCISI,
public domain

However, two Frenchmen came close to solving the puzzle. PIERRE CHI-RAC (1650-1732, born Conques, France, and died Marly-le-Roi, France) was physician to King Louis XV.

The Reign of Terror during the French Revolution came after him. King Louis XV is regarded as ineffectual and hastened the decline of French royalty, which led to the French Revolution of 1789.

Chirac in 1698 tied off a dog's coronary artery and found that the heart immediately stopped beating. He had discovered the source of the heart's mechanical ability to pump but unfortunately did not recognize what he had discovered and never took his observations any further.

Jean-Baptiste de Senac (1691-1770, born and died Gascony, France) also lived during the reign of Louis XV. He noted in 1749 that the left ventricle sometimes developed a thin wall and bulge, known today as an aneurysm, and commented upon ossified coronary arteries. Like Lancisi, Senac came very close to recognizing the relationship between blocked coronary arteries and heart attacks with subsequent damage and heart muscle thinning. He could have solved the problem but never made the connection that the two were causally related.

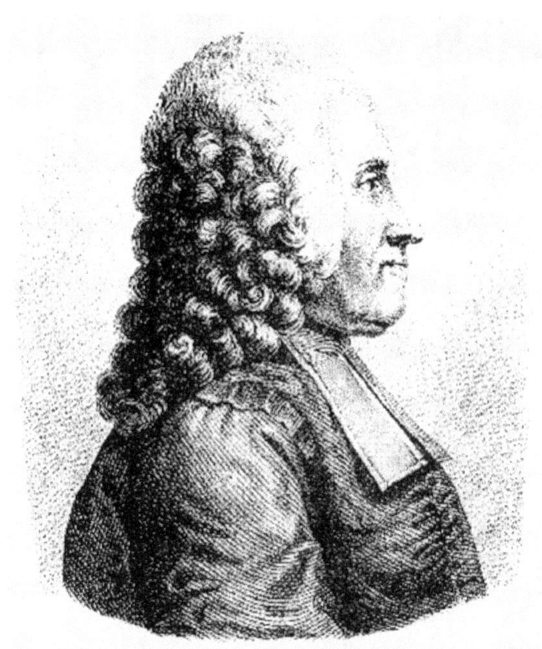

JEAN-BAPTISTE DE SENAC,
Science Photo Library License

In 1757 a German named JOHANN FRIEDRICH CRELL (1707-1747, born Leipzig, Germany, and died Hemschedt, Germany) had his papers published posthumously on Coronary Atherosclerosis. He also noted an autopsy finding of coronary arteries "hard as bone" with a soft substance inside containing a soft mass similar to a sebaceous cyst. This soft substance, in retrospect, was probably the first anatomic description of cholesterol deposits within the artery (i.e. atheromata, or fatty collections). Unfortunately, his observations were ignored by the medical profession for years, and he died before his publication so he could not either defend nor advocate for his findings. Obviously, his death prevented him from reporting on more patients. Nor did Crell associate his findings directly as the cause of myocardial infarctions (heart attacks). He came close to solving the mystery, but "no cigar."

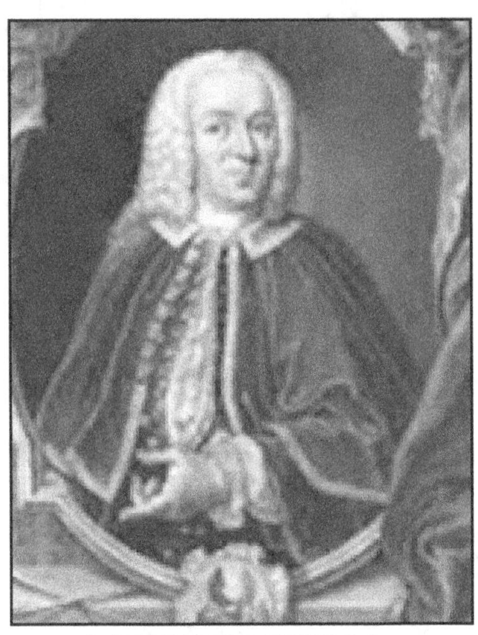

JOHANN CRELL,
public domain

In 1761 GIOVANNI (GIAMBATTISTA) MORGAGNI (1682-1771, born Forli, Italy, and died Padua, Italy) described hardening of the arteries of the heart but never connected his finding to heart damage caused by a heart attack. He was an early proponent of trying to link the clinical symptoms to the autopsy findings to explain disease.

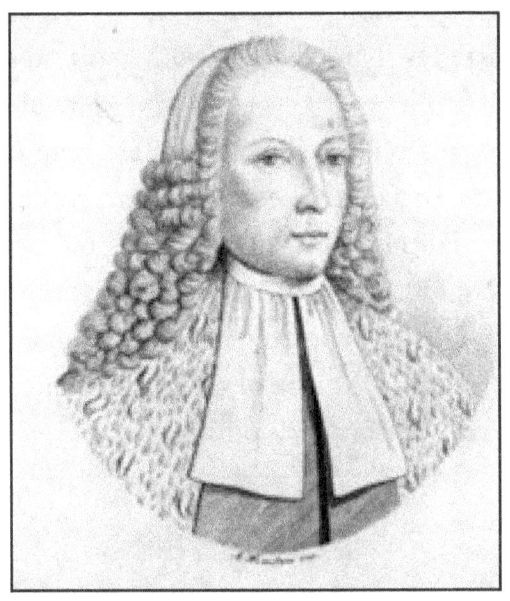

GIOVANNI BATTISTA MORGAGNI
National Library of Medicine, public domain

Thus, many times and many physicians in the 1700s came close to proving the mystery of coronary artery disease's link to angina and heart attacks, as the answer was right beneath their noses, but no one stopped to smell the roses properly.

IN WHAT COUNTRIES WERE DISCOVERIES MADE AND WHAT DETERMINED WHERE THESE SCIENTIFIC LEADERS LIVED?

Part of the reason it took so long to solve the link between coronary artery disease and symptoms of angina and heart attacks was that Europe was in nearly constant turmoil for three centuries, and the money to fund scientific experiments often shifted from country to country depending upon the individual country's fortunes. Thus, a discontinuity occurred from one discovery to the next.

The scientific cardiac leadership originally was in Italy in the 16th and 17th centuries. Subsequently Italy sank into political disarray and poverty. In the 17th and 18th centuries France, England, and Holland were the countries making contributions with Italy only to a lesser extent, but then France suffered from the ravages of their revolution and the Napoleonic Wars and had no money to support science. In the 19th century England, Germany, Austria, and to a lesser extent again France, Holland, and for the first time the U.S., performed most of the research. By the 20th century the leadership was clearly with England, Germany, and the U.S., the three richest countries in the world.

The determinants of where the research was performed and who made the contributions to coronary artery disease understanding can be explained to a major extent by political turmoil and wars, which hindered progress. Most science was financed by the Crown or very wealthy nobility, but money was short when armies had to be raised and fed. During the French Revolution and the Napoleonic Wars that followed, armaments and paying soldiers were more important to rulers on both sides who had most of the money via taxes than spending money on scientific advancement. After all, if few scientists had scientific curiosity, how could one expect the nobility and royalty to push research with their national treasury? France stopped being one of the main scientific centers when it succumbed to anarchy of its revolution and then the defeat of

Napoleon Bonaparte in battle in 1815, concluding 23 years of nearly continuous war. Sadly, his wars consumed the French Treasury.

These national issues diverted money, intellectual investment, and resources for research to other national needs. Poverty into which countries like Italy descended was also inconsistent with research support and caused Italy, the original leader, to take a back seat to other Western European countries. Diseases such as the plague, tuberculosis, cholera, and typhus also curtailed scientific inquiry, as funds were needed elsewhere and populations who supplied tax money often dwindled in numbers from the scourges. Even Germany, eventually one of the leaders of culture and science, could only become one of the leaders after it unified in 1871, as Germany previously was only a patchwork of principalities and duchies and continually squabbling or fighting with its neighbors and principalities.

But a major question remains. Pieces of information were discovered. Astute minds should have been able to connect the dots, but they did not. Why?

The road to understanding the unity of coronary disease with angina pectoris and heart attacks was like chasing butterflies—just when you thought you had the butterfly, it flew away and you didn't!!!!

The problem was that most doctors from the 17th through the 19th centuries were confused about the anatomic cause of angina pectoris and what it could lead to and often did not even associate this symptom as even originating from the heart. Confusion was compounded by the fact that 1) some patients died suddenly with angina, 2) some patients lived long lives with their anginal symptoms, and 3) others seemed "cured" with time as the symptoms might disappear. So it was difficult to associate this with a consistently significant malady that could cause a heart attack. Not recognized was that in many patients the symptom went away because a heart attack caused death of the heart muscle supplied by a narrowed coronary artery, which reduced the blood supply only to a portion of the heart muscle and not to the entire heart. Sometimes it did not cause enough permanent damage and spared death if the remaining live heart muscle was sufficiently functional.

PROBABLY MOST IMPORTANTLY, a heart attack was not a common medical problem in the 16-19th centuries, as most people did not live long enough to develop either angina or a heart attack as statistically these conditions do not usually manifest until most people are in their late 50s through their 70s or even 80s or more. Unfortunately, the average life expectancy in the Western world until 1900 was only forty years of age and did not rise to age fifty until the beginning of the 1900s. Thus, few people lived long enough to make coronary artery disease an important public health problem. Coronary artery disease remained a rare medical problem (known today as an "orphan disease," when few have the problem) until the mid-1950s, when it became and has remained the most common cause of death followed by cancer in the Western world.

It was far more likely that someone between 1700 and 1900 would die in war of injuries, from famine, from infection such as tuberculosis or even from syphilitic heart disease than die of a heart attack. To make matters more confusing, the great Laennec, who invented the stethoscope and was the father of cardiac physical diagnosis, remained influential for several subsequent generations of physicians and transmitted that in his belief angina was nothing more than a benign nervous disorder, not related to the heart. How wrong he was!

STEP FOUR: LATER STEPS ASSESSING THE OUTSIDE AND INSIDE OF CORONARY ARTERIES AND ATTEMPTS TO LINK DISEASED CORONARY ARTERIES TO CARDIAC MUSCLE PATHOLOGY

An English surgeon, JOHN HUNTER (1728-1793, born Killbride East, Lanarkshire, Scotland, and died London, UK), became famous during the Seven Years' War between England and France (1756-1763) and is credited with transforming surgery from a trade into a profession. He was also the brother of William Hunter, who obtained DaVinci's papers. Among John Hunter's accomplishments was performing an autopsy in the late 1770s on a patient of Dr. John Fothergill (1712-1780, born Wensleydeale in Yorkshire, England, and died London, England). Hunter was known for advocating and lecturing on the benefits of mouth-to-mouth ventilation for the "suddenly apparently dead," an early proponent of what would become known as CPR.

Coincidentally, Fothergill was not only a friend of Hunter but also a friend of Benjamin Franklin. Fothergill's patient was 63 years of age and had previously suffered from angina pectoris. Hunter found a white scar (clearly a heart attack scar) in the heart muscle and two calcified coronary arteries at autopsy..

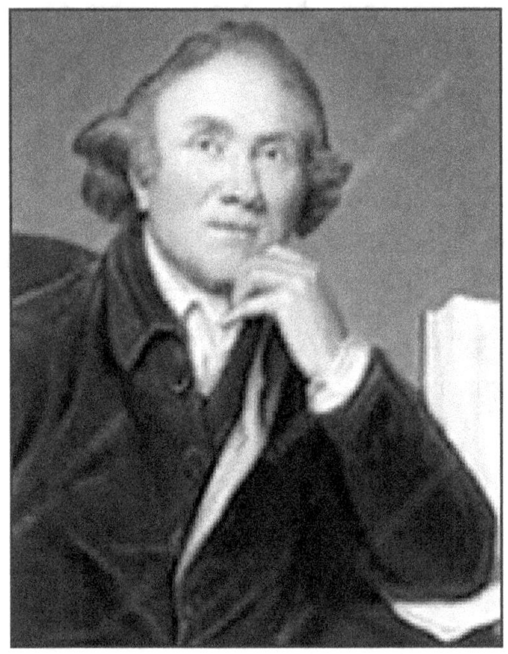

JOHN HUNTER
National Library of Medicine, public domain

"as hard as bone" with calcium. Unfortunately, he never used his scalpel to cut into the artery to see what was inside, unlike Crell who did, presumably a clot and/or cholesterol plaque, or both, so he did not make the connection between the death of the patient and the diseased coronary artery or even the patient's previous angina pectoris and its progression to a heart attack (as a reminder, the coronary artery, although at least 70% narrowed in angina patients, is completely blocked 100% when causing a heart attack). Ironically, Hunter also suffered from angina and died suddenly of a heart attack while arguing with a colleague at his hospital.

A further irony to this story is that two physicians and friends of John Hunter did make the connection between coronary artery disease and heart attacks (myocardial infarctions). They were EDWARD JENNER (1740-1823, born Berkely, UK, and died Berkely, UK) and CALEB HILLIER PARRY (1755-1822, born Cirencester, UK, and died Bath, UK).

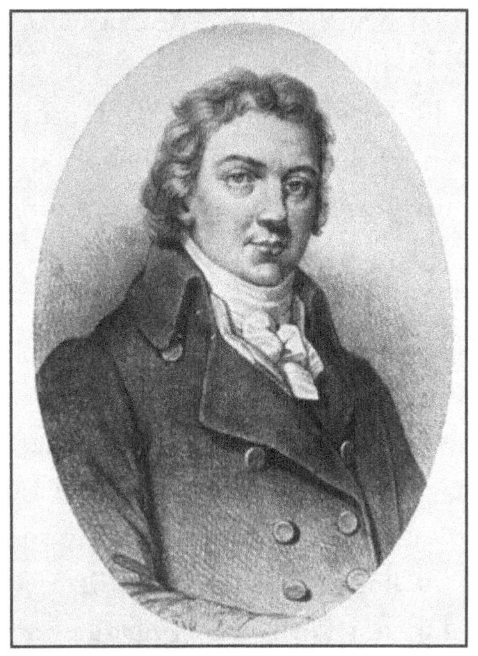
EDWARD JENNER
National Library of Medicine,
public domain

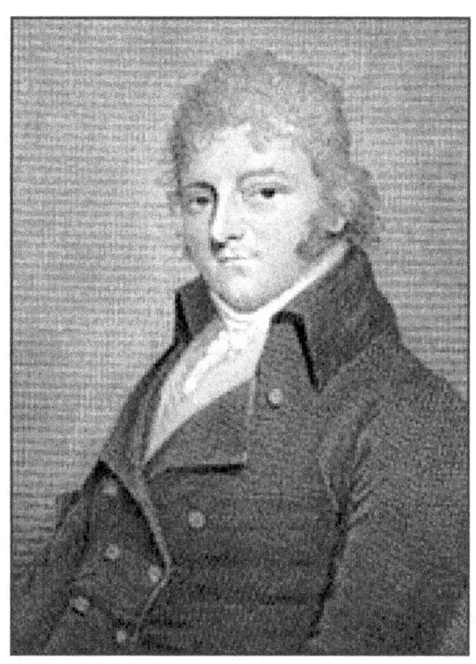
CALEB HILLIER PARRY
National Library of Medicine,
public domain

Jenner was of small pox vaccination fame. Parry was the father of the future
rear admiral and arctic explorer William Edward Parry. Together they were certain that coronary arteries were the cause of angina pectoris and cardiac death
but were afraid to publish their theory until their friend John Hunter died for
fear that if he read their paper, Hunter would be in despair, triggering a fatal
heart attack. Jenner and Parry were prescient, but it took a long time for others
to listen and follow up on their thesis. Jenner wrote, "And if we can suppose
that the coronaries may be so obstructed as to intercept the blood which should
be the proper support of the muscular fibers of the heart, that organ must become thin and flaccid (i.e. has suffered a heart attack) and unequal to the task of
circulation" (i.e. the left ventricle has gone into heart failure). So they waited
until 1799 to publish their hypothesis after John Hunter died ("true friendship").
They also had been asked by Hunter to perform his autopsy, which they did.
The autopsy of Hunter also disclosed two hard coronary arteries and a white
myocardial scar. Obviously they found atherosclerotic coronary artery disease
and a myocardial infarction. However, they, too, failed to prove the connection
since they also did not cut into the coronary artery to see what lay inside. Al-

though certain of the cause of heart attacks being blocked coronary arteries, they did not actually prove it. Their theory waited another 119 years for proof and an additional thirty years for the medical profession's acceptance of these findings. It remains inexplicable why these two brilliant men did not use a simple scalpel available to them to incise the coronary artery and peer inside. Certainly they would have seen a blockage due to a plaque or even a clot, which would prove their hypothesis. BUT THEY DIDN'T!!

In 1809 another Scotsman, ALLAN BURNS (1781-1813, born and died Glasgow, Scotland, UK), also a surgeon, made an important observation. He noted that the symptom of angina pectoris with exertion but relieved by resting closely resembled the "fatigue" symptoms of extremity muscles in a moderately tight ligated limb upon exertion but receding with the tourniquet's release. Although his observation totally explained the link between coronary artery disease and angina, he only hinted at it and did not take his theory further nor did others for some time.

A surgeon from England named JOSEPH HODGSON (1799-1869, born Pennith near Birmingham, UK, and died London, UK) made an important discovery. He lived during the Victorian Era of Queen Victoria, who ruled from 1837-1901. Her job was to reign, not to rule, and the English monarch became mainly a figurehead during this era. In the reign of Queen Victoria, England continued to grow militarily and economically and became the first global industrial power. England abolished slavery in 1838 with Caribbean plantation owners receiving compensation "from the crown," although former slaves received nothing. In that same year the *S.S. Great Western* steamship crossed the Atlantic from Bristol to New York in a record fifteen days. The mail delivery changed, no longer requiring rich and poor alike to pay to receive a letter, only to send one. In 1845 the Irish potato famine from a fungal disease of the potato plant started and lasted four years, causing mass hunger and disease with one out of every eight Irishman dying as a result and causing mass immigration from Ireland to the New World. In 1854 the Crimean War between Russia against France, England and the Turks occurred. One and a half million soldiers fought in this war, with 367,000 deaths ensuing. This was the era of change. The construction industry in England was revolutionized when Henry Bessemer in 1856 developed a new process to manufacture steel, allowing large construction of bridges, boats, and railroads. In 1859 Darwin published his *Origin of the Species*. In 1863 the London underground subway was opened and in 1869 the Suez Canal opened.

Interestingly, many of the discoveries about the heart were made by surgeons as well as by medical doctors. Hodgson theorized that the coronary arteries led to heart damage in 1815, and he published three autopsy cases of hardened and obstructed coronary arteries as evidence of his theory. Eureka!! He had discovered the Holy Grail. Unfortunately, his theory was not widely accepted and totally ignored for another eighty years.

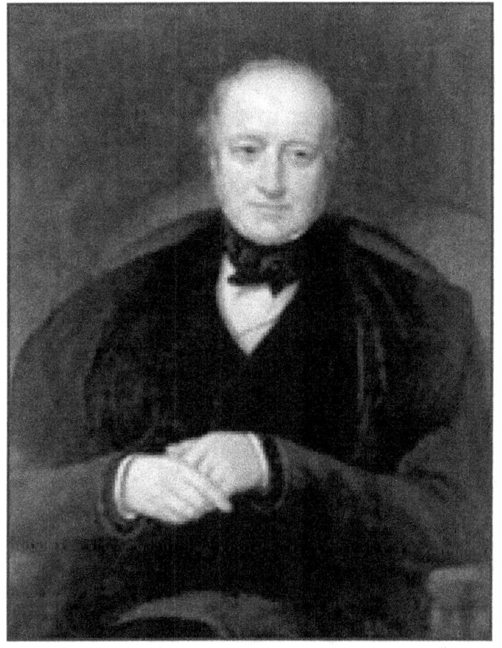

JOSEPH HODGSON,
public domain

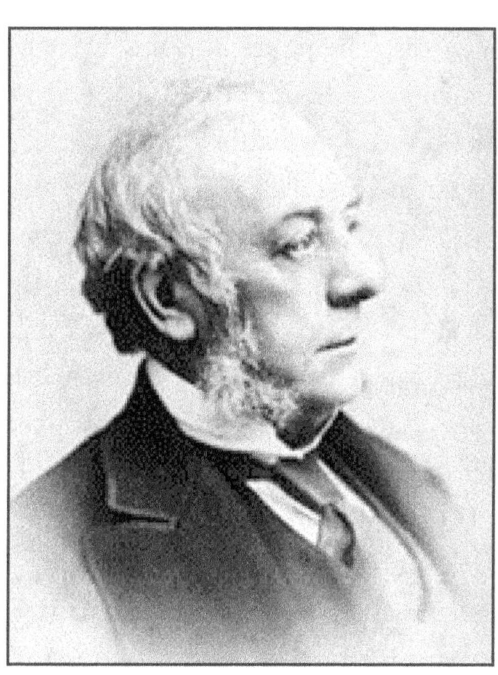

JOHN ERICHSEN,
Creative Commons John Partridge,
artist permission: Welcome images.org

Another British surgeon, JOHN ERICHSEN (1818-1895, born Copenhagen, Denmark, and died Folkstone Kent, UK), in 1840 tied off a dog's coronary artery and witnessed the dog's death in twenty minutes but he did not carry these experiments further, although he was on the trail of discovery.

With German unification in 1871, the German mind finally awakened as Germany became a major military, educational, and economic power in

STEP 5: THE PUZZLE IS SOLVED AND THE FINAL PIECE FALLS INTO PLACE – THE NINETEENTH CENTURY WAS THE AGE OF EXPERIMENTATION AND DISCOVERY, ESPECIALLY WITH THE AWAKENING OF THE GERMAN MIND

Europe (both in Germany but also in German-speaking Austria, especially Vienna). The puzzle was finally to be solved.

In 1880 KARL WEIGERT (1845-1904, born Ziebice, Poland, and died Frankfurt, Germany) wrote a paper and almost absentmindedly wrote in his paper in 1880:

"Atherosclerotic changes of coronary arteries not infrequently thrombotic or embolic in origin form in the branches of arteries. If the obstruction forms slowly, or at least in such wise that collateral channels exist, but not enough to keep up nutrition, a slow atrophy occurs with destruction of muscle. The muscle fibers that disappear are replaced by fibrous connective tissue." He recognized the link between coronary artery disease and left ventricular scarring and damage!!!

Julius Friedrich Cohnheim (1839-1884, born Demmin, Germany, and died Leipzig, Germany) next came along. Cohnheim studied under Ludwig Traube (see Chapter 1: Physical Diagnosis) and dedicated his own papers to Traube's memory. He also studied under the famous pathologist Virchow, including research on embolisms (blood clots traveling from one place to another) as well as a paradoxical embolism through the wall between the right and left atria, known as the foramen ovale, published in 1889 and previously not thought possible. Later he studied circulatory disturbances with Karl Ludwig (1816-1895). Cohnheim worked with Karl Huber and, like Erichsen earlier, he tied off the coronary artery of a dog and observed sudden death within twenty minutes (published 1881). Moreover, he correctly hypothesized the link and causality between coronary artery atherosclerosis and myocardial scarring and sudden unexpected death, whereas Erichsen did not interpret further his findings. However, Cohnheim and others incorrectly assumed that humans, if cut off from the origin of a major coronary artery supply, would also not survive the heart attack and die suddenly just as the dog did. On the other hand, he recognized that tying off smaller branches often allowed survival or were even without any clinical consequence. Furthermore, he concluded that slow or incomplete obstruction (now recognized as the cause of angina pectoris) led to patchy fibrosis and sometimes with no symptoms but sometimes with congestive heart failure, depending on how much tissue was involved. He believed, correctly, and was later proved to be correct by Richard Gorlin and his group at the Peter Bent Brigham Hospital in Boston in the twentieth century that the pain of angina was due to an accumulation of toxic chemical products due to the lack of oxygen, the term for it being "anoxemia." Gorlin, in the 1960s, showed this substance to be lactic acid (see below).

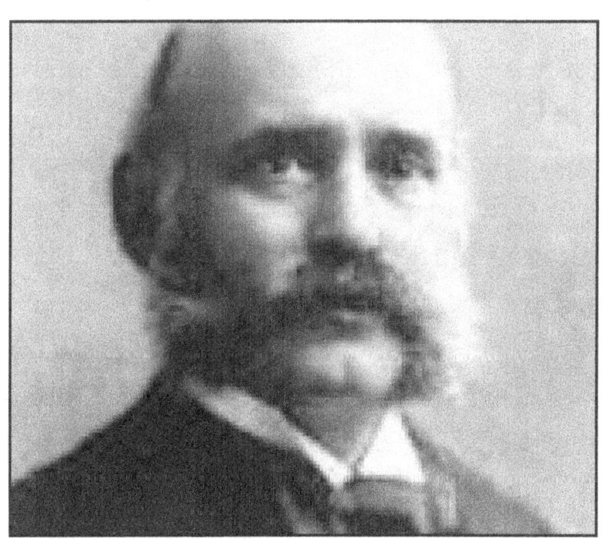

KARL WEIGERT
public domain

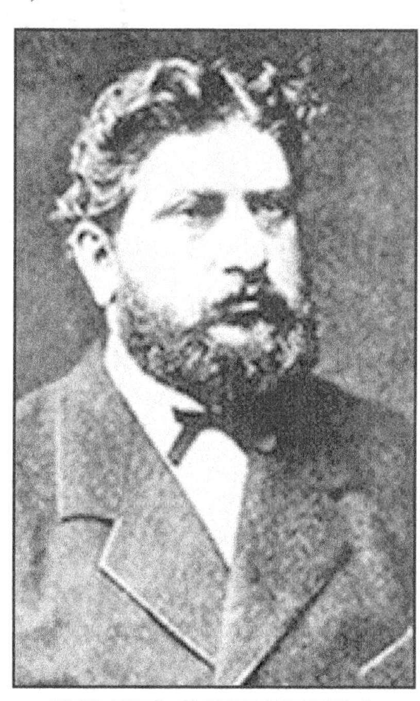

JULIUS COHNHEIM
National Library of Medi-
cine, public domain

ERNST VICTOR VON LEYDEN (1832-1910, born Danzig, Poland, and died Charlottenburg, Germany) in 1884 published a paper recognizing a group of elderly patients with or without previous angina who died suddenly and had coronary artery plaques. Some of the patients recalled lesser attacks or even more severe episodes from which they recovered totally.

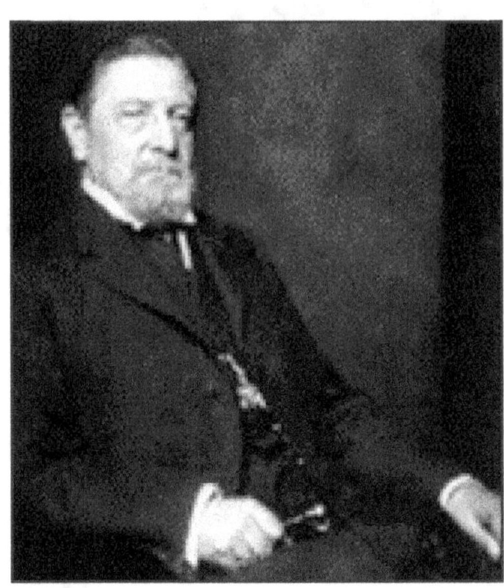

ERNST VON LEYDEN
National Library of Medicine, public domain

The coronary artery hypothesis was now proved, i.e. that coronary arteries filled with plaque (part of which was fat and cholesterol) led to the symptoms of angina pectoris when the narrow channel provided insufficient blood for the needs of the heart muscle and that totally clogged coronary arteries could produce heart attacks with subsequent heart muscle death.

So Jenner and Parry linked angina to heart attacks in 1799 but did not provide the needed proof. Multiple investigators, including famous German scientists writing in the 1880s, corroborated and proved Jenner and Parry's thesis. But after 1884 the hypothesis was neglected and forgotten for nearly thirty years until James Herrick from the U.S. came along with his two papers in 1912 and 1918. Even he had difficulty convincing the medical profession that blocked coronary arteries caused angina and heart attacks.

WHY WAS THE CORONARY ARTERY THEORY IGNORED AND SUBSEQUENTLY NEGLECTED?
The answer is complex but includes:

1. Cohnheim's experiments tying off a dog's coronary artery upstream and causing the dog's death was remembered more than his experiments that found when smaller branches were tied off, it was still compatible with survival.

2. Virchow and Rokatinsky (see below) were the two giants of pathology of the 19th century. They incorrectly believed that heart scarring (myocardial fibrosis) was due to primary heart muscle inflammation as the primary insult and not a secondary phenomenon due to deprivation of the heart muscle from its blood supply, so many ignored Cohnheim et al.

3. The invention of the stethoscope and the ability to diagnose many heart diseases premortem preoccupied doctors with valvular rather more than coronary artery disease.

4. Many doctors wrongly thought that if there were no audible abnormal findings by stethoscope, then the heart must be healthy. Coronary artery disease is often silent for many years until or even despite a heart attack occurring.

5. Medical journals at the time were filled with articles unrelated to the coronary arteries and more often about infections such as tuberculosis, typhus, cholera, and malaria, which were perceived more important issues of that time.

6. No cars existed until the 20th century, so people were physically in better condition because they walked more than today, helping coronary artery health. Exercise helps prevent heart attacks. This may have also contributed to fewer heart attacks until the 20th century, when the auto became so important culturally as well as for transportation.

7. Because myocardial infarctions rarely present before the late 50s of age, there were not many heart attacks numerically seen by doctors until the 1950s, as the average life expectancy was only forty years of age at the beginning of 1800 and only fifty years of age at the beginning of the 1900s. In short, most people did not live long enough until recently to acquire symptoms of coronary artery disease and died earlier of other medical problems.

8. Basically, disease of the coronary arteries was the orphan disease of its time being terrible but also terribly rare.

9) Finally, the unity of coronary artery disease was not considered as "sexy" as other medical subjects by investigators and clinicians alike until the mid-1900s. Scientists were either captivated by the physical findings made available by Laennec's stethoscope or were seduced by the new science of bacteriology invented by Pasteur and Koch and its byproduct of aseptic techniques invented by Lister.

TWO STRANGE NEW INVENTIONS HELPED TO REFOCUS THE MEDICAL PROFESSION ON CORONARY ARTERY DISEASE

The first was the discovery of x-rays and the invention of the x-ray machine by WILHELM ROENTGEN (1845-1923, born Lennep, Prussia, and died Munich, Weimar Republic, Germany). A real Disruptor, Roentgen justifiably earned a Nobel Prize for Physics in 1901 for his discovery of x-rays in 1895 (which he named). His discovery arguably led to the most important inventions in the modern era of cardiac imaging, including chest x-rays, later cardiac catheterization and CT scans. His first radiograph using x-rays was on his wife Anna Bertha's hand. Interestingly, the adoption of his findings occurred extremely rapidly with a large number of scientific investigations published by 1896. In the U.S. fifty institutions were performing radiation research within three months of Roentgen's discovery, including early fluoroscopy by Francis Henry Williams in 1896 (1852-1936, born Uxbridge, Mass., U.S., and died Boston) only a year after Roentgen's discovery. He became the first radiologist at the Massachusetts General Hospital in Boston. The discovery of x-rays led to fluoroscopy of the heart, which allowed physicians to see the outline of the heart and some motion with the ability to determine if the heart was enlarged or even in congestive heart failure and eventually to cardiac catheterization and coronary angiography, which were indispensable in the development of operations on the heart.

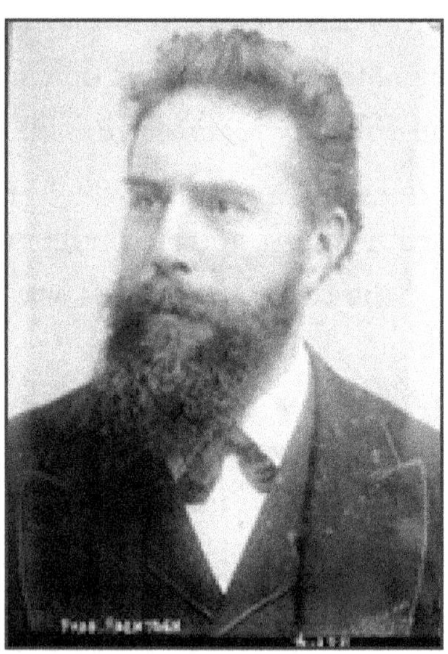

WILHELM ROENTGEN,
from Library of Congress George Bain Collection, no restrictions

Augustus Desire Waller (1856-1922, born Paris, France, and died London, England) was the first to record an electrical signal from a human heart via surface electrodes in 1887 but was unable to record the atrial activity. Waller's leads were placed on a human chest and back. Only a ventricular depolarization was recorded, not a full EKG. Nevertheless, Einthoven gave him credit for Einthoven's invention of the EKG (also known mainly today in the U.S. as ECG) machine.

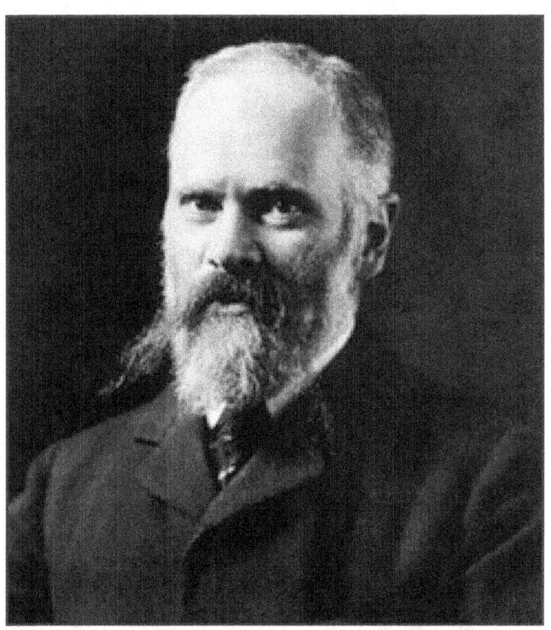

AUGUST DESIRE WALLER,
from the Wellcome Trust Collection and in public domain via Creative Commons

The second important invention and disruption in refocusing the medical profession on coronary artery disease was the invention of the EKG machine by WILLEM EINTHOVEN (1860-1927, born Semerang, Indonesia, and died Leiden, Netherlands). He was a true Disruptor. He was not a practicing physician although he went to medical school but a practicing physicist. His machine with further developments on its availability, affordability, and portability has allowed widespread use by physicians to detect heart rhythm disturbances and heart attacks to this day. Although having witnessed Waller record a human electrical lead, it was Einthoven who invented the first fully usable clinically EKG machine in 1901. He decided to improve upon the results of Waller. Einthoven reported clinical findings using his EKG machine in 1903. Einthoven set down the rules for choosing a lead system, where to place the leads, and the names of the deflections (P, Q, R S, T and later U), and speed of the paper recording the EKG, all still being used today. His system was completed by 1908. Einthoven's EKG machine only had lead II, III, AVR, and AVF, i.e. the limb leads. During heart attacks, these only allow the undersurface of the heart being damaged to be diagnosed (known an inferior infarctions). A great advance in cardiology came when in 1932 leads on the chest were added by Charles Wolferth (1887-1965, died Gladwynne, Pennsylvania, U.S.) and Francis Wood (1901-1990, born Wellington, South Africa, and died Haverford, Pennsylvania, U.S.), allowing heart attacks on the front of the heart also to be diagnosed, which are the most lethal of heart attacks.

Although EKG machines are now easily portable and even battery-powered and compact, Einthoven's original machine weighed 594 pounds and took five people to operate and move it. He would be pleased if he were still alive to see how his EKG machine has been made so much more usable, although the basic principles have not changed. For his accomplishment, Einthoven received a Nobel Prize in 1924. Perhaps Waller, who died in 1922, would have received one also had he still been alive in 1924, as the Nobel Prize requires recipients to be alive when it is bestowed.

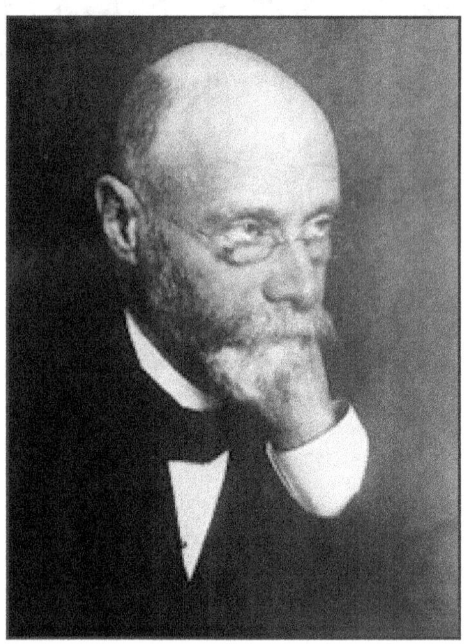

WILLEM EINTHOVEN
from the Library of Congress, George G. Bain collection, no restrictions

SELLING THE CONCEPT TO THE MEDICAL PROFESSION

The final proof that coronary artery disease caused heart attacks and convincing the medical profession of its importance required James Herrick's research publications in 1912 and 1918 and his scientific and professional salesmanship of the concept to the medical profession. Remember that the German scientists in the late 1880s proved the link among coronary artery disease, angina, and heart attacks, but 37 years would elapse before the concept was widely accepted by the medical profession. It took the right salesman to convince the medical world.

Dr. James Herrick was this person. James Brian Herrick (1861-1954, born Oak Park, Illinois, U.S.A., and died Chicago, U.S.A.).

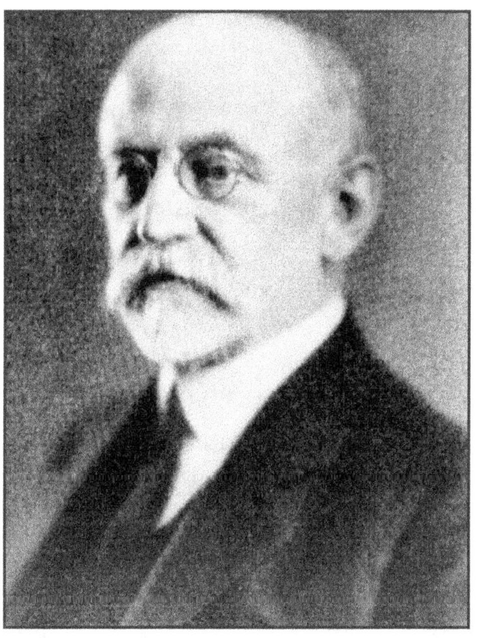

JAMES HERRICK,
Science Photo Library License

His first paper of 1912, just before the start of World War I, created almost "no ripples in the medical community," as he said although he as a scientist finally asked the right question. People took notice, however, when he published his second paper in 1918 and then another in 1919, opening doctors' eyes to the possibility of coronary artery disease, not only causing heart attacks but that people could actually survive heart attacks. The 1918 paper included a report of three patients who had suffered a heart attack and survived the initial insult (one patient was the one from the 1912 paper) for days or weeks after the incident, proving that heart attacks were not uniformly or immediately fatal. The paper included early EKGs up to 178 days after the event as well as pathologic studies showing totally occluded coronary arteries. His contribution was not only that humans could survive a heart attack but that even clotting off of large branches was compatible with survival. The cardiac community finally opened its eyes and awakened to the fact that not only did diseased coronary arteries produce heart attacks, but that a patient could survive for some period of time after the event. Herrick had also performed animal experiments ligating coronary arteries without animal succumbing.

In 1944 Herrick wrote that his 1912 (Herrick, JB JAMA 1912: 59:2015-20: Clinical features of sudden obstruction of the coronary arteries) paper "fell like a dud." He went on to write "there are reasons for believing that even large branches of the coronary arteries may be occluded—at times acutely occluded—without resulting death, at least death in the immediate future." Finally the 1918 paper aroused a huge interest. If death was not uniformly immediate after a heart attack, the possibility of finding a way to prevent the heart attack altogether and treating it remained realistic for future research and discovery.

The previous confusion about surviving a heart attack caused by an occluded artery in retrospect was understandable. Different branches of the coronary tree not only supply different important areas but even different-size areas of heart muscle, thus producing different outcomes. Early dog experiments usually tied off the large left anterior descending branch down the front of the heart, which was so important that most dogs died quickly, and scientists assumed that humans physiologically would react the same if a major coronary artery were suddenly blocked. In 1919 Herrick was not sure if all angina was cardiac in origin and even sided at that time with others that most angina pectoris episodes arose not from the coronary arteries but from the aorta. Even today it is sometimes difficult to differentiate what seems to be cardiac angina pectoris from chest superficial muscle pain, pain of the heart outer covering called the pericardium, or gastrointestinal causes. So imagine doctors struggling in the early twentieth century to figure out a patient's cause of chest pain without sophisticated diagnostic tests of today. Even with today's many physiologic and anatomic diagnostic tools, there are many cases of angina pectoris not caused by cholesterol in the coronary arteries but due to spasm of normal coronary arteries, atypical coursing of the coronary artery within the heart muscle known as coronary bridging, or problems with the invisible tiny branches of the coronary arteries in a condition known as microvascular angina or microvascular ischemia (ischemia means inadequate blood supply). So one can imagine that in the early 1900s even common atherosclerotic coronary artery disease as a cause of angina would be difficult to assess and evaluate, let alone determine what organ caused it.

By 1931 Herrick finally concluded that most cases of angina pectoris arose from the coronary arteries, nineteen years after his first paper in 1912, although it really took new technology to completely prove the thesis.

First describing the EKG findings during a heart attack was Harold Pardee (1886-1973, born New York, NY, and died NY, NY, U.S.A.). Although often forgotten by present-day doctors, his description of the "tombstone" appearance of a heart attack EKG became known as the "Pardee Sign," although his name attached to this has been forgotten by most doctors in the present era. Further technological advances including using the EKG during some form of exercise (originally the Master's Two-Step EKG, Arthur Master (1895-1973, born NYC, U.S.A., and died NYC, U.S.A.))

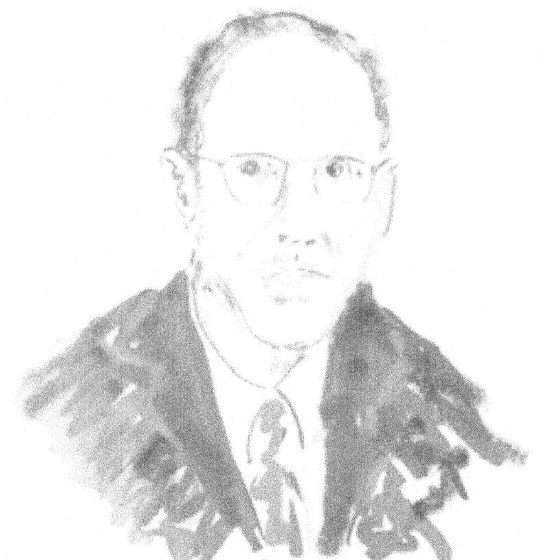

ARTHUR MASTER, original drawing by Dr. Roy Nuzzo
Author's personal collection

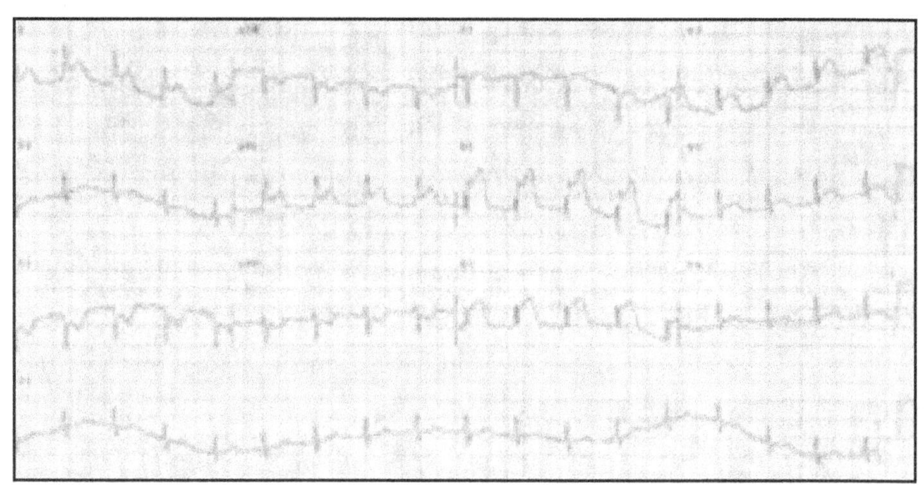

EKG showing "Pardee Sign" with tombstone elevation of leads v1-v4 – Pardee's original EKG showed these changes in limb leads ii, iii, AVF.

in 1950 looked for chest pain and EKG changes not present before exercising as a sign that the patient's chest discomfort was due to a blocked coronary artery. Later, treadmill and bicycle EKGs using the Bruce protocol (1963), developed by Dr. Robert Bruce (1916-2004, born Somerville, Mass., U.S.A., and died Seattle, Washington) produced EKG changes with exertion since the heart required more oxygen than able to be supplied by a narrowed coronary artery or arteries often with chest discomfort. These are known as stress tests and attempt to produce symptoms and EKG changes when the threshold is crossed between the supply of oxygen to the heart being inadequate for the demand.

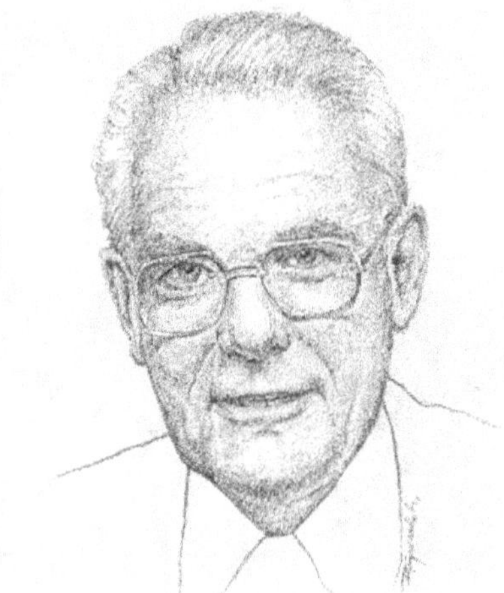

ROBERT BRUCE,
permission by Creative Commons and Cardionetwork with hand drawing from photo by David Gavasheli

Subsequently, nuclear stress testing, stress echoes and coronary angiography (see below section on heart catheterization) have made the diagnosis of angina easier and the cause more precise. Modern testing has allowed cardiologists to understand the mechanism of angina and the precise anatomic origin in the coronary artery tree where it is arising, although none of these tests are perfect.

Finally, the frosting on the cake was placed by Mason Sones (1918-1985, born Noxapater, Mississippi, and died Cleveland, Ohio), who first developed coronary angiography in 1958, which allowed physicians to see the inside of coronary arteries and how much narrowing the plaque was causing while the patient was still alive and not on an operating table or, worse, on a pathologist's dissection table.

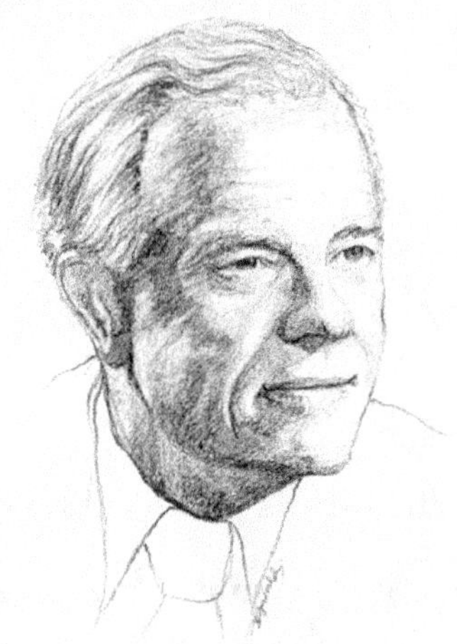

MASON SONES by David Gavasheli
Hand drawn from public domain photo

Over eighty years before RICHARD GORLIN (1926-1997, born in Jersey City, New Jersey, and died in Manhattan, New York) and his group demonstrated in 1963 that pacing the right atrium at increasing heart rates would cause angina pectoris symptoms and EKG changes with the toxic chemical produced with ischemia being lactic acid, Julius Cohnheim had postulated the very same. Gorlin's group found that lactic acid levels would rise with ischemia (inadequate blood supply to the heart muscle) and fall when ischemia abated. Julius Cohnheim had been correct.

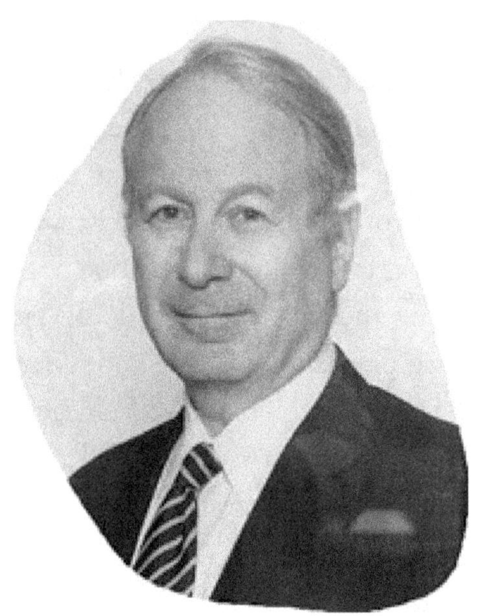

RICHARD GORLIN, courtesy of Dr. Stephen Winters
from his private collection

GLOSSARY CHAPTER 2

Myocardial infarction – heart attack with closed coronary artery causing death of heart muscle tissue, usually only 10-40% of the entire heart muscle

Coronary artery – three arteries arising from the aorta above the main outlet valve from the heart, the aortic valve. On the left there is the left main, which quickly divides into the left anterior descending down the front and circumflex around the left outside and back of the heart. On the right is the right coronary artery supplying the undersurface.

Coronary artery disease – also known as atherosclerotic coronary artery disease is the buildup of material in the coronary artery, including fat and cholesterol

Left ventricle – main pumping chamber on the left side of heart receiving blood from the left atrium above it and pumping through the aortic valve blood into the aorta to be distributed to the body

Plaque – buildup of material in an artery including fat and cholesterol but also cells and a gluelike "ground substance"

Interventricular septum – wall between the right and left ventricles

Pores – small holes thought by Galen to connect the two ventricles (they are not present)

Occlusion – total blockage

Stenosis – narrowing

Arteries – blood vessels that bring oxygenated blood to the organs

Vein – blood vessels take deoxygenated blood back to the heart to be refreshed

Pulmonary circulation – the pulmonary artery leaves the right ventricle, where smaller branches known as capillaries receive oxygen from the lungs and then bring this blood via pulmonary veins to the left atrium and then the left ventricle

Histology – microscopic study of tissue of the body

Cellular pathology – study of abnormal individual body cells

Angina pectoris – symptom of chest pressure with effort when the heart's need for oxygen outstrips the supply due to a narrowing or stenosis. The symptom usually is relieved with rest.

Atherosclerosis – fatty buildup in arteries

CHAPTER 3
EARLY MEDICAL THERAPEUTICS

I was an intern in internal medicine in Boston in 1968 when "on call" was every other night, often without any sleep. One morning when I arrived on the floor to make rounds (the medical term for examining and assessing a hospital patient's status each day) on my patients, the charge nurse said to me, "Are you angry at me, Dr. Guss?" I was bewildered that she would ask me such a question because I certainly was not upset at all with her. When I asked her what she meant, she responded, "I called you about 3 A.M. and said Mrs. Jones was having VPCs" (extra beats from the bottom of the heart). "You told me to 'give her some more digitalis.'" Fortunately she was not on this medication, which is often contraindicated for this condition. She said, "Dr. Guss, I told you that she was not on digitalis so you said to 'give her two milliliters per' and hung up on me." (This last suggestion does not even make grammatical let alone medical sense.) Thank God the nurse was smarter than I was (also she was awake and lucid), so Mrs. Jones survived the event just fine. Lack of sleep for the doctor can be dangerous for the patient!! Residents no longer work the grueling every other night on call. We "old" doctors often discuss with our contemporaries whether the tradeoff produces physicians as well trained and with the same training experience as our generation of doctors.

Despite the cause of angina and myocardial infarctions remaining a mystery, some physicians had ideas about treatment for angina and congestive heart failure, which often is caused by a heart attack. Thus, the 1700s and 1800s were the beginning of cardiac therapeutics. At that time therapeutics meant medications. Today it may include devices as well.

DIGITALIS – WILLIAM WITHERING (1741-1799, born Wellington in Shropshire, UK, and died Sparbrook, Birmingham, UK). Withering was alive during the American Revolution, when King George III was the British monarch. Withering used digitalis leaf, a ground powder from the leaf of the foxglove plant, in 1776 to treat a patient with severe swelling of the body (medical term: anasarca), legs, and feet. This swelling is known as edema (in the eighteenth century called "dropsy"). It worked well, and he found the heart rate also slowed. His idea came from observing patients who used this treatment from English folklore and one elderly female patient of his who was on death's door but took foxglove and had a miraculous cure. In the 20th century, digitalis became the "go-to" drug to treat congestive heart failure and to slow atrial fibrillation heart rates. Subsequently, synthetic compounds were produced and digitalis leaf was replaced and its use eventually abandoned in the early 1970s.

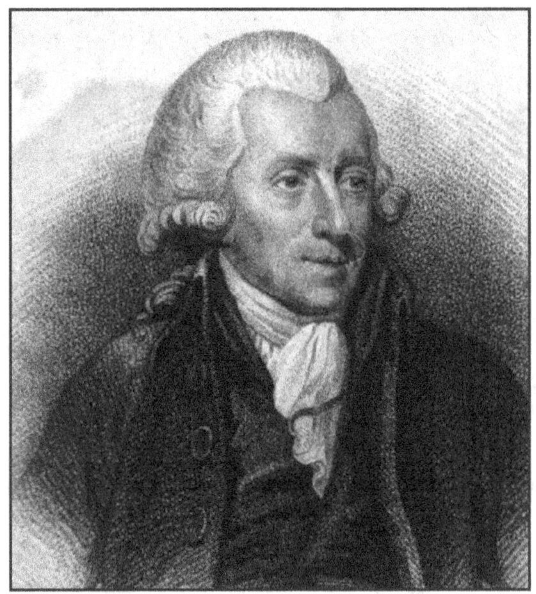

WILLIAM WITHERING
National Library of Medicine, public domain

NITROGLYCERIN – THOMAS LAUDER BRUNTON (1844-1916, born Roxburgh, UK, and died London, UK) discovered a medical use for amyl nitrite (a derivative of nitroglycerin). He lived during the great industrial revolution in England at the time "Britannia ruled the waves." Being the major sea power of the world and the main colonial ruler in the world, this was the time of the height of British power and intellectual breakthroughs.

Brunton reasoned that amyl nitrite might help angina by opening arteries of patients and in 1867 published that placing five to ten drops on a cloth and quickly inhaling the fumes caused the episode of angina pectoris to quickly disappear. He came to this conclusion after watching experiments by Dr. Arthur Gamgee, whose results have remained unpublished, that amyl nitrite lessoned the "arterial tension both in animals and man." Brunton noted that digitalis and brandy were of little use but chloroform relieved temporarily the pain during "partial stupefaction." He also noted that the attack would come on gradually and "the pulse would become smaller and the arterial tension greater as the pain increased in severity." During the attack "the breathing is quick, the pulse small and rapid, and the arterial tension high," as recorded on his sphygmographic pulse tracings. "As the nitrite is inhaled, the pulse becomes slower and fuller, the tension diminished, and the breathing less hurried."

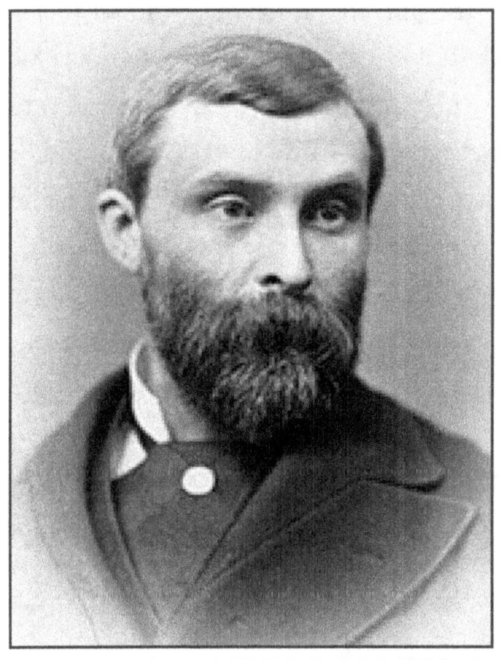

THOMAS LAUDER BRUNTON
National Library of Medicine,
public domain

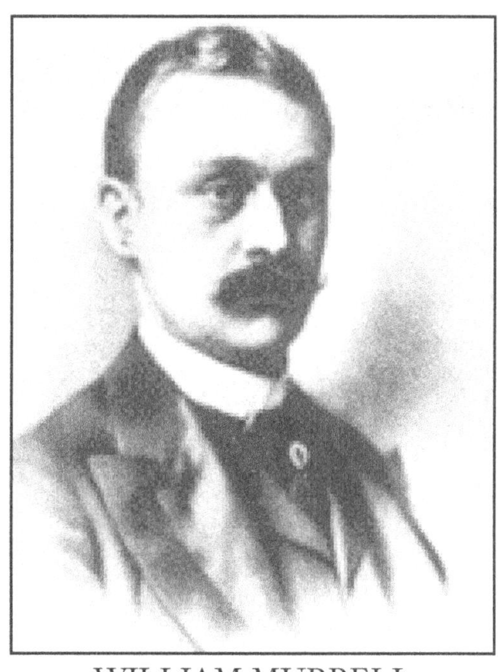

WILLIAM MURRELL
National Library of Medicine,
public domain

Brunton experimented with nitroglycerin liquid, but WILLIAM MURRELL (1853-1912, born London, England) was the first to publish his findings of nitroglycerin using a 1% solution dripped onto a gauze and touching it to the tongue as a successful angina remedy in 1879. He administered nitroglycerin to 35 patients after reporting on others who had tried it earlier. He published that the amyl nitrite and nitroglycerin had similar actions so he thought it might be helpful for angina pectoris. Like Brunton, he used a syphmographic tracings of the pulse and noted taking the medication caused after six or seven minutes a quickening of the heart-beat and taking "a dose of medicine during an attack would cut it short…Patient had adopted the plan of carrying his medicine with him in a vial and taking a dose if an attack seized him in the chest…. It never failed to afford relief."

DIURETICS – WILLIAM STOKES (1804-1878, born Dublin, Ireland, and died Howth near Dublin, Ireland) used a compound of mercury to treat edema (swelling). He may not have associated this swelling with congestive heart failure, but most cases were certainly due to congestive heart failure. Mercury (Thiomerin) around 1950 continued to be used by intramuscular injection as a diuretic (fluid and salt-removing medication) until the mid- to late 1960s, when it was replaced by another diuretic, ethacrynic acid, thought safer because no mercury was contained in it. The replacement turned out to be more effective as a diuretic, but ethacrynic acid in intravenous doses occasionally caused hearing loss and has since been replaced by other diuretics, especially by furosemide (Lasix), which not only did not have this side-effect in the usual clinical doses but could be given in much smaller volumes iv (1-4cc compared to 50-100cc) compared to ethacrynic acid and given orally, too, making administration quicker, safer, and easier. Stokes is the same physician of Adams-Stokes Attacks, which will come later in this book, and described complete heart block before the days of EKG machines.

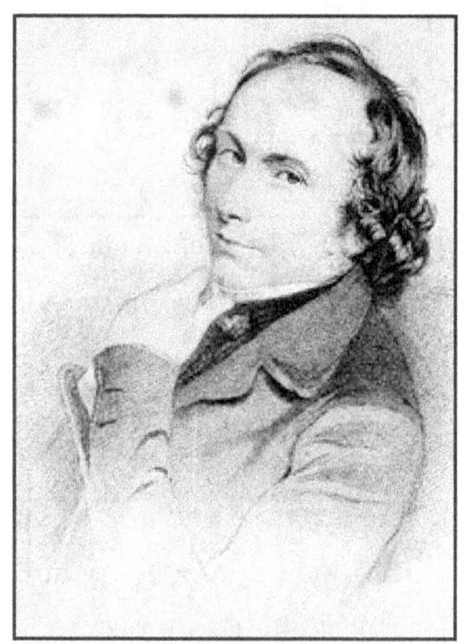

WILLIAM STOKES,
public domain

Aspirin is used today to treat and prevent heart attacks by its anticoagulation effects against platelets, which can cause clotting. It was first used in 1763 in a form of dried Willowbark powder to reduce fever (remember Hippocrates used a form of it to ease the pain of childbirth). JOHANN ANDREAS BUCHNER (1783-1852, born Munich, Germany) isolated the active ingredient of the Willowbark and named it Salicin in 1828. CHARLES GERHARDT (1816-1856, born Strasbourg, France, and died Strasbourg, France) added an acetyl group to Salicin but never marketed it. Finally, FELIX HOFFMAN (1868-1946, born Ludwigsburg near Stuttgart, Germany, and died Switzerland), who was working at Bayer Pharmaceuticals, noted less gastrointestinal irritation with an acetyl group, and it was introduced commercially by Bayer in 1899 for pain and fever. The name Aspirin is derived for A for acetyl, S for Spir from the plant Spirase Ulmaria and IN commonly used as a suffix for drugs at that time. Ironically it was advertised as having no effect on the heart, only to become one of the most important cardiac medications in the 20th and 21st centuries to prevent and treat heart attacks for its antiplatelet clotting effect.

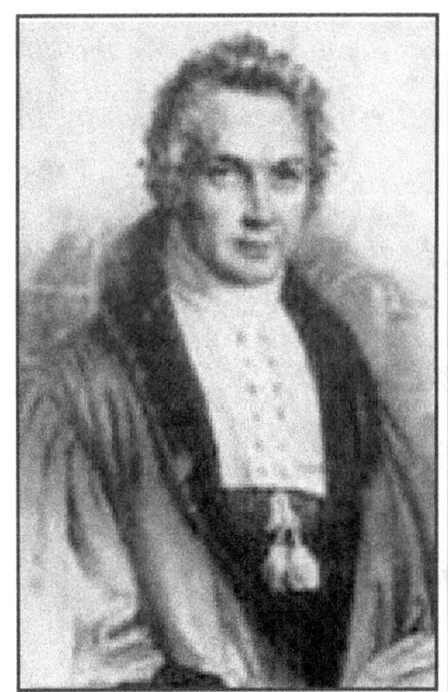
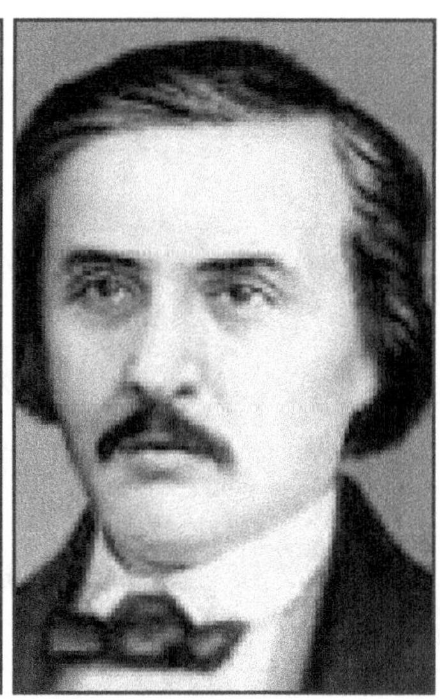
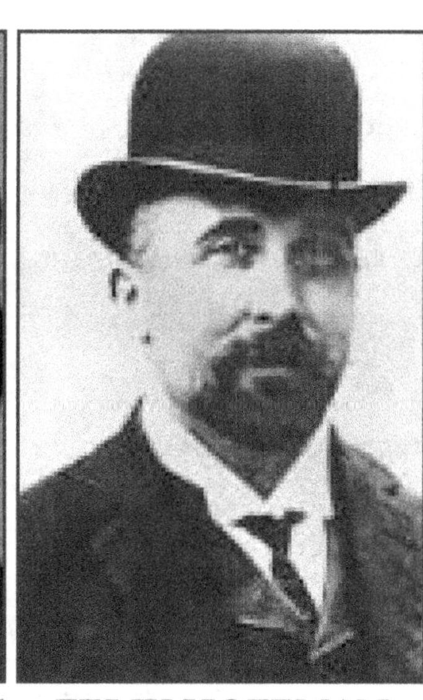

JOHANN BUCHNER
public domain

CHARLES GERHARDT
public domain

FELIX HOFFMAN
public domain

Therapeutics means different things to different doctors, and I always told medical and cardiology residents: "Beware! There is rarely only one right way of treating" (Sir

William Osler gave a similar warning long before I did). An unusual example of my dictum occurred when I was in my second year of internal medicine training (you need to complete internal medicine training before starting a specialty training such as dermatology or cardiology) when a patient came into the Beth Israel Hospital in Boston with very severe congestive heart failure, including severe edema (swelling) of the legs from the feet up to his scrotum. Despite having many excellent and even world-renowned cardiologists on staff at the Beth Israel Hospital, the family was very (almost obnoxiously so) insistent on an outside consultant and voiced their desire to retain Dr. Michael DeBakey to see their family patriarch. When I explained that this would be impossible since he was in Houston, Texas while we were in Boston, one of my interns piped in with "How about Dr. Paul Dudley White?" (1886-1973, born and died Boston, Massachusetts, U.S.). Dr. White, the world-famous cardiologist at the Massachusetts General Hospital across town and cardiologist to former President Eisenhower, was also known as an early advocate of exercise and low-fat diets. I threw the problem back on my wise guy intern, telling him to call the M.G.H. and make arrangements, thinking that the chances of Dr. White coming to our hospital might occur when there was a cold day in hell. To my surprise his secretary said that he was about to leave for the airport to fly to a speaking engagement but would stop at the Beth Israel Hospital on his way. Indeed, he arrived in under an hour, spoke to and examined our patient and then wrote a consultation in very beautiful handwriting and flowery language during an era when notes were known for contractions and abbreviations of 80% of the words in order to save time by interns and residents. White recommended the use of Southey tubes, which none of us had ever heard of nor had they been used as far as I can determine for over thirty years. As an aside, I found an article while researching this book from 1937 that mentions Dr. White's advocacy of using the small bore hollow metal tubes to drain recalcitrant fluid (i.e. Southey tubes). We thanked Dr. White but continued to use diuretics after he left. I made a copy of his note, which I framed and to this day still have, sometimes regretting that I did not keep the original and place the copy in the chart. Honesty is always the best policy, and the memory of that day remains etched in my mind as an original even if my paper note by him is only a Xerox copy.

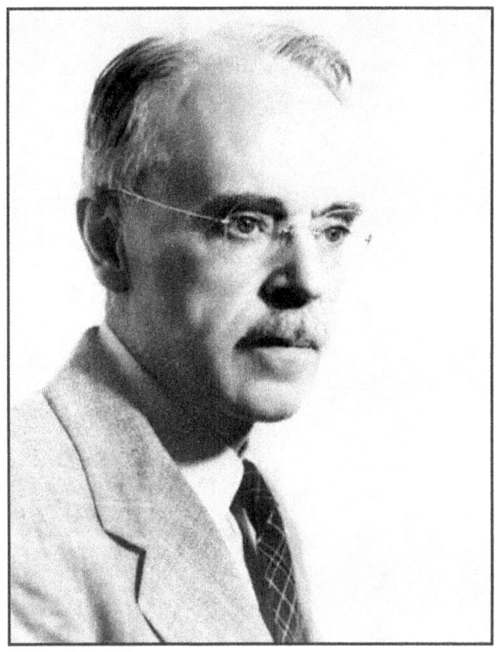

PAUL DUDLEY WHITE
permission: Lasker Foundation

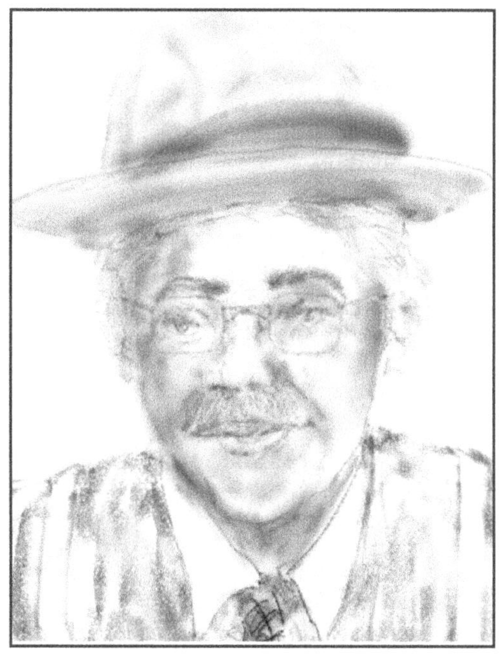

PAUL DUDLEY WHITE,
drawn by Dr. Roy Nuzzo

GLOSSARY CHAPTER 3

Anasarca – swelling of most of the body with fluid

Edema – swelling, usually of extremities with fluid

Diuretic – medicine given orally, IV, or by muscular injection to have the kidney rid the body of excess fluid and sodium (salt)

EKG = ECG – electrocardiogram

Anticoagulation – "thinning the blood" in lay parlance but really preventing blood clotting, not changing the thickness of blood

Platelets – one of the blood cellular components that helps the body form needed clots after injury but can lead to strokes and heart attacks when uncontrolled. The platelet clot is light gray and called "white clot," whereas other blood chemicals form "red clots."

CHAPTER 4
THE DEVELOPMENT OF THE BLOOD PRESSURE MACHINE (SYGMOMANOMETER)

Although seemingly straightforward, taking a blood pressure reading can be fraught with pitfalls. Under normal circumstances, blood pressures should be the same in both arms, but true differences will not be noted unless one takes the time to take the blood pressure on both arms multiple times to be sure that any discrepancy is consistently found because the blood pressure normally changes with mood and activity from moment to moment. When taking systolic blood pressure first on one arm and then the other, a difference of over 10 mmHg systolic pressure must be confirmed and is abnormal. By taking the blood pressure sequentially on both arms several times until one is sure that right and left arm discrepancies are real, results are more reliable. By not measuring the blood pressure on both arms, one can miss a significant plaque in one of the arteries traversing the chest to the arm, a torn aorta with blood blocking off one arm and known as a dissecting aneurysm or even a congenital narrowing in the aorta between where the right arm blood flow and the left arm blood flow takes off, known as a coarctation. A patient who became my patient was transferred to our hospital with the diagnosis of an infection on his aortic valve, which opens to allow blood out of the heart on the left side. However, when I detected that the blood pressures were higher on the right compared to the left arm, I quickly realized that the problem was not an infection but an aortic dissection, or tearing of the aorta above the aortic valve, which is life threatening if not quickly operated upon, requiring an emergency echocardiogram and emergency surgery, as every hour that passes brings another 10% mortality. Fortunately, he had both and echo and surgery and is alive today and doing well.

STEPHEN HALES is the father of measuring blood pressure, although he called it "force." Of course, his measurements were not in humans but in animals since his tubes had to be placed into the artery directly, and this could not be safely or sterilely performed in humans during his time. So blood pressure measurements awaited a noninvasive machine development.

KARL LUDWIG (1816-1895, born Witzenhausen, Germany, and died Leipseig, Germany) in 1847 measured blood pressure in animals using an external cuff attached to a mercury column and a kymograph (a wave writer with a paper on a drum to record movement) to record the measurements, but this was only the first step toward blood pressure measurements, which eventually would be made noninvasively in humans.

Samuel Von Basch (1837-1905, born Prague, Czechoslovakia, and died Vienna, Austria) in 1891 invented the first noninvasive blood pressure machine for humans (sphygmomanometer). It was not easy to use, so it is no longer used by doctors and medical personnel. But it was a beginning.

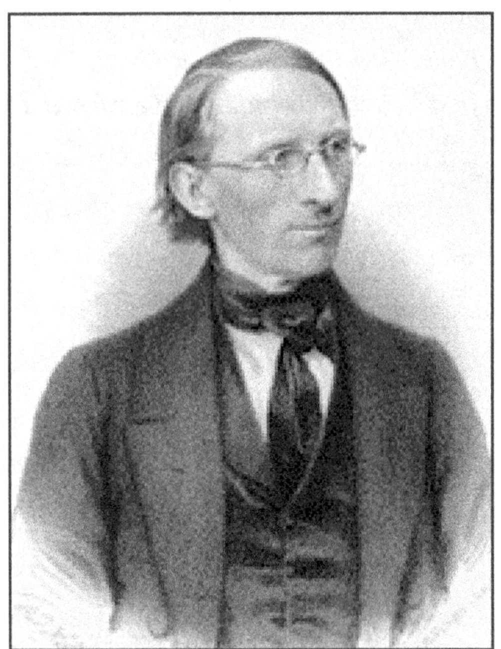

KARL LUDWIG, National Library of Medicine, public domain

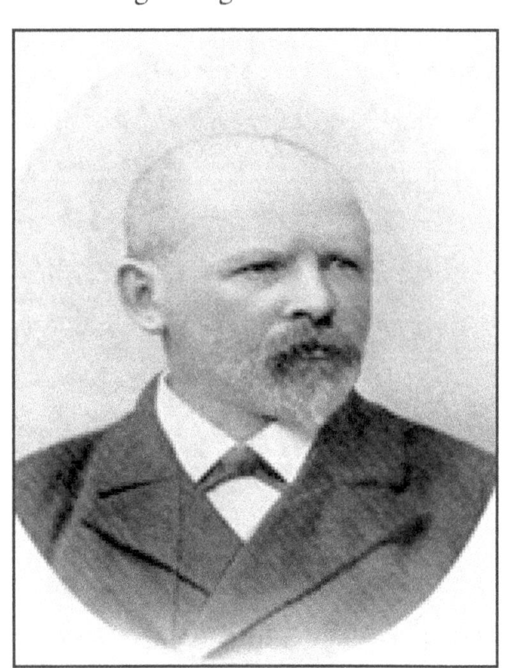

SAMUEL VON BASCH, public domain

SCIPIONE RIVA-ROCCI (1863-1937, born Almese, Italy, and died Rapallo, Italy) made the first practical blood pressure machine.

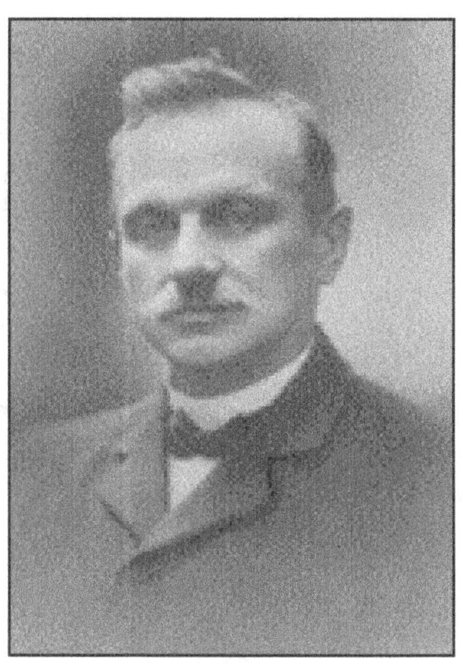

It was Riva-Rocci who invented an easy-to-use cuff-based blood pressure machine in 1896. His mercury sphygmomanometer became the standard for nearly one hundred years. He measured only systolic blood pressure by seeing or feeling the pulse (inspection or palpation) and noting at what measurement it visually appeared or could be felt. The cuff encircled the arm with rubber bulbs filled with water or air to manually compress the artery, and then gradually it was released until blood flowed. He measured peak systolic pressure, where the pulse again was pulsating when the finger felt it as the cuff was gradually being released, but this device did not allow diastolic blood pressure measurements. Dr. Harvey Cushing (1869-1939, born Cleveland, Ohio, and died New Haven, Conn.) was a famed neurosurgeon and pioneer of brain surgery, especially of the pituitary gland. He visited Riva-Rocci in Italy and took back a drawing and a model of the Italian device and popularized its use in the U.S., first at Johns Hopkins Medical School. The arm cuff became widened from the original 5cm, and this made its measurements more reproducible.

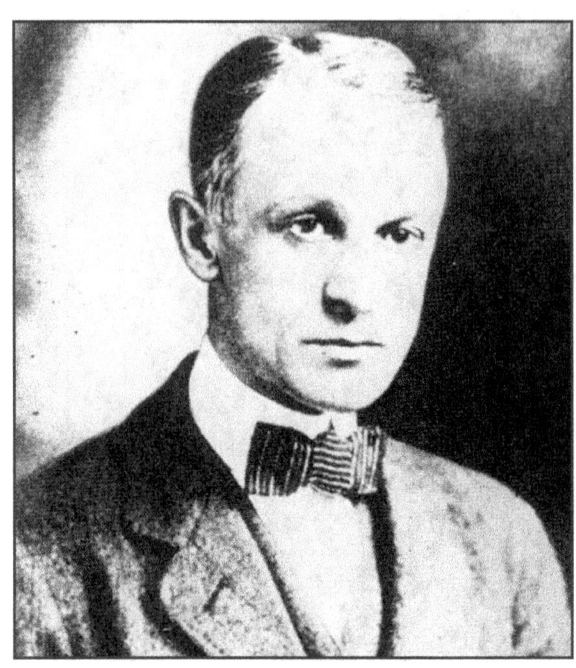

HARVEY CUSHING,
Science Photo Library License

In 1905 NIKOLAI KAROTKOFF (1874-1920, born Kursk, Russia, and died Saint Petersburg, Russia), only three years after completing his medical training, pointed out that the blood pressure sounds could be heard with a stethoscope instead of only feeling for a pulse with one's fingers. He presented his findings at a seminar in St. Petersburg at the Military Medical Academy. His discovery allowed for an easily measurable systolic and diastolic pressure, thus ushering in the auscultatory measurement of blood pressure used today. It was simple, reproducible, and accurate. Karotkoff was in the Russian Army in 1904-1905, during the Russo-Japanese War, and served in the most disputed area, Harbin, China. His discovery was later presented at his 1910 defense of his dissertation for a Doctor of Medical Sciences and the reviewing professor, S. P. Fedorov, wrote that "Karotkoff's discovery revolutionized the existing field of heart and vascular diseases." He was interested in vascular war wounds he had seen and wanted to find a way of measuring and predicting the surgical survival of a wounded limb with an aneurysm if the artery supplied was tied off. Cardiologically he also noted that one-third of the time interval that occurred between two heartbeats was the amount of time required to eject the blood (i.e. systole), an astounding observation and deduction for his time.

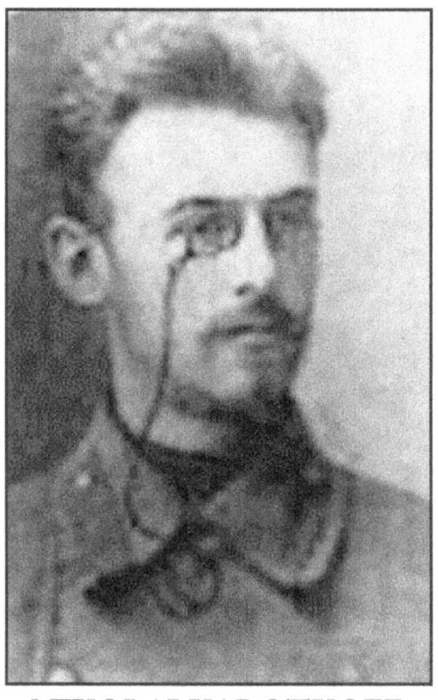

NIKOLAI KAROTKOFF,
public domain

GLOSSARY CHAPTER 4

Systole – the phase of the cardiac cycle when the left ventricle pumps blood to the body

Diastole – the phase of the cycle when the left ventricle relaxes and fills with blood

Sphygmomanometer – machine for taking blood pressure

CHAPTER 5
THE DEVELOPMENT OF HEART CATHETERIZATION AND CORONARY ANGIOGRAPHY

In 1986 Robert Chambers was convicted of strangulating his girlfriend Jennifer Levin in Central Park. He was a wealthy Manhattanite who attended the best schools up to his age of twenty at that time. He maintained he was not trying to kill her but that it was "rough sex" when she died. His defense went upon deaf ears by the jury, who convicted him of second-degree manslaughter and sentenced him to fifteen years in prison and then another nineteen years after having two more convictions occurring after his first release. This is background for an experience I had around 1990, when I was 47 years old and performing a cardiac catheterization on a sixty-year-old female psychologist who seemed ancient to me then at my then tender young age but would seem like a youngster to me today at my current age of eighty. After the first injection into the left coronary artery, she passed out. I quickly acted and gave her at least four vigorous compressions of CPR to her chest. She quickly regained consciousness and normal vital signs. I looked at her angiogram quickly and saw no bubbles injected. I told her I was not sure what had occurred, but she would be fine and observed in our CCU overnight. I went to check on her at the end of the day, when my other procedures were completed, in order to reassure her that she would be fine and would be discharged the next morning but that her chest might be sore from the CPR (cardiopulmonary resuscitation) compressions. She responded, "That's okay, Doctor. I thought you and I were having rough sex!!" Nothing in her face suggested she was pulling my leg. I walked the fifty feet out of the CCU but pivoted and took one step back to ask her if she was joking but then quickly pivoted again and left without approaching her. I said to myself, "I don't want to know if she is kidding me since it would ruin the story." You can decide for yourself.

WHAT IS CARDIAC CATHETERIZATION?

Cardiac catheterization is the procedure of placing flexible hollow tube into a vein or artery and directing the tube retrograde (back toward the heart) until it enters the right or left side of the heart (right side of heart via a vein and left side of heart via an artery). It is used for measuring pressures in the four heart chambers, measuring the amount of blood pumped out by the heart per minute (called cardiac output) or with each beat (called stroke volume), photographing the arteries supplying the heart muscle with blood known as coronary arteries to look for obstruction within them, photographing blood clots in the arteries supplying the lungs, and photographing how the main heart chamber, the left ventricle, is pumping and whether there are areas of damage.

Some would argue that cardiac catheterization started with Stephen Hale's placing tubes into horses and other animals' arteries. True, this was the first tube placed into a blood vessel, but he did not push his tubes further to gain access into the heart itself. Others would maintain that CLAUDE BERNARD (1813-1878, born Saint-Julien, France, and died Paris, France) is the Father of Cardiac Catheterization for his 1844 experiments measuring temperature and pressure inside animal hearts with a tube. I agree. He even coined the term "cardiac catheterization." Bernard was an experimenting scientist and a forerunner of cardiac catheterization, which has been so important in the 20th and 21st centuries. Bernard's major contribution was an understanding of the physiology of circulation and its relationship to nerves, specifically the sympathetic nervous system, which speeds or slows the heartbeat and controls the blood vessels' ability to dilate (enlarge). Bernard is also referred to as the "Founder of Experimental Medicine." This is quite an amazing ending to what began as a pedestrian beginning. Bernard flunked his university baccalaureate degree in 1831. His lottery number came up in 1833 to be drafted into the French Army for seven years. Fortunately, his family was allowed to pay for a substitute to take his place. In his mind he was determined to be a play write for his living. Fortunately for humanity his writing skills were not as good as his medical research ability and he gave up writing in 1834, after his professor read his play and suggested going to medical school instead. He then finally passed his baccalaureate exam and entered school to study medicine. After this rocky beginning, by 1851 he had won three prizes from the Academy of Sciences. He made great discoveries in gastrointestinal tract physiology, including discovering that excess sugar in the blood was brought to the liver to be converted into glycogen to be saved for a "rainy day" or temporary "famine." He determined that glycogen was again converted into sugar for the body to use for energy production. In the field of cardiology he showed that after cutting the sympathetic nerves, enlargement of blood vessels (vasodilatation) occurred and blood flow increased to the area supplied by those nerves. To this day, surgery on the sympathetic nervous system is sometimes performed due to the knowledge Bernard advanced. Bernard's animal research technique was a first step toward human heart catheterization. Treatment of high blood pressure has recently had proponents in some cardiology circles advocating radio-frequency catheters "cutting" (ablating) the sympathetic nerves to the kidneys to treat high blood pressure that is refractory to medications, and the FDA is very close at the time of writing this chapter to give its blessing to the procedure, which will be used by interventional cardiologists.

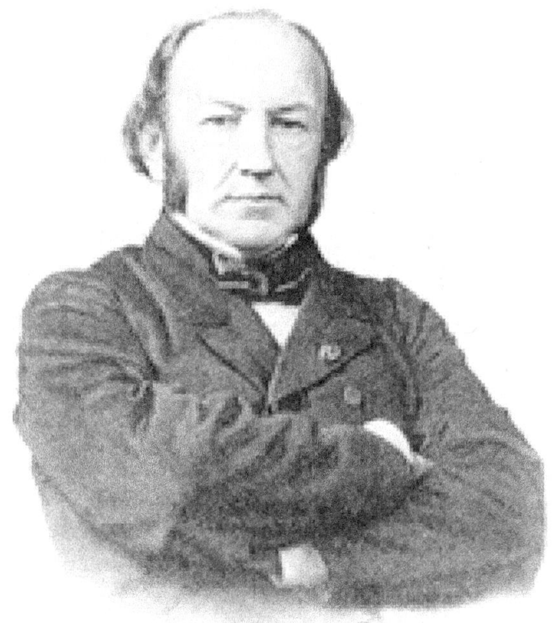

CLAUDE BERNARD,
public domain

Friedrich Jamin (1872-1951) and Hermann Merkel (1873-1957) were German physicians who published in 1907 an atlas of the coronary arteries taken with direct x-ray contrast injections. However, these were made from postmortem hearts and cannot really be considered a cardiac catheterization, only a beginning.

In 1908 Fritz Bleichroeder (1875-1938, born Berlin, Germany, and died Berlin, Germany) put a tube in the femoral vein and pushed it toward the heart, but no radiological evidence or even right-sided pressure measurements were made to prove whether or not he actually entered the heart. He was interested in carbohydrate metabolism and first performed the procedure on dogs before performing it on his laboratory technician Joseph Portmann in his hospital using a ureteral catheter (urological catheter used to instrument the bladder).

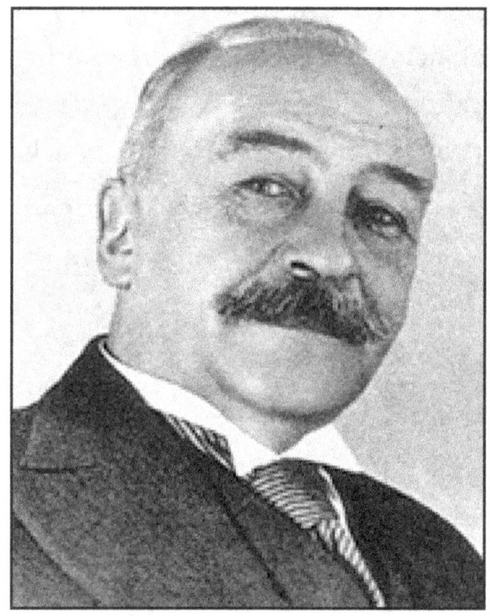

FRITZ BLEICHRODER,
public domain

Without Roentgen's study of x-rays and their offspring, the x-ray machine, no clinical heart catheterization would have been possible. However, in 1929 Werner Forssmann (1904 -1979, born Berlin, Germany, and died Schopfheim, West Germany) performed a groundbreaking experiment, on himself!!!!!!!

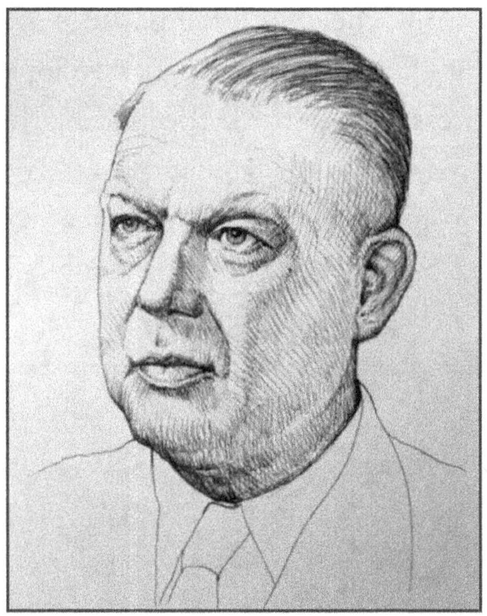

WERNER FORSSMANN, hand drawing by David Gavasheli from original photo, public domain from author's personal collection

Forrssman was a surgical resident at the time and was aware of the earlier works of Claude Bernard. He was especially influenced by the experiments of Auguste Chauveau (1827-1917, born Villenneuve-la-Guyard, France, and died Paris, France), who experimented on horses. Chauveau chose to experiment on the horse because its heart resembled the human circulatory system and because its resting slow heart rate made measurements easier and more accurate. He introduced catheters and measured the pulse and pressure on both sides of the horse's heart. Forssmann knew of his research.

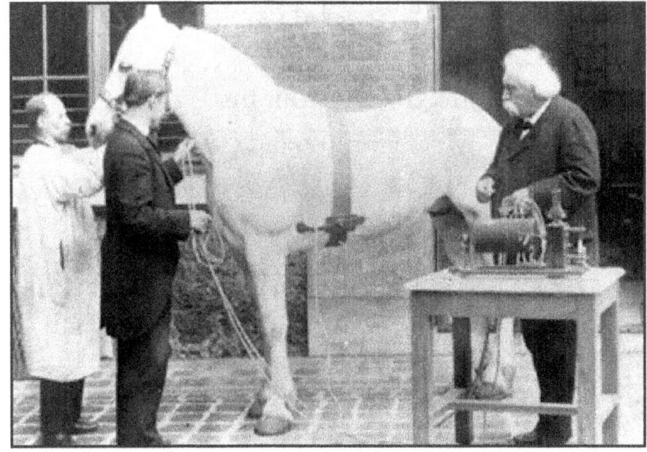

Left: Professor AUGUSTE CHAUVEAU, Creative Commons, public domain

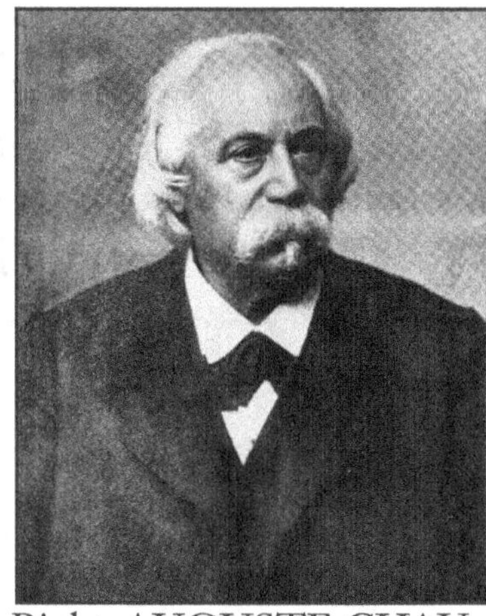

Right: AUGUSTE CHAU-VEAU, National Library of Medicine, public domain

Forssmann was also influenced by Etienne-Jules Marey (1830-1904, born Beaune, France, and died Paris, France), who developed instrumentation for measuring pulse and pressure. He worked with Chauveau in many of the experiments. (Coincidentally he was instrumental in the development of the motion picture which, ironically, was the way that we reviewed coronary angiograms for the first 25-plus years of coronary angiography until digital storage became available and replaced the cine.)

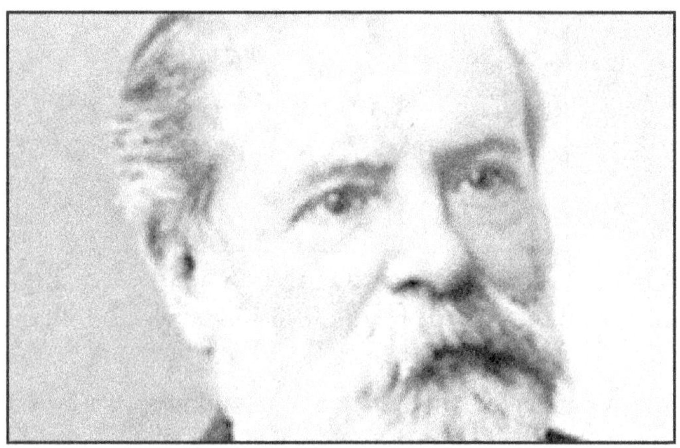

ETIENNE-JULES MAREY
National Library of Medicine, public domain

In 1929 Forssmann secretly made an incision (known as a "cut down") on his own left antecubital vein (just above the elbow bend) and threaded a 65cm (25.5 inches) rubber sterile urinary catheter tube toward the heart. He required some help and enlisted the aid of the nurse in charge of sterile equipment, Gerda Ditzen, who said she would help him on the condition that she was the subject, not Forssmann. He agreed but never intended to carry out his agreement. After he anesthetized the arm of Nurse Ditzen, he only pretended to make an incision on her vein (after all, she could not feel what he was doing since the skin was numb) but made it on his own instead, as he had intended all along, and inserted a urinary catheter into his own arm vein. He then freed her up from the table restraints and together they walked a distance to the x-ray machine on the floor below, after she called x-ray to alert them to what would happen next. Forssmann had an x-ray of his chest taken showing the catheter had not reached the heart but only the left shoulder, so he pushed his urinary catheter in his arm vein 35cm further (total of 65cm from the entry point) and had another x-ray taken, which showed the catheter at the superior vena cava – right atrial junction (without a pressure measurement or x-ray contrast injected, it is impossible to say with certainty whether the catheter actually entered the heart into the right atrium or remained in the superior vena cava just above the right atrium, as the superior vena cava drains the head and arms of blood and connects to the right atrium). To most people's surprise (including his own), he survived. He only felt a little warmth and mild nausea. Instead of his surgical chief recognizing what an accomplishment had occurred and how this would bring fame to his own department and to perhaps himself as well, he fired Forssmann from his residency! This was another example of Restrainers vs.. Disputers (Forssmann). Forssmann eventually went into urology (quite ironic, as urologists are known for using the same catheter Forssmann used but in a different part of the body). He had performed the first, at that time known, human cardiac catheterization, but in a limited way. He was exonerated when he was awarded the Nobel Prize for Medicine in 1956 for this creative, heroic and possibly dangerous experiment.

Unfortunately for his future reputation, he joined the Nazi Party, rose to become a major, and was captured as a POW by the U.S. Army but released in 1945. He became a country doctor with his wife, also a urologist. They had six children. While he was still in prison as a POW, Andre Cournand, who was next on the scene and also received the Nobel Prize along with Forssmann and his own colleague Dickinson Richards in 1956, read Forssmann's paper and was inspired to perform more catheterization experiments.

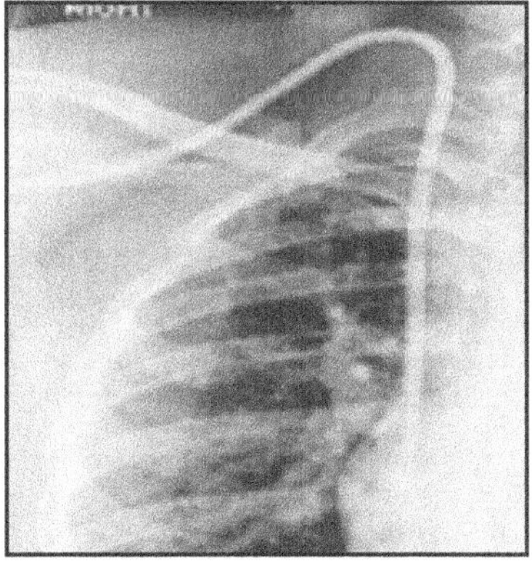

The above radiograph from the author's practice and personal collection is similar to what Forssmann published but is a catheter placed from the right arm, whereas Forssmann used his left arm.

However, little known to scientists and certainly not to the Nobel Committee for Medicine, Otto Klein (1891-1968, born in Pilsen, Czech Republic, and died Buenos Aires, Argentina) actually performed the very first documented right heart catheterization in the world, not Forssmann. Klein placed his catheter into the right atrium and right ventricle of patients and estimated the cardiac output (amount of blood in liters pumped by the heart per minute). He performed his experiment in 1929, before Forssmann performed his, and was unaware of Forssmann's work, just as Forssmann was unaware of Klein's experiment. Klein presented his research in a lecture in Prague in November of 1929 and at the Congress of the German Society for Internal Medicine in Wiesbaden in April of 1930. His findings in 1930 were on eleven patients on whom he measured the cardiac output and passed his catheter into both chambers on the right side of the heart. He was not allowed to continue his studies by his professor Nonnenbruch, who was in charge of the II Medical Department at Charles University in Prague, and his findings were forgotten for many years and never discovered by the Nobel Committee while Klein was still alive. Klein's professor was also a Restrainer, just as was Forssmann's chief. To make matters worse, in 1938 Klein was forced to resign from the Charles University Faculty because he was Jewish. In 1939, just a few days before Hitler invaded Czechoslovakia (as a Jew, he saw the handwriting on the wall), he immigrated to Argentina, where he died in 1968. He tried to convince the Boston medical establishment in 1939 on a visit to the U.S. to allow him to continue his research but was turned down by the myopic medical establishment Restrainers. This is another example of fellow scientists either being jealous or having a lack of imagination, which Osler warned his fellow physicians in his famous Harveian Lecture in the 1890s (see Chapter 1). Cournand and Richards in 1956 received the Nobel Prize, along with Forssmann. Many consider Klein the forgotten father of diagnostic cardiac catheterization. He deserved to share the Nobel Prize with Forssmann, Cournand and Richards for cardiac catheterization but never received his recognition. However, in 2000 and 2005 two international symposia were held in Prague, where he received posthumously celebration of the 70th and 75th anniversaries of his groundbreaking work. I wonder if Cournand (see below) was aware of Klein's work. Perhaps he was but hopefully not. If he had known, hopefully he would have informed the Nobel Committee that Klein should also be recognized. Since Nobel Prizes can be only given to living scientists, by the time Klein's work became public knowledge he had already died.

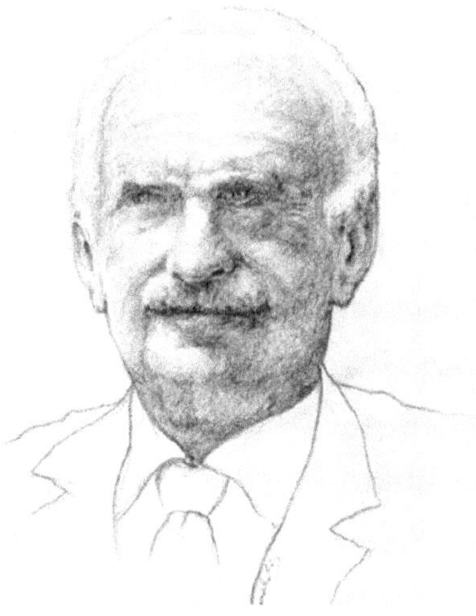

Original drawing by David Gavasheli, personal collection of author

Andre Cournand (1895-1988, born Paris, France, and died Great Barrington, Massachusetts, U.S.) read Forssmann's paper and thought that catheterizing the right side of the human heart would help him measure cardiac flow in various parts of the lung, which interested him and his partner Dickinson Richards (1895-1973, born Orange, NJ, U.S., and died Lakeville, Connecticut, U.S.). Cournand wanted to move to the U.S. and in 1930 secured a training program under Richards at Columbia University's division at Bellevue Hospital in NYC. Cournand became an American citizen in 1941.

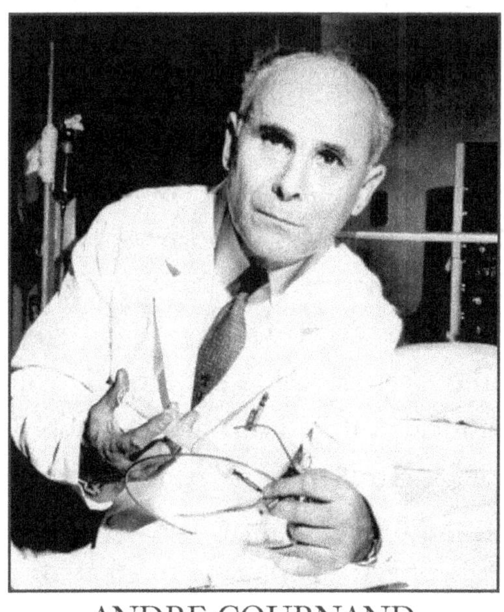

ANDRE COURNAND

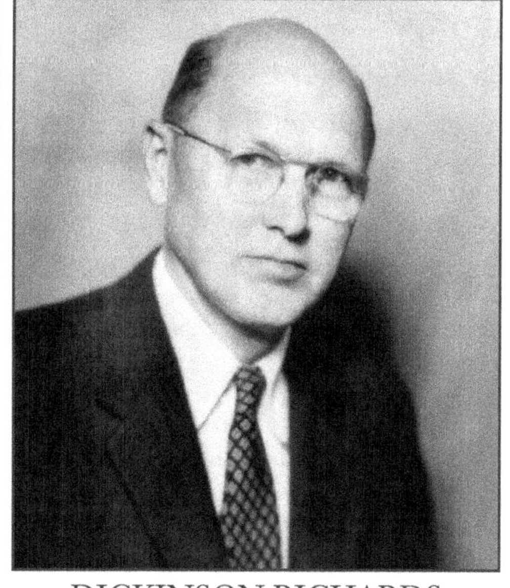

DICKINSON RICHARDS

Both photos: National Library of Medicine/Science Photo Library License

Cournand and Richards performed physiologic experiments using catheters on the right side of the heart in 1941, and both were awarded the 1956 Nobel Prize for Medicine along with Forssmann. Working together Cournand and Richards performed heart catheterizations on the right side of the heart via arm vein cutdowns to measure pressure and cardiac output from within the heart. Whereas Forssmann was the first to perform a right heart catheterization, Forssmann intended to use it for medication delivery or cardiac output measurements and was not interested in chamber pressure measurements. The real developments physiologically and in clinical disease were made by Cournand and Richards, who paved the way for other cardiac hemodynamic measurements. By 1944 they had measured the pressures in all the right heart chambers and pulmonary artery. They recognized that the pressures were much lower on the right side of the heart compared to the comparable chambers on the left. They published in 1945 a large series of patients who had a catheter safely left in the pulmonary artery for 24 hours and two patients up to 48 hours.

The remaining right heart measurement, known as the pulmonary capillary wedge, did not come until 1947 (published 1949), made at the Peter Bent Brigham Hospital in Boston when Harper K. Hellems (1920-1999, born Sinks Grove, West Virginia, and died Jackson, Mississippi, U.S.) and Lewis Dexter (1910-1995, born Concord, Massachusetts, and died Boston, Massachusetts), the head of the laboratory, were the first to measure the pulmonary capillary wedge pressure in thirteen patients using a hollow catheter with just an end hole. This was and continues to be an extremely important measurement, allowing the filling pressure in diastole of the left ventricle to be measured from the right side of the heart indirectly. The pulmonary capillary wedge pressure, now renamed the pulmonary artery occlusive pressure, is a surrogate and closely approximates the left atrial pressure without entering the left atrium, which technically is more difficult from the right side of the heart and also approximates the end diastolic pressure of the left ventricle (the relaxing pressure in diastole when the left ventricle fully relaxes), which at that time of Hellems and Dexter's experiments had not been catheterized in humans for fear of its dangers. Hellems and Dexter carefully pushed their catheter into the very end of a small pulmonary artery branch, which blocked forward blood flow and pulmonary artery pressure until the pressure recording looked like the left atrial pressure (only previously measured in animals).

The oxygen saturation from blood taken was fully saturated (i.e. close to 100%, whereas the pulmonary artery saturation is usually in the 70s%). The importance of this measurement from their discovery is of enormous importance, as it allows cardiologists to know the pressure in the relaxing phase left ventricle (diastole)—as the wedge pressure is the same as the left ventricle pressure in diastole except that it is taken from the right side of the heart without putting a catheter into the left side of the heart. This allows physicians to assess the overall health of the left ventricle from the right side of the heart to determine whether the left ventricle is suffering from congestive heart failure and whether the left sided mitral valve is severely thickened and narrowed.

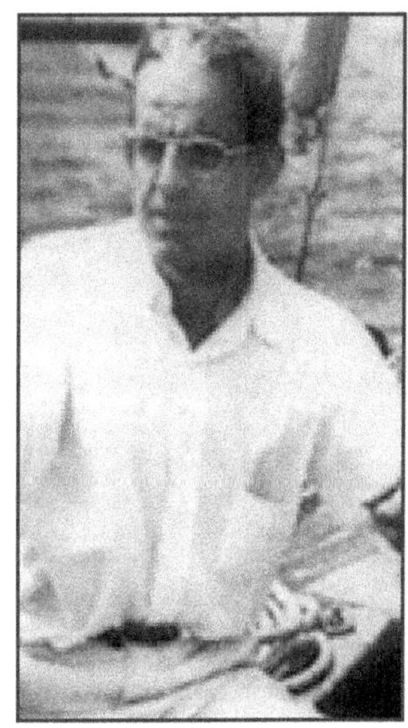

Lewis Dexter

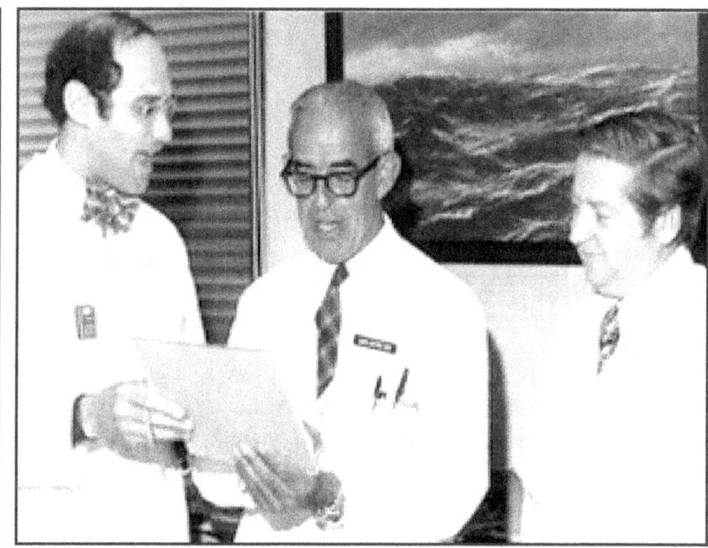

Dr. Dexter in center with Dr. Joseph Alpert on his right, Dr. James Dalen on his left

Both photos courtesy of Dr. Joseph Alpert's private collection, Tucson, AZ

In the early days of cardiac catheterization, catheters were inserted after cutting down on and isolating an artery or a vein. Often this was difficult and always tedious and slow. Repair occasionally left no pulse beyond the incision, requiring a vascular surgeon to come to the rescue to repair the artery. In 1953 Sven Seldinger (1921-1998, born Mora, Sweden, and died Dalarna, Sweden) of the Karolinska Institute in Stockholm, Sweden, developed a percutaneous technique (by a skin puncture with no incision) for introducing catheters into veins and arteries without making a cutdown. His technique allowed easier access and avoidance of surgical incisions by interventional radiologists and interventional cardiologists. Ironically, evidently his professor did not think much of his research and nor worthy of giving him his Ph.D. for his research!! Yet not long after his research was academically turned down, his technique has been adopted worldwide by literally thousands of cardiologists and radiologists and continues to be used today.

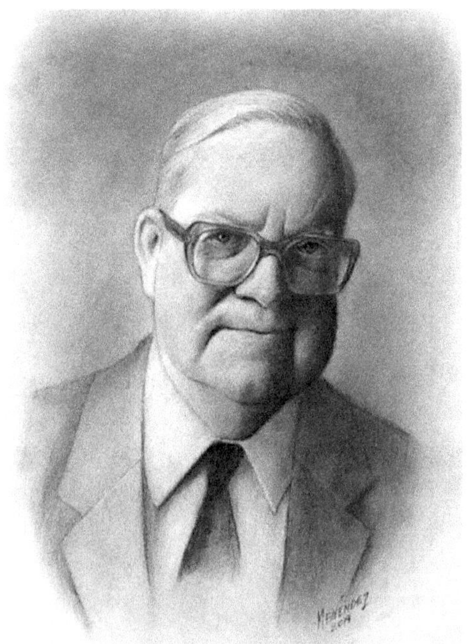

SVEN IVAR SELDINGER
Original drawing and permission to use by Moses Menendez, MD

The first true left heart catheterization (a catheter actually entering the left side of the heart into the left ventricle) of a human was by Henry A. Zimmerman (1915-2007, born Holsopple, Pennsylvania, U.S., and died Vero Beach, Florida, U.S.) in 1950 with his colleagues Roy W. Scott and Norman O. Becker from Western Reserve University (the catheter entered the left ventricle from the aorta through an incision in the left forearm in the antecubital artery). Interestingly, although fairly routine today in any type of patient, they were only able to enter leaking aortic valves and could not cross the valve to enter the left ventricle in five normal patients. Two patients died in their study, presumably they were quite ill when instrumented as the procedure is fairly benign in trained hands (Circ. 1950:1. P357-59).

Many people over time improved the technology of the catheters, the x-ray machines, and contrast materials used, but the advance that made treatment for heart attacks, coronary artery stenting, aortic valve replacements without surgery (TAVR) and even coronary bypass surgery possible was the accidental discovery by F. Mason Sones in 1958 (1918-1985, born Noxapater, Mississippi, U.S., and died Cleveland, Ohio. He was probably the greatest cardiology Disruptor of the 20th century) of selective coronary angiography. While working in the radiology suite in 1958. His catheter was placed in the ascending aorta (as the large artery exits the heart) near the aortic valve and was accidently whiplashed into the mouth of the right coronary artery when the contrast was given by a power machine injection intended for the aorta above the aortic valve. He was horrified and felt certain the patient was going to die but lo and behold, he was then gratified to find that his patient survived.

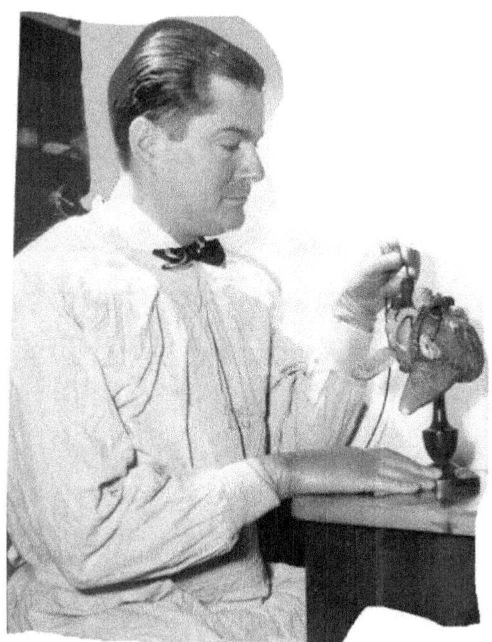
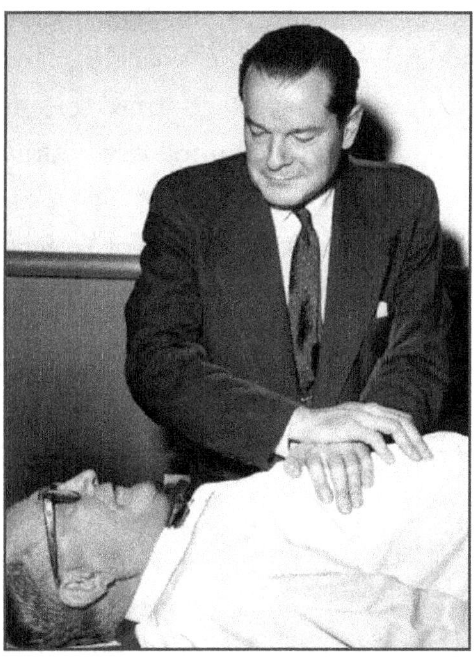

HENRY ZIMMERMAN
permission: ClevelandMemory.org

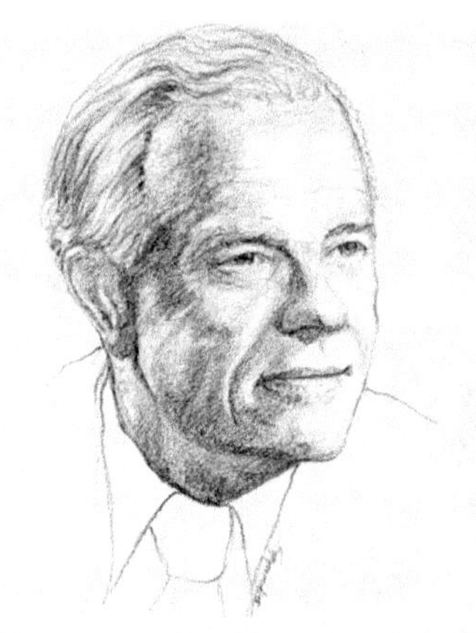

F. MASON SONES, original drawing by David Gavasheli, from photo in
public domain, personal collection of author

Instead of the expected ventricular fibrillation, the patient developed asystole
(stoppage with no electrocardiogram EKG complex), which with coughing restored
his normal rhythm quickly. This was the beginning of coronary arteriography (also
called coronary angiography), which opened the door to other advanced treatments
such as coronary artery stenting. Two days later (and against the advice of Dr. Cournand, who received the Nobel Prize for his work on right heart catheterization two
years earlier), Sones performed selective coronary angiography intentionally on a
patient with a leaky mitral valve. Although dogs went into ventricular fibrillation
and died with such injections, Sones surmised correctly that humans were different
as his patients lived. The era of Selective Coronary Angiography was born.

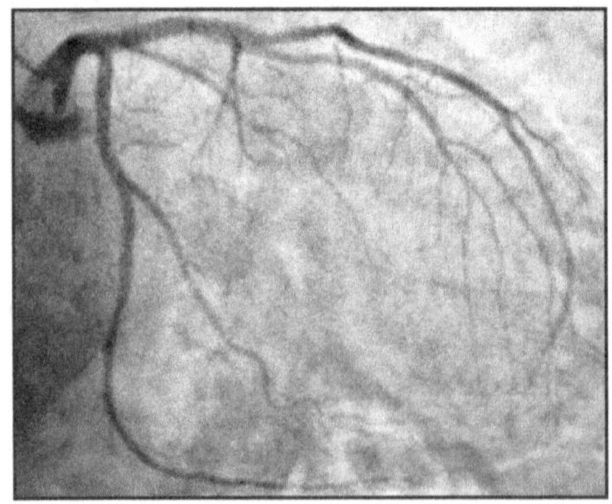

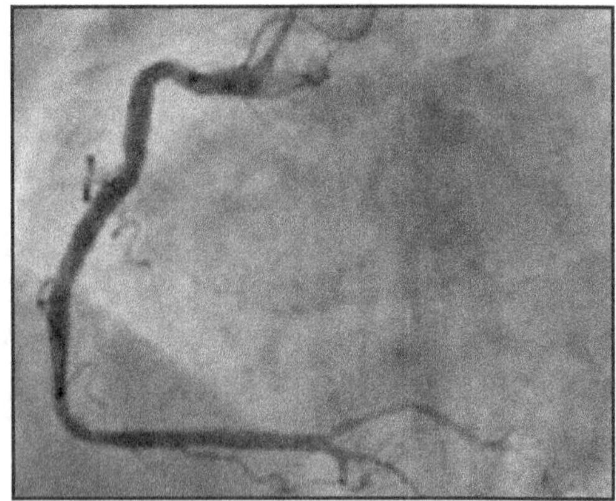

Coronary arteriogram of nearly normal left coronary artery The blush of
contrast is just above the aortic valve.

normal right coronary artery similar
to Sones' first. The arrow shows the
catheter in the artery mouth.

From the author's personal collection

Further developments on the right heart catheters for bedside use were made by Jeremy Swan (1922-2005, born Sligo, Ireland, and died Los Angeles, California) and Willian Ganz (1919-2009, born Kosice, present-day Slovakia, and died Los Angeles, California) in 1970 by placing an inflatable balloon on the tip of a very flexible hollow-end hole catheter so that it could be literally "floated" in the flow current of blood in the right heart through the right atrium, right ventricle, and into the pulmonary artery even without x-ray guidance for use in humans in the lab or at bedside in an intensive care unit. A modification of their catheter was first used in dogs in 1953 by Dr. Swan, who said he developed this idea while watching sailboats in Santa Monica Bay with his children. This eventually allowed for clinical use outside the cardiac catheterization laboratory such as in the CCU (cardiac care unit) to more accurately monitor critically ill patients, their cardiac outputs, and the pressures within the right side of the heart. Thanks to the invention of the Swan-Ganz catheter, which bears the names of the two inventors, most trained doctors can place and utilize a catheter for pressure measurements of the heart, not just invasively trained cardiologists.

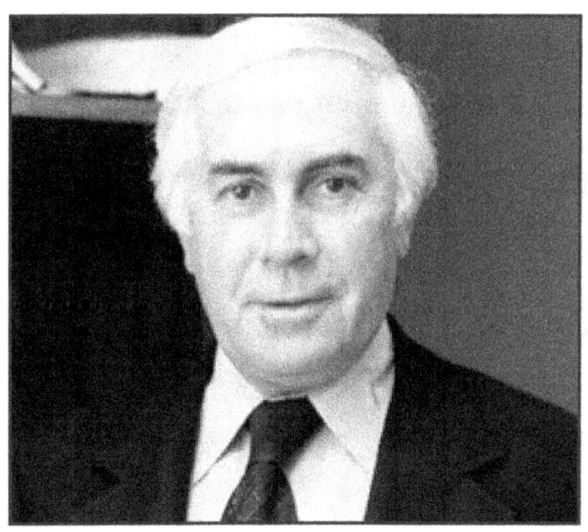

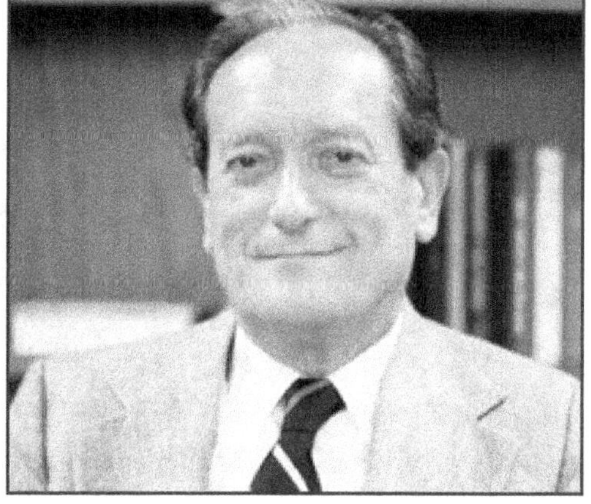

JEREMY SWAN   WILLIAM GANZ

Both photos permission of Edwards Lifesciences Co.

Melvin Judkins (1922-1985, born Los Angeles, California, and died Riverside, California, another great Disruptor.) in 1967 made his great contribution and in so doing advanced cardiology log rhythmically by developing pre-shaped catheters for coronary angiography, which were introduced percutaneously primarily via the femoral artery at the groin crease using the Seldinger technique rather than by arterial cutdown above the right elbow used by Mason Sones. The two approaches became known as the Sones technique (via cutdown) and the Judkins technique (via puncturing the skin from outside (percutaneous)).

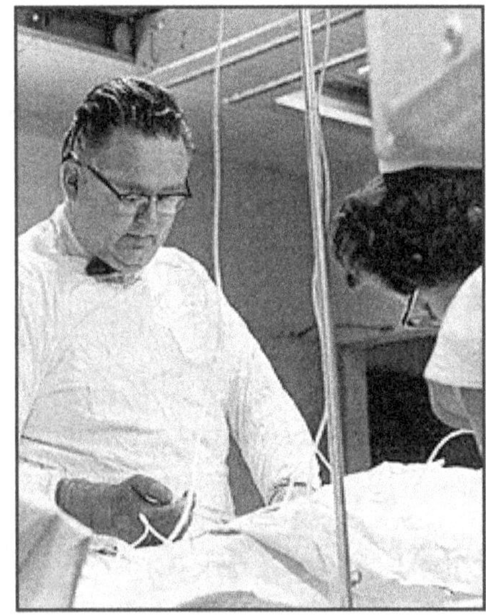

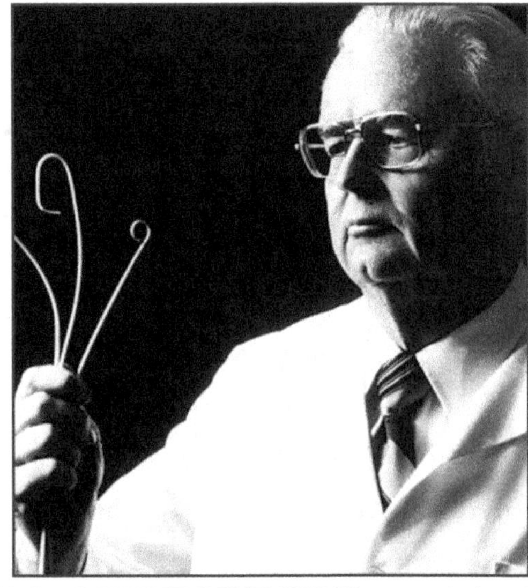

Left: MELVIN JUDKINS, license via Creative Commons

Right: MELVIN JUDKINS, permission by Oregon Health & Science University Hospital, Dotter Interventional Institutez

Incidentally, Sones catheters were not pre-shaped and required sometimes tricky manipulation to enter the mouth of each coronary artery (right and left). One catheter usually sufficed for both arteries with the operator using various maneuvers of pushing and twisting, although not always easily entering the intended mouth of the intended coronary artery. The Judkins catheters most of the time can be pushed without steering into the right or left coronary artery using a different-shaped catheter for each artery, although changing the catheter for a different-size angle near the artery entrance is sometimes required. The Judkins technique made coronary arteriography easier, safer, and faster for most invasive cardiologists without the need for a surgical cutdown and time-consuming arterial repair after the procedure.

Harold T. Dodge (1925-1999, born Seattle, Washington, and died Seattle, Washington) in 1956 published with his team how to calculate the volume of the left ventricle from x-ray contrast injections into the left ventricle on cineangiography (left ventriculography). From these he calculated how to calculate what for 65 years has become an extremely important measurement, the percent of blood pumped by the left ventricle into the aorta per heartbeat, known as the ejection fraction (normal 55-65%) and a close estimate of volumes in systole and diastole. This allows cardiologists to determine whether the left ventricle is pumping normally or has been damaged and weakened in its pumping phase, systole.

Dr. Sones was one of the most unforgettable characters I have ever met. I had the privilege in 1974, when I was a cardiology resident, to visit his lab with our head of the University of Pennsylvania cardiac catheterization laboratory, Dr. James Shelburne, and my future cardiology practice partner for 47½ years, Dr. Arthur Fisch, also a cardiology resident with me. Dr. Shelburne was looking for new equipment for the U of P lab and took us both to Cleveland with him. Whereas we used totally aseptic techniques in Philadelphia with sterile gowns, masks, gloves, and caps for our arterial cutdowns, Dr. Sones wore no mask or cap and actually had a cigarette straddling (almost dangling) on one corner of his two-by-four-feet instrument table, which is found in all cardiac catheterization laboratories and from which he took a puff after most injections. We observed that day that we were probably over precautioned in our lab at U of Penn, as Sones had no more infections than did we despite our assiduous sterile technique. When one of Dr. Sones' patients whom he was catheterizing became hypotensive (i.e. had a very low blood pressure), we expected that a measured amount of stimulant medication would be given to raise the blood pressure back to normal. Instead of a strictly measured amount and quantitative dose, Sones had a stainless-steel bowl six to eight inches in diameter and about three to four inches high filled with (to us) was an unknown liquid or liquids of no particular measured concentration and a 10cc syringe. We never did find out exactly how much and of what medication or medications he was using when he nonchalantly drew up the liquid and injected it into his catheter, giving his patient some of what he referred to as "soup." The patient's blood pressure quickly rose back to normal as Dr. Sones had anticipated, and he casually continued the study.

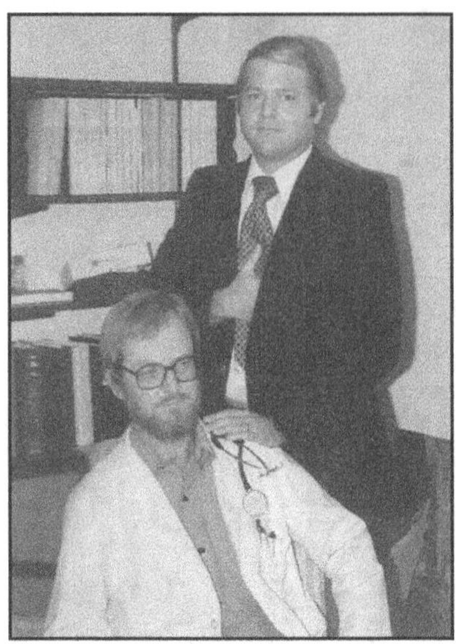 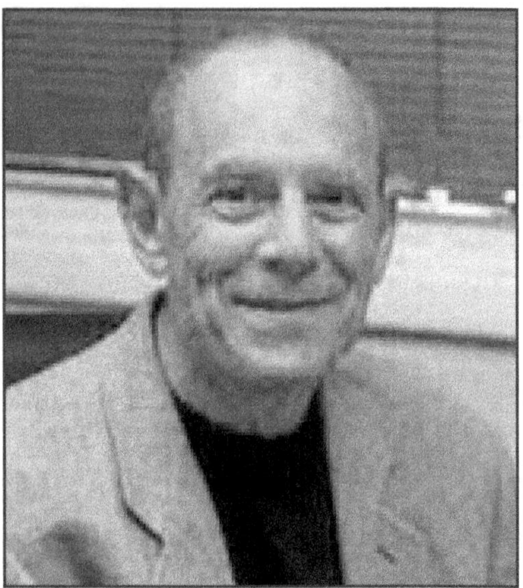

Left: Dr. James Shelburne (sitting), who took me as a cardiology fellow to see Dr. Sones in his lab at the Cleveland Clinic. His codirector, Dr. Joel Manchester, standing. By permission of Dr. Shelburne, from his personal collection

Right: Dr. Arthur Fisch, who accompanied us on the trip to Dr. Sones' laboratory and also practiced with the author for 47½ years. From author's personal collection

GLOSSARY CHAPTER 5

Cardiac catheterization – placing a hollow tube into the heart's left side via an artery or right side via a vein

Catheter – hollow flexible tube with either a single end hole of sometimes with small side holes near the tip, which prevent catheter recoil with injections

Sympathetic nervous system – the nerves that determine the "fight or flight" response

Vasodilation or vasodilatation – causing an artery or vein to enlarge

Femoral artery and vein – artery or vein at the groin crease

Cutdown – making an incision on an artery or vein

Antecubital artery and vein – artery or vein just above the elbow on the inside of the arm when the palm is facing the ceiling

Superior vena cava (SVC) – vein returning blood from the head and arms and upper chest wall

Right atrium (RA) – upper chamber on right side of heart

Right ventricle (RV) – lower chamber on the right side of heart that pumps blood to the lungs for a renewal of oxygen

Left atrium (LA) – upper chamber on left side of heart receiving oxygenated blood

Left ventricle (LV) - lower chamber on left side of heart that pumps oxygenated blood to the entire body

Pulmonary capillary wedge pressure (PCW) – also known as pulmonary artery occlusive pressure – pressure measured when blood pressure in a small pulmonary artery is only sampled from backflow of blood as the catheter prevents forward blood flow. It measures from the right side the pressure in the left atrium and left ventricle in diastole (relaxing phase of the ventricles).

Percutaneous – via a puncture through the skin

Ascending aorta – the part of the aorta above the aortic valve immediately next to the left ventricle that delivers blood in the chest toward the head and rest of the body

Asystole – when cardiac electrical activity ceases

Ejection fraction – % of blood from the left ventricle at the beginning of the diastolic relaxing phase that is pumped out with each heartbeat (normal 55-60%)

Coronary angiography or arteriography – taking pictures of the arteries supplying the heart muscle using x-ray contrast material (iodinated) to "light up" the artery

Coronary care unit (CCU) – special area of a hospital for caring for very sick cardiac patients

Hypotension – abnormally low blood pressure

Left ventriculography – a cine picture of the left ventricle pumping out its blood usually taken with a catheter inside the left ventricle to deliver the contrast material

CHAPTER 6
NEW APPROACHES FOR TREATING HEART ATTACKS

This section is about two stories and lessons. You will quickly see that the section is related to the theme of Chapter 2 both because this is about coronary artery disease, how it affects the heart, what causes heart attacks and how scientists often ignored or did not believe what some researchers had found. It is about the struggle between the Disruptors who advance progress and the Restrainers who resist change. Scientists like political leaders often must relearn history.

This section is about a drug that can abort a heart attack, how it was discovered, how it was first tried, and how the results were ignored by the medical profession for two decades, similar to the long hunt for linking coronary artery disease to heart attacks in Chapter 2 and the long lag time between discovery and acceptance by the medical profession of 32 years, discussed in Chapter 2.

Long before the first coronary angioplasty was performed for treating a heart attack, Dr. WILLIAM TILLETT (1882-1974, born Charlotte, North Carolina, U.S. and died Essex, Connecticut, U.S.) in 1933 discovered a drug to dissolve blood clots, streptokinase, while at Johns Hopkins School of Medicine in Baltimore, Maryland. It was purely by accident that he made his discovery. However, serendipity not only requires discovery but recognizing the importance of what one has found. Tillett was such a man. He thought that streptococci bacteria might contain the ability to dissolve clots, but the experiment he set up showed absolutely nothing—zilch, nada. He continued to think about his "failure." Fortunately, he did not discard his test tubes of his experiment and came back on another day to have his "Eureka moment," finding that only the tube with streptococcus bacteria dissolved blood clots. (At another time he also discovered C-reactive protein, which indicates inflammation and is widely used today by physicians to predict future heart attack risk.) He and his student Dr. Sol Sherry were intrigued by the strange molecule produced by the streptococcus bacterium that could dissolve clots. Tillet called this new compound "streptokinase" (an enzyme from the strep bacterium), and in 1947 Tillett asked Sherry to investigate possible therapeutic uses for streptokinase.

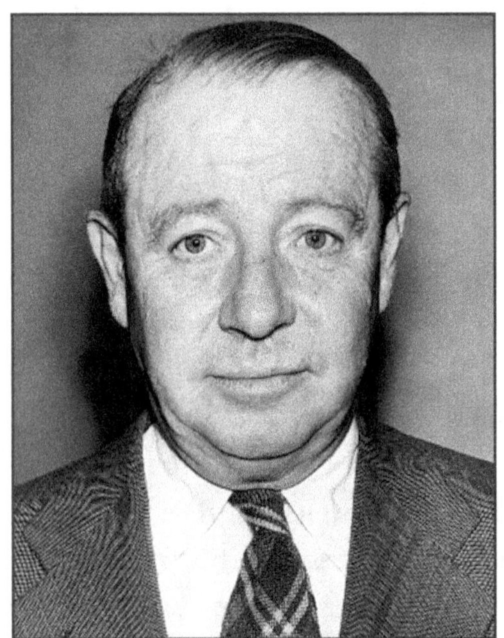

WILLIAM TILLETT
permission: Lasker Foundation

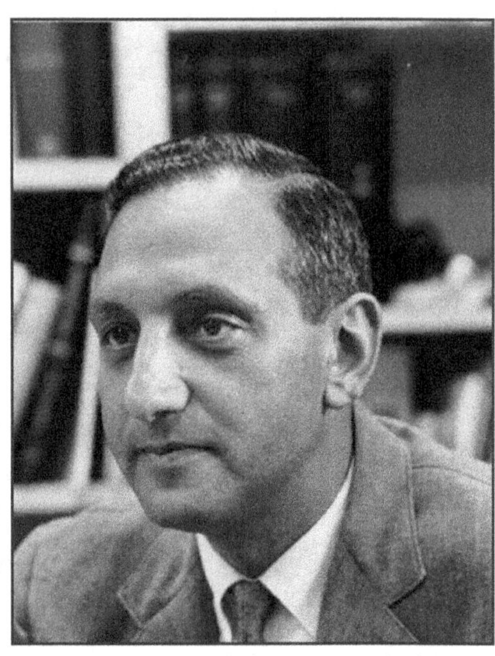

SOL SHERRY, by D. Gavasheli permission: Becker Medical Library
Wash U School of Medicine

Tillet's student SOL SHERRY, a hematologist, not a cardiologist (1916-1993, born New York City and died Philadelphia, Pennsylvania, U.S), began administering streptokinase intravenously (iv) for heart attacks and was convinced that heart attacks were about a clot on top of an atherosclerotic plaque. Sherry and Fletcher performed a small study in 1958 before the era of CCUs and even extensive cardiac catheterization laboratories to prove his hypothesis on 24 heart attack patients. He found an 87% survival, and although a small study his results were much better than data from other concurrent studies (one source stated that his results were "inconsistent." I don't know if this source was biased or ignorant). Fortunately Sherry recognized the need to focus on "cure" rather than "palliation" during heart attacks. Science is replete with investigators who had the answer long before colleagues would listen (Disruptors vs. Restrainers). Remember the fiasco of science when Galen ruled without challenge? Unfortunately the cardiologic world ignored Sherry's findings for another twenty years just as they ignored the German scientists who proved the coronary artery hypothesis in the late 1800s, requiring 32 years before James Herrick convinced cardiologists of the its importance (see Chapter 2). Cardiologists were also afraid of bleeding or allergic reactions due to streptokinase, but this does not explain the neglect of Sherry's findings. So, the clotting hypothesis was soon forgotten, and a twenty-year setback for heart attack patients occurred. Sherry was the unsung hero of heart attack cause and treatment. Dr. Sherry went on to an illustrious career, including the study of lung clots (pulmonary emboli) and dissolving them with streptokinase after being ignored by the cardiology community. Ignoring Dr. Sherry reminds one of Sir William Osler's warning in his lecture to the William Harvey Society in London in 1906, which I have already quoted.

However, there were two physicians who were aware of Sherry's work and did not ignore it unlike the rest of the cardiology world. We can thank Dr. K. Peter Rentrop and Dr. Marcus DeWood for their insight and vision or we might still be struggling to discover a way to treat a heart attack early in its course. (Parenthetically, at this time the cardiology researchers were focused on limiting the size of a heart attack rather than stopping it in its tracks.) We can especially thank Dr. Rentrop, who also had the courage to take his coronary angiographic observations and go a step further in treatment, rediscovering how to use streptokinase to treat heart attacks by direct intracoronary infusion of streptokinase. Mason Sones' accidental discovery in 1958 of selective coronary angiography with its subsequent developments and improvements of contrast agents, catheters, and x-ray equipment were also now available to Rentrop and DeWood to prove their hunches that heart attacks were due to clots, as it allowed both of these investigators the ability to show that clots were the direct cause of heart attacks and observe the clot while the heart attack was actually occurring.

In October 1977, K. Peter Rentrop (1940, born Cologne, Germany) cared for a 45-year-old truck driver with severe chest discomfort that began 45 minutes before coming to the hospital. His EKG demonstrated a heart attack of the under wall of the left ventricle known as an inferior wall infarction. His coronary angiogram showed a 60-70% narrowing of the right coronary artery, which caused his heart attack, although the artery was now partially open 30-

40%. Although treated conservatively at the time, including three weeks of hospitalization, he continued to have chest pressure with exertion after discharge and was readmitted in June of 1978. During his second admission catheterization was again performed, during which he developed recurrent chest pain but no EKG changes, and the right coronary artery showed good filling of contrast material, meaning that blood was freely flowing through it. But a few minutes later the patient once again developed chest pain, now with an EKG showing evidence of a new inferior infarction on top of the old one, and the right coronary artery was 100% blocked by angiography due to a clot that had formed to totally block the channel. Nor did this obstruction resolve with thirty minutes of intravenous nitroglycerin, so Dr. Rentrop could be confident that this was not arterial spasm but a clot (thrombus). Dr. Rentrop then pushed a very thin metal wire through his catheter tube, which was sitting at the mouth of the right coronary artery, and carefully fished it through the coronary obstruction, which offered only mild resistance to the wire, because fresh clots are the consistency of jelly. When he removed the wire and injected x-ray contrast again, he could see that he had created with the wire a narrow channel allowing blood to flow through (visualized with his contrast agent) and regression of his patient's pain and EKG changes. He sent his patient for bypass surgery, and his patient did well. Dr. Rentrop had performed the world's first angioplasty on an acute heart attack patient a year after Dr. Andreas Gruentzig performed one on a stable patient (1976) although Dr. Rentrop used only a wire, not a balloon to abort the heart attack and allowing his patient to proceed non-emergently a few hours later to bypass surgery, as no balloon catheters were readily available to perform a balloon angioplasty to enlarge the channel to a more normal size (stents were also not as yet invented). His patient suffered no significant heart muscle damage. Thus, Rentrop proved that a heart attack could be caused by a clot. A chronic blockage would not be soft enough to admit the wire he used to restore even a modicum of blood flow down the artery if it had been a remote heart attack rather than one in progress. Subsequently Rentrop treated fifteen patients with a modification of his wire technique but this time with small taper tipped tubes inserted within his main catheter and pushed through the obstruction sequentially to gradually increase the size of his formed channel in the totally blocked channel. In nine of fifteen acute myocardial infarction patients, he succeeded in blood flow restoration. He treated his patients within six hours from the start of their heart attacks with improvement of heart muscle pumping not seen in thirteen control patients treated medically. He published the results of his first seven patients in 1979.

In addition, Dr. Rentrop, also being aware of Sherry's work, reasoned that intracoronary streptokinase rather than intravenous streptokinase should be used, on the theory that the concentration where it was needed would be greater at the site of the thrombus (10,1000-20,000 units as a bolus with 1000-2000 units a minute up to an hour) and equally effective with less allergic reactions from the smaller total dosage. His initial results were successful and reported in August of 1979 (shortly after he performed his angioplasties for heart attacks), on acute heart attack patients with success in four of five patients in restoring blood flow and forming a partially open channel. He made a decision to add his intracoronary streptokinase results at the end of his American Heart Association talk in November, 1979 on mechanical wire and tapered catheter enlargement of coronary artery channels although this part of his talk was not listed in the program printed synopsis for that meeting. He told me he received a resounding applause from the audience with cardiologists from the Massachusetts General Hospital in Boston (Drs. Robert Leinbach and Herman Gold, see chapter 17 on intra-aortic balloon pump) soon repeating his intracoronary streptokinase results and Dr. Lance Gould from Houston sending a cardiology resident to Germany to look at Dr. Rentrop's angiographic results. He unexpectedly added his addendum since he correctly feared that his findings would be rejected for presentation at the ACC 1980 Spring meeting. As important as his "pilot" findings were on intracoronary streptokinase, a letter shared with me by Dr. Rentrop to him by the American College of Cardiology dated November 5, 1979, rejected his important initial observations from his small trial of intracoronary streptokinase for presentation at the March 1980 Scientific Session of the American College of Cardiology. I cannot say whether the small sample of the study determined the reviewers assessment or whether the previous closed mind of the academic cardiology world was still prevailing. In either case it was the Disruptor vs. the Restrainers pushing back on progress.

Dr. Rentrop moved to the U.S. and took a new position at Mt. Sinai Hospital in New York City, where in 1984 in the *New England Journal of Medicine* with his

Mt. Sinai and NYU-collaborators (Dr. Arthur Fox and Dr. Fred Feit) he published a series of patients with acute myocardial infarctions using intracoronary streptokinase for treatment. Sixty-one patients had a total blockage. Treatment with intracoronary streptokinase caused a reopening of the channel in 32 of 43 patients given (74%), whereas only one of eighteen (6%) opened without streptokinase. There was at six months no statistical difference found between the treated and untreated groups in terms of survival. Unfortunately, the success in terms of muscle saved with treatment was not evaluated in his study. Further studies with more patients were recommended to assess this new therapy. Studies from other centers using Rentrop's technique quickly followed, and his treatment protocol became widely used by cardiologists in the United States (including by the author and his partners).

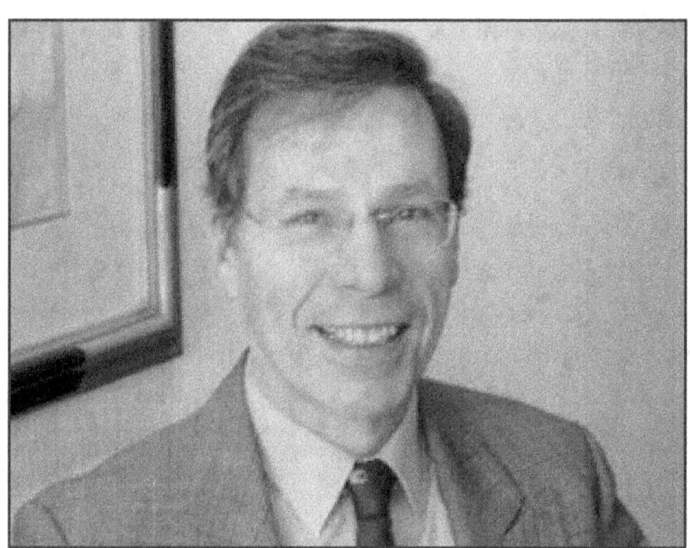

PETER RENTROP,
by permission of Dr. Rentrop from his personal collection

Marcus DeWood, in Spokane, Washington, was also intrigued by the clotting hypothesis as the cause of heart attacks and published an article in the *New England Journal of Medicine* in 1980 while working with his cardiothoracic colleagues. They performed a study of 59 patients catheterized within four hours of their heart attacks who then were sent to the operating room, where surgeons fished out a clot from the involved artery (found also at catheterization as a total blockage) removed with a small tube with a small balloon at its tip to pull out the clot, known as a Fogarty catheter (also used by vascular surgeons to pull out clots from blood vessels). Fifty-five of their 59 patients (88%) who underwent heart catheterization within four hours of their pain had a total blockage of an artery on their arteriogram and a clot fished out at surgery (some patients are fortunate enough to dissolve their clots without medication or surgical intervention due to the body's own clot-dissolving chemicals). DeWood and Rentrop confirmed what Sherry had discovered twenty years before, i.e. acute myocardial infarctions were mainly caused by red fibrin clots blocking the arterial channel. (It is felt that 80% of heart attack clots are caused by red fibrin clots and can be dissolved, whereas 20% are caused by white platelet clumps and can not be dissolved by clot busters.) The cardiology world finally awakened, very similar to the delay in accepting coronary artery narrowings as the cause of angina and leading to heart attacks, which took thirty years to convince the cardiology world after the German scientists provided the proof in the early 1880s but required Jamers Herrick to be the salesman between 1912 and 1918 of this concept to the cardiology profession (see Chapter 2).

The large multi-center GISSI study of 1986 using intravenous streptokinase provided the confirmation of the worth of streptokinase and clots causing heart attacks. Intracoronary streptokinase was soon replaced, first once again by a more easily administrated intravenous streptokinase and then by intravenously tPA which, although more costly than streptokinase, could be given more quickly as a smaller volume and without the fear of the allergic reactions and low blood pressure that streptokinase often provoked. It worked as well as the intracoronary streptokinase infusions, and the technique being IV rather than intracoronary was easier to administer and much less stressful on the cardiologist operator's heart as well. Thus began the Age of Clot Busters with Rentrop, DeWood, and the GISSI study finally exonerating Sol Sherry.

Eventually coronary angioplasty and stenting replaced thrombolytic agents such as streptokinase and tPA to treat acute heart attacks except in rare cases or because of specific indications, including the inability to perform coronary artery angioplasty and stenting within a one-and-a-half-hour window after arrival to the hospital. Dr. Rentrop told me on a phone conversation that at that time he performed his wire and tapered tube angioplasties he approached Dr. Andreas Gruentzig (see below), the father of coronary balloon angioplasty, who was now in Zurich, Switzerland with his idea. Dr. Gruentzig told Dr. Rentrop, "We will divide the world. I will do the chronic narrowing cases, and you do the acute heart attacks."

I remember spending many early morning hours (i.e. middle of the night) with one of my partners, Dr. Richard Watson, in the cardiac catheterization lab infusing intra-coronary streptokinase into the occluded coronary artery, which was causing the heart attack. It was a time of two hours of boredom interspersed with minutes of terror and panic as some patients' hearts went into ventricular fibrillation with restoration of blood flow and required CPR and electrical shocks to bail us out of the jam. Even when everything went smoothly, we always wondered whether we arrived at the patient soon enough to make a difference in saving heart muscle let alone the patient's life.

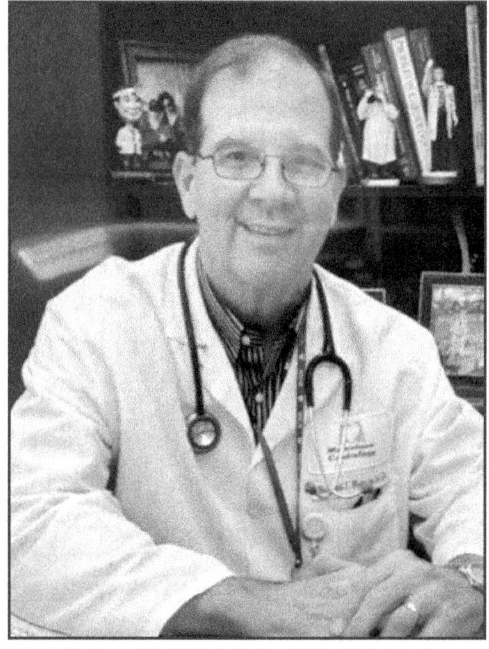

DR. RICHARD WATSON
Author's personal collection

GLOSSARY CHAPTER 6

Pulmonary embolus – clot in a lung artery usually coming from abdominal, pelvic, or leg veins known as embolization

Inferior infarction – heart attack of the undersurface of the heart that rests on the diaphragm separating the chest from the abdomen

Angioplasty – opening or widening an artery usually with a balloon but sometimes with a tiny wire or sequentially slightly larger tubes to widen a channel

Thrombus – blood clot

Acute myocardial infarction – a heart attack causing permanent damage to a segment of the left ventricle's muscle (and occasionally the right ventricle)

Fibrin – a protein formed from fibrinogen during formation of blood clots. It forms a mesh-like shape, impeding blood flow in a blood vessel

CHAPTER 7
THE DEVELOPMENT OF CORONARY ANGIOPLASTY AND CORONARY ARTERY STENTS

I was about to perform an angioplasty and stent on a 68-year-old patient with a blocked artery down the front of the heart known as the LAD and, in some circles called "the widow maker." I knew from years of performing these procedures that oversedation could be dangerous, so I always chose to mildly sedate and distract patients by talking to them, thus keeping them relaxed. It seemed to work well during my thirty years of performing over five thousand angioplasty and stent procedures. I told my patient that while watching a documentary on television about George Bush and John Kerry at Yale that I discovered that Kerry was a year behind me in college and was on the debate team. Despite having a very successful debate year as a freshman with no losses, I was required to try out my sophomore year with a speech. I "winged" it, either out of over-assuredness or assuming a good debater would be on the team the following year. But I was cut from the team. The documentary, which I saw over forty years later, shocked me to discover that John Kerry must have taken my place on the debate team. This discovery occurred the evening before the Bush-Kerry 2004 election, and I assure the readers that my discovery did not affect how I voted in that election. My college roommate called me after the election and chided me for not practicing my speech well enough and said, "If you had practiced your speech, you would be president of the U.S. now and John Kerry would be practicing cardiology in NJ." I related this story to my patient while he was lying on the table, sterilely draped, and waiting for me to begin. He was quiet for half a minute (it seemed much longer) and then said to me, "Doc, I don't know what kind of president you would have made, but you have my vote to proceed with this procedure." The stenting went well, and he went home the next day.

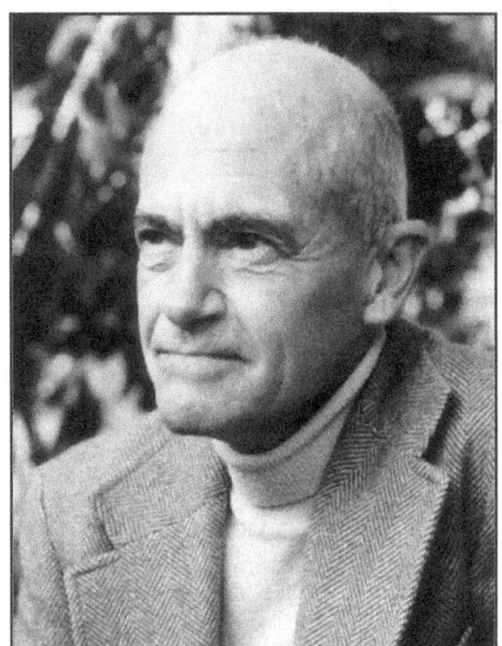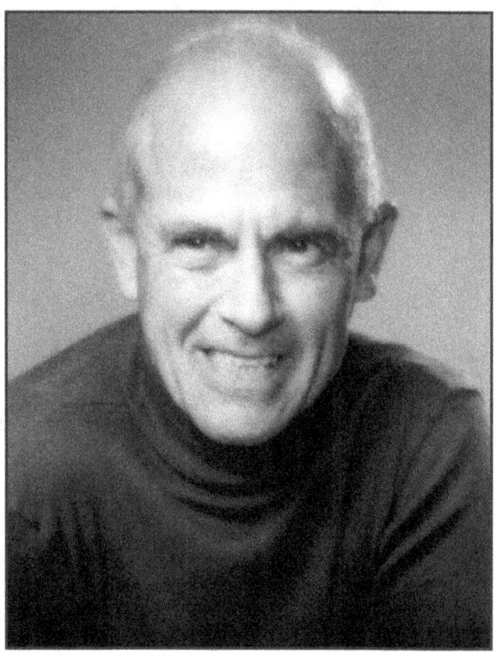

CHARLES T. DOTTER

Both photos permission by Oregon Health & Science University Hospital,
Dotter Interventional Institute

Coronary angioplasty is an invasive cardiac procedure, not surgery. Using catheters (hollow tubes) through which x-ray contrast is injected, effective due to its iodine component, the coronary arteries can be visualized and areas of narrowing identified. This first part is known as coronary arteriography or coronary angiography, as both terms mean photographing a coronary artery, the procedure Mason Sones developed back in 1958. Through the initial guide catheter inserted via the femoral artery at the groin crease into a short slightly larger diameter plastic tube known as a sheath (in the past five to seven years using the artery where the arm meets the hand at the wrist on the thumb side (radial artery) has become the preferred entrance site to allow speedier ambulation after the procedure), a smaller-diameter catheter is inserted. Through this catheter, which is advanced to the mouth of the coronary artery on the left or right depending upon which target artery is the goal, a very thin metal wire is inserted and steered through the arterial narrowing in the coronary artery with the wire tip positioned downstream from the arterial plaque, narrowing the coronary artery. Then over this wire and through the original guiding catheter a very small-caliber catheter with a 2-4mm-diameter inflatable balloon on its tip and usually 20mm long is pushed and positioned inside the areas of coronary artery, narrowing and inflated to literally push the plaque outward against the artery wall to enlarge the channel (lumen) and compress it against the artery wall. This is the angioplasty catheter with balloon. When a small hollow stainless-steel wire mesh (a scaffold) is wrapped around the deflated angioplasty catheter balloon, the procedure becomes a stenting procedure. The stent is opened against the artery wall when the balloon is inflated, compressing the fatty plaque between the stent wire mesh and the artery wall. Nearly always the artery is first enlarged with only a balloon catheter, which is then removed and replaced with the very narrow catheter, which not only has a balloon on it but also a metal stent compressed upon the balloon. When this balloon is inflated, the stent expands against the coronary artery wall. The balloon catheter is then deflated and removed, leaving the stent as a scaffold to keep the artery open, hopefully permanently. So much for the introduction to angioplasty and stenting. How and when did it come about?

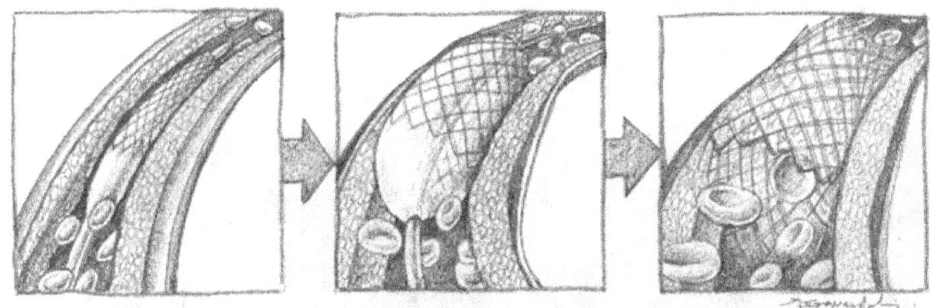

METAL STENT DEPLOYMENT ON BALLOON
by D. Gavasheli, from author's personal collection

The Father of Interventional Radiology and percutaneous transluminal angioplasty of the lower extremities, i.e. catheter therapy, was CHARLES DOTTER (1920-1985, born Boston, Mass., and died Oregon, U.S.), a Disruptor who accidently opened a totally blocked right iliac artery (deep in the body between the belly button and the groin) while passing a catheter up stream to film the abdominal aorta (i.e. the aorta in the mid-abdomen) in 1963. In 1964 Dotter and his resident Melvin Judkins (1922-1985, born near Los Angeles, California, and died Riverside, California, U.S.) subsequently, intentionally used a catheter to open a leg artery of a woman with gangrenous toes in a short narrowed segment of the thigh artery (superficial femoral artery) using dilating catheters with a tapered tip. This was similar to what urologists have used for decades to enlarge a narrowed urethra or catheterize a man with an obstructing prostate and similar to what Peter Rentrop later used in the coronary artery during an acute heart attack. The procedure caused her foot to warm immediately. Without Dotter and Judkins' pioneering and creative clinical research, the field of coronary angioplasty would have never developed since the cardiologists drew on the knowledge and skills obtained by Dotter and Judkins and applied this knowledge to the coronary arteries. Judkins, another Disruptor, made his greatest contribution to cardiology by developing preformed catheters and using the Seldinger technique from the groin rather than using a cutdown to access arm's brachial artery. Today similar catheters that he first used, although smaller in diameter, are frequently used via the radial artery at the wrist. Due to Judkin's technique, coronary angiography could be performed on most patients without the surgical skills required of the Sones technique (cutdown on the arm), and the field of coronary angiography exploded. It was now performed by many more cardiologists than ever before. Judkins published his research in 1967. Today cardiologists speak of performing their procedures either via the Sones (artery cutdown) or Judkins (percutaneously, i.e. through the skin) techniques.

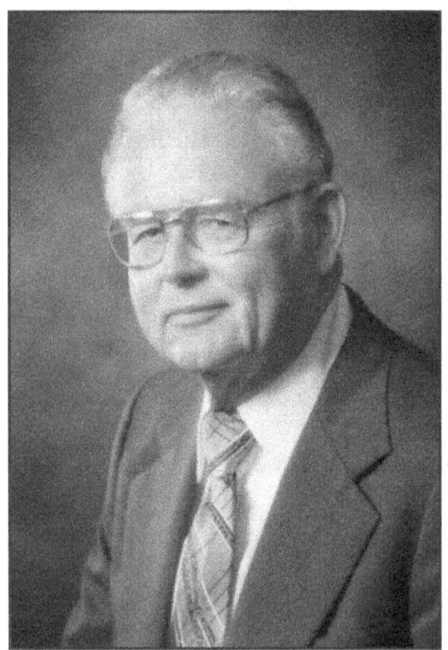
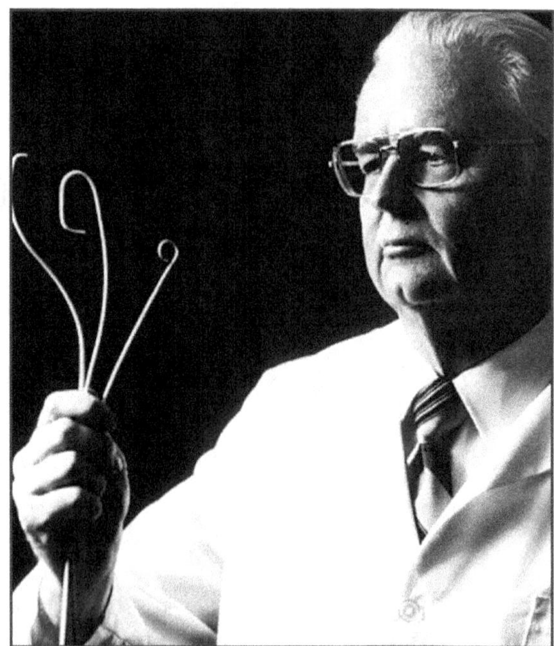

MELVIN JUDKINS, left and right, by permission
Oregon Health & Science University Hospital, Dotter Interventional Institute

The first balloon coronary angioplasty was performed by Andreas Gruentzig (1939-1985, born Dresden, Germany, and died Forsyth, Georgia, U.S.) while working in Zurich, Switzerland. He took advantage of the previous work of Dotter and Judkins with which he was familiar. He practiced on leg arteries before tackling the coronary system. He was one of the great 20th-century cardiac Disruptors, being hindered in Germany by his hospital from pursuing his research (Restrainers). So he moved to Zurich. He used preformed catheters for the coronary artery and the percutaneous femoral approach. He and his wife in their kitchen initially made their own balloon catheters to dilate the obstructed coronary artery, gluing the balloon to the catheter shaft, and used these in his Swiss cardiac lab.

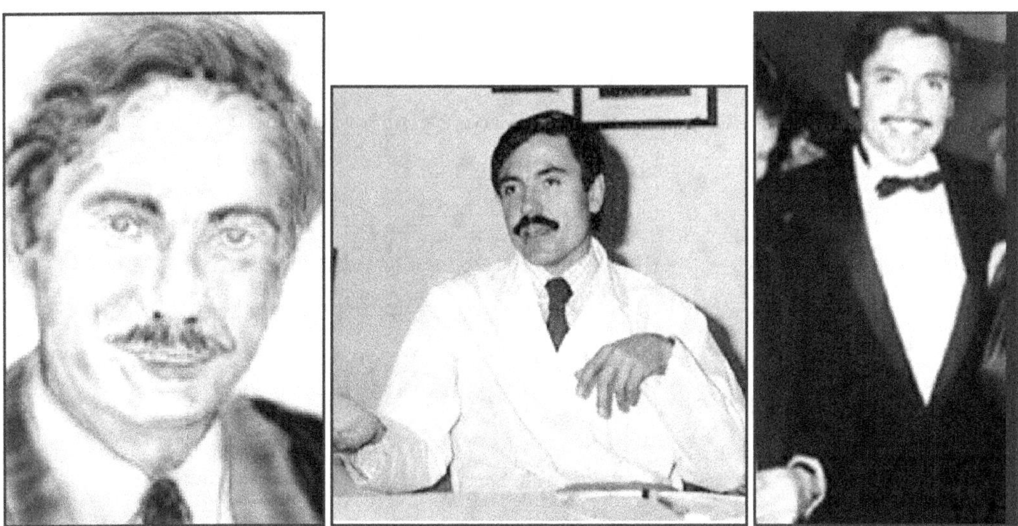

ANDREAS GRUENTZIG original drawing by Dr. Roy Nuzzo, courtesy of Dr. Gary Roubin's private collection, author's personal collection

Being aware of the work of Dotter, Gruentzig learned first how to perform angioplasty of peripheral leg blood vessels before tackling the coronary arteries. Because of Dotter's groundbreaking work, Gruentzig was inspired to perform similar blood vessel openings on the coronary arteries using a balloon mounted on the end of a small diameter hollow tube (catheter). His first balloon coronary angioplasty was performed in September of 1977 in Zurich, Switzerland, on an awake patient's left anterior descending coronary artery (the front branch), which had an 80% narrowing of the artery channel diameter, and the successful procedure relieved the angina pectoris of his patient. Ten years later, when the patient underwent a follow-up coronary angiogram, the artery was fully open. Gruentzig presented his first four cases at the 1977 American Heart Association meeting, and "the rest is history," as they say. About a year before he met his tragic death while flying his own jet, I spent two days in the fall of 1984 shadowing him at Emory University Hospital in Atlanta, Georgia, where he moved his lab. He was gracious to me with his time and was happy to answer all of my many questions as I watched him perform coronary angioplasties (also known as PTCA or percutaneous coronary angioplasty (including on one of my patients whom I referred to him)). Gruentzig was outgoing, charming, and had a wonderful joie de vivre and a great sense of humor. I still remember that he was on a diet at the time and kept himself from hunger by eating carrots all day when I was with him (of course, he offered me some). It is said that he had two of his cardiac fellows perform coronary angiography on himself in 1985 and, after the procedure, instead of taking the day off returned to his office while constantly applying pressure to his groin to be sure no bleeding occurred. Inspired by him after my visit and after obtaining further training under a tutor back home in New Jersey (my tutors, Dr. Russell Broncato at St. Joseph's Hospital in Patterson, NJ, and Dr. Virender Sethi at Hackensack Hospital, NJ), I subsequently entered the field as a coronary angioplaster or what now is termed an "interventional cardiologist." Tragically, Dr. Gruentzig died while flying his own twin-engine plane back from Sea Isle, South Carolina, to Atlanta in a storm in 1985. Dr. Gruentzig's pioneering work and teaching prevented thousands if not millions of patients from undergoing open heart bypass surgery for revascularization of their hearts. His procedure saved countless lives. But to this day there still remains disagreement and controversy in the field despite a multitude of studies whether angioplasty and now stenting is preferable to coronary artery bypass surgery, or even continued medical therapy in medically stable patients.

My friend Walter, whom I arrived with for his balloon angioplasty with Dr. Andreas Gruentzig in Atlanta, Georgia, in the fall of 1984, used to tell our friends at parties that "Guss came with me to Atlanta and watched Dr. Gruentzig perform a few angioplasties and told me that it did not look so hard. So he went back to New Jersey to become an angioplaster." Although it was more complicated than that and took some prolonged training, there was a modicum of truth in Walter's statement.

I remember performing one of my first angioplasties on my own patient, whose case would have been quite easy a few years later as the equipment evolved and improved. At that time the diameter of the catheter and deflated balloon was much larger, making it much more difficult to place the balloon into the area of narrowing where the balloon was to be expanded as the plaque became an obstacle. In this particular early case of mine, no matter how I struggled, the catheter would not cross the narrowing in the artery, and the patient was having chest pain each time the balloon catheter was partially in the obstructing plaque, now preventing all passage of blood downstream to the artery supplying the heart muscle beyond. I remember thinking, Why did I ever leave dermatology (I have two of three years' training in skin diseases) for interventional cardiology and its stress on my heart? Finally, the catheter and balloon moved. The worry was always that the equipment being so large in diameter (we call it "profile") would injure irreparably the artery, making emergency surgery necessary. I did not get out of every jam I encountered, but the one I am now describing fortunately finally yielded, allowing my balloon on the catheter to reach the proper position to inflate and relieve the obstruction. The patient went home the next day. I went home that day, first to shower off my profuse sweat before afternoon office hours.

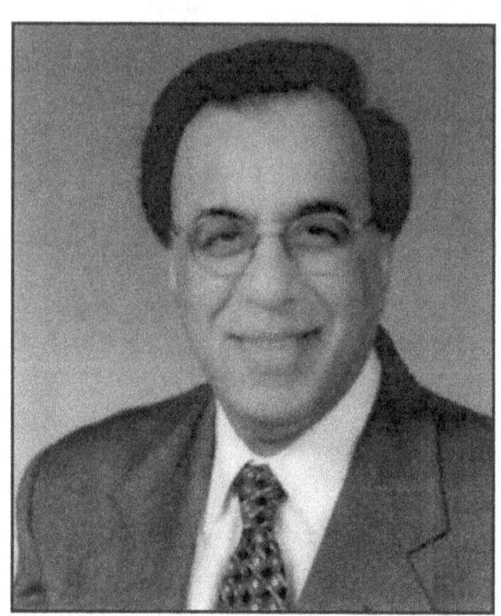

Virender Sethi, author's personal collection

During my long career consulting and performing coronary angioplasty and coronary stenting procedures, I would often have the following conversation after patients would ask me whether to have angioplasty, bypass surgery, or continued medical therapy. Since no cardiologist can see into the future and predict whether a serious complication will occur in any single angioplasty/stenting or bypass surgery case, we can only cite the literature and present statistics. To try to help patients understand our dilemma and that our advice is not perfect, I used to bring out my crystal ball paperweights that were given to me as gifts from patients from my credenza to the desk and say to many patients, "You see these crystal balls? They used to foretell whether to recommend stenting, bypass surgery, or medical treatment. Obviously, if they predicted a severe complication in any of these, I would recommend the alternative choice of therapy. However, not too long ago they stopped working, and I had to put flowers, or cityscapes into them."

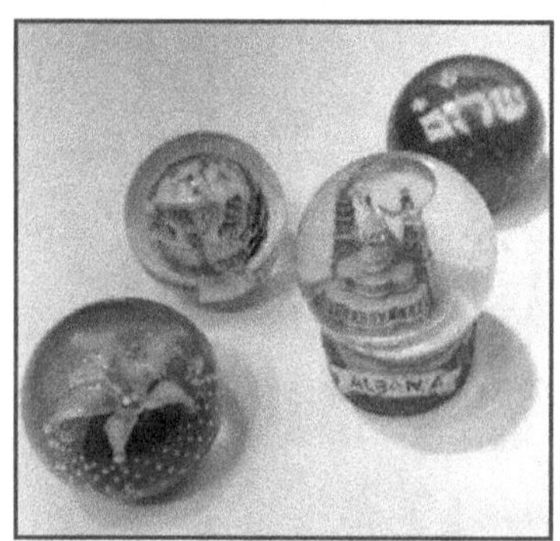
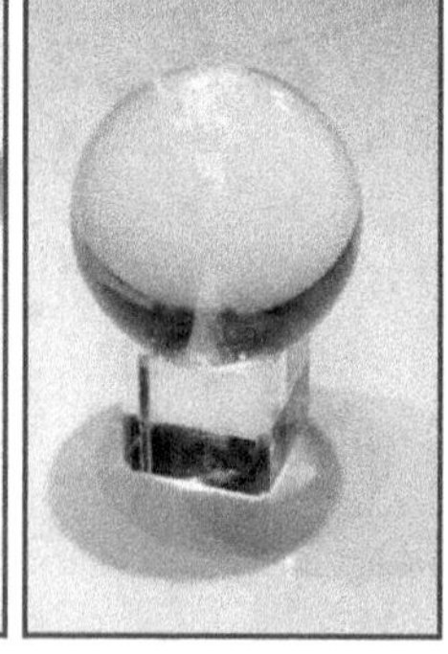
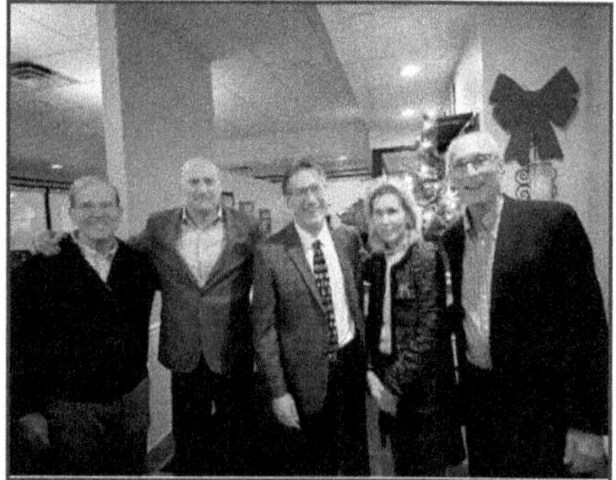

Morristown Cardiology angioplasty team: Drs. R. Watson, C. Rosen, D. Santiago, A. VonPoelnitz, S. Guss

Then I'd go on to say, "Actually, had your appointment been an hour ago, we could have used this clear crystal ball. Unfortunately, it suddenly went on the 'fritz' about a half-hour ago." I think the patients better understood the uncertainty of medical decision-making after having this explanation.

Early angioplasty (now called "plain old balloon angioplasty," or POBA) pioneers and teachers at national and international meetings and courses for the rest of us who subsequently became interventionalists include but are not limited to such greats as (many of whom were unforgettable characters as well as creative and often "cowboys" of their craft) Geoffrey O. Hartzler (1946-2012, born Goshen, Indiana, U.S., and died Lake of the Ozarks, Arkansas, U.S.), who was the first to perform balloon angioplasty during a heart attack (1980) (not just the use of a wire or dilating catheter performed by P. Rentrop a year earlier) and then publish his results of a series of such patients. He advocated using balloon angioplasty to treat a heart attack, which is now standard treatment.

Richard K. Myler (1936-2013, born Springfield, Massachusetts, U.S., and died Belmont, California, U.S.=ioll) was the first to perform an angioplasty in the U.S. in 1978 with Dr. Simon Stertzer from NYC Lenox Hill Hospital).

Gary Roubin was the first to develop an FDA approved stent (see below). Patrick Serruys taught the cardiac world to use stents. John Simpson invented the first over the wire balloon catheter in 1981. Martin Leon (1950, born NY, NY) was a pioneer of angioplasty and stenting, principal investigator of 75 trials, and the lead investigator for the PARTNERS trial leading to approval of the first U.S. TAVR device.

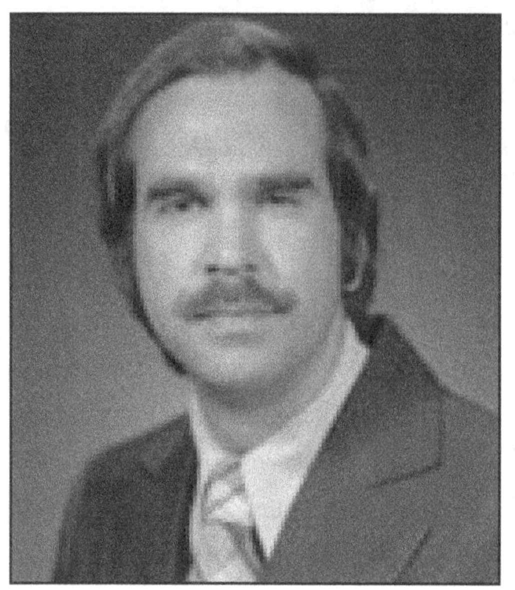

GEOFFREY HARTZLER
permission: Mayo Clinic

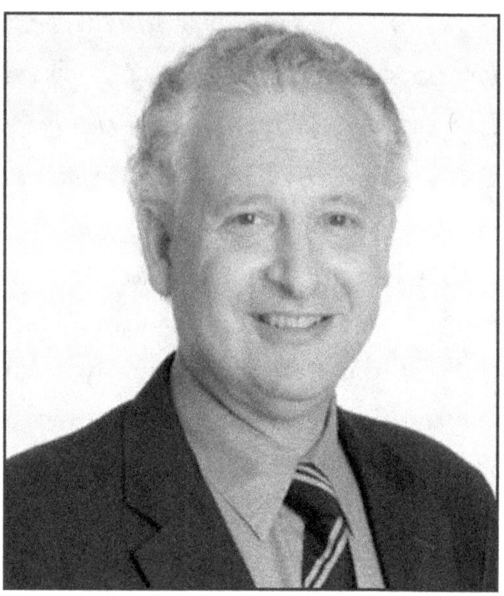

MARTIN LEON
permission: American College of
Cardiology

It should be mentioned that the earlier field of cardiac catheterization and coronary angiography had become predictably safe, and the field of interventional cardiology attracted a different cardiac personality than that of only the diagnostic catheterizing cardiologist (also called invasive cardiologist). The risk of angioplasty in the early years before stents was related to 1) early designed equipment, which was less predictable in outcome—bulkier, less trackable through the artery, less compliant balloons; 2) risk of shutting down the coronary flow during the procedure requiring emergency bypass surgery due to a clot or tear in the coronary artery inner layer known as a dissection; and 3) mortality, which went from 1:1000 in catheterization i.e. coronary angiography to 1/100 during angioplasty. Early angioplasty catheters were larger in diameter (profile) and stiffer than those of today, often making them more difficult to traverse very narrowed or tortuous blood vessels and across calcified lesions.

Although coronary angioplasty revolutionized cardiology, there was a frustration due to a sponge-like effect, which immediately caused re-narrowing of the channel in 5-10% of patients (known as elastic recoil), immediate clotting in a small number (under 1%), and nearly 50% of all patients had re-narrowing of the artery within six months (a term known as restenosis and occurring because of over-healing at the balloon inflation site due to balloon injury of the coronary artery with the several inflations). The healing cells moved in to heal but, instead of repairing, actually caused a re-narrowing of the channel as much and often even more than caused by the original plaque. The appearance of bare metal stents (like a coiled spring or metal scaffold or metal mesh) compressing the plaque centrifugally against the artery wall to prevent recoil and to enlarge the channel reduced the restenosis problem from 50% to 20% of patients. Subsequently, coating the stents with a drug (naturally, these stents are now called "drug eluting stents, DES), which gradually washes off the stent in four to eight weeks and prevents the injury response, reduced the restenosis down from 20% to only 5% of patients. DES use has become the norm.

The first coronary artery stent was placed by Jacque Puel (1946-2008, born Rodez, France. and died Toulouse, France) in Toulouse, France. in December 1985. The cardiologist who was supposed to perform the procedure was out of town, so Dr. Puel filled in admirably. The second person to deploy the same type of stent (called the Wallstent) was Urich Sigwart (1941-, born Wuppertal, Germany) in Lausanne, Switzerland, in 1986 with a publication in the prestigious *New England Journal of Medicine* in March of 1987. The manufacturing company Medinvent was started by a Swedish engineer, Hans Wallen (hence the name Wallstent). The company had anticipated that both men would perform the stenting procedure on exactly the same day, but Sigwart's case was delayed in Lausanne due to "administrative difficulties" despite the Medinvent Company inviting both doctors to place the first stent simultaneously. Once again we see an example of Disputers vs. Restrainers. Complications and deaths doomed this stent to the dustbin of cardiac interventional history. The Wallstent was self-expanding (i.e., the sheath on top of the stent was removed, the material allowed expansion against the artery wall with no balloon inflation, whereas most coronary stents are now balloon expandable). The Wallstent did last long enough for me to hear Dr. Sigwart eloquently lecturing about his experience with this stent at several meetings. Dr. Peul was not a speaker in the U.S. since he did not speak English.

Dr. GARY ROUBIN (1948, born Brisbane, Queensland, Australia) worked with Dr. Cesare Gianturco (1905-1995, born Naples, Italy, and died Urbana, Illinois) to develop the first implanted balloon expandable stent in the U.S. in September of 1987, which was the first FDA-approved stent in May of 1993 (a metal spiral coil was placed on a deflated balloon and expanded against the coronary artery wall when the balloon was inflated). Dr. Roubin, in his book on the history of his stent, emphasizes that cardiologists do not like the term "blow up the balloon" but prefer "inflate the balloon" to avoid a negative connotation. A coronary stent holds open a coronary artery about to collapse or to prevent spongy recoil after balloon angioplasty similar to a scaffold in a mine preventing the walls from collapsing on the miners. The term stent is not new and was originally used in the 1800s, when a dentist, Dr. Thomas Stent, made a paste that hardened after shaping to hold open a patient's mouth so that the dentist could work without oral obstruction. The term "stenting" became used with time to mean "hold things apart or in place." The term was first used in cardiology, according to Dr. Roubin, by Dr. Julio Palmaz in 1988 (more to come about his coronary stent) for the coronary artery appliance to hold the artery open, i.e. a coronary artery stent.

With the help of Cook Medical and working with Dr. Gianturco starting in 1985, Dr. Roubin used extremely rigorous and scientific protocols for animal experiments to prove the worth and safety of his device before testing it on a human. This attention to detail Dr. Roubin credits Dr. Gruentzig in his teaching his cardiology fellows and followers of whom Dr. Roubin was both a resident under Dr. Gruentzig and then his protégée and friend. Originally the stent idea began with Dr. Gianturco, who was a radiologist. He developed a large stent for veins while working at MD Anderson Hospital in Houston, Texas to prevent tumor compression of abdominal veins. Working together, Dr. Gianturco suggested the shape of the coronary artery stent to be called the Gianturco-Roubin Stent from a roll of stainless-steel electrical wire, which he took out of his pocket and coiled around a small rod for shaping when he demonstrated his idea to Dr. Roubin. The stent was then placed on top of a catheter's balloon and compressed to maintain a low profile until the balloon would be inflated at the site of the injured closing artery. The inspiration for Dr. Roubin to develop this coronary stent was the ongoing issue of acute coronary artery closure, usually due to a clot or tear in the artery inner of three layers from the balloon trauma of coronary angioplasty, which would cause vessel closure and require emergency bypass surgery at best to save the day and a heart attack and death at worst. (As an aside, Dr. Roubin speculated that Dr. Gruentzig would not have died in his plane crash had stents been available in 1985, when he crashed his plane. Dr. Gruentzig cared deeply about his patients' outcome and always took responsibility for a complication and was involved in the post care. The day he died was after a successful angioplasty on a patient who later in the day closed his artery and suffered a heart attack, requiring emergency bypass surgery. Despite a developing storm, Dr. Gruentzig, according to Dr. Roubin, felt obligated to fly back to help his patient and his patient's family. A stent might have prevented the need for bypass surgery if it had been available in 1985. Dr. Gruentzig might have still been alive had he not felt compelled to fly back to Atlanta from the South Carolina coast on that fateful and fatal day.) Finally, the proper stainless-steel diameter of the stent struts was determined after experimenting for the Gianturco-Roubin Stent in 1986. Dr. Roubin's idea to develop a stent to prevent blood vessel shutdown came to fruition. The stent that Dr. Roubin and Dr. Gianturco invented was called the Giantourco-Roubin Stent, but this stent quickly became mainly used as a "bailout" device for emergency artery closures during the angioplasty procedure and was never intended to be used as a permanent device placed electively as we now place stents. Once the Palmaz-Schatz Stent entered the scene and the restenosis rate of the Gianturco-Roubin Stent was greater than that of the Palmaz-Schatz Stent, the Palmaz-Schatz Stent became the "go-to" stent used by most cardiologists as a more permanent solution to the restenosis and even acute closure problem.

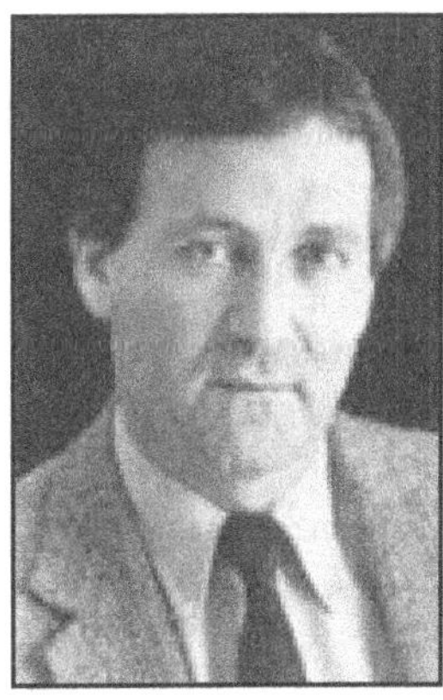

GARY ROUBIN, courtesy and with permission of Dr. Roubin's private collection

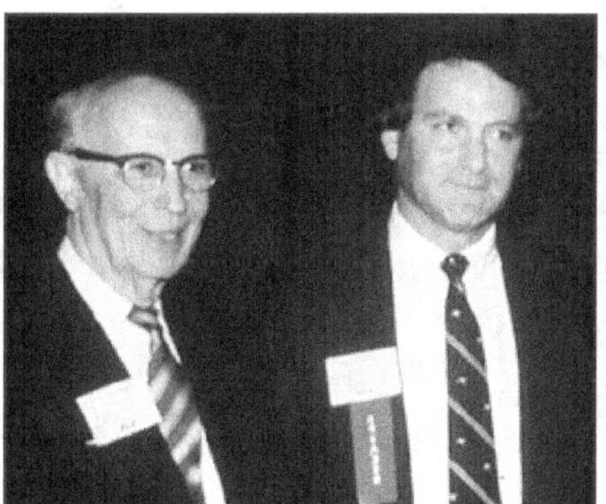

Dr. GIANTURCO AND DR. ROUBIN, with permission of Dr. Roubin's private collection

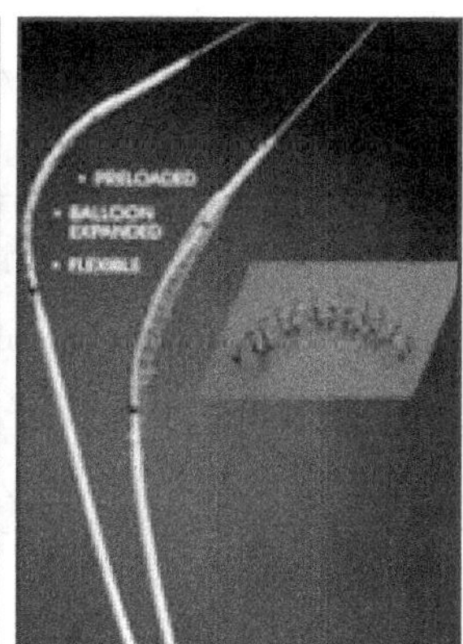

GIANTURCO-ROUBIN STENT, with permission of Dr. Roubin's private collection, wrapped on balloon, balloon inflated, expanded stent

The Palmaz-Schatz Stent, which was initially rejected by the FDA in December 1993, became FDA approved and available in August 1994 and had a lower re-narrowing (restenosis) rate than just balloon angioplasty and/or the Gianturco-Roubin Stent. It quickly captured the market. JULIO PALMAZ, a radiologist (1945-, born in La Plata, Argentina), perfected his stent at the U of Texas, San Antonio. He first conceived of the idea in 1978 after seeing a presentation by Dr. Andreas Gruentzig at the American Heart Association meeting. With the help of RICHARD SCHATZ, a cardiologist (1952-, born Queens, NY), together they developed a flexible balloon expandable stainless-steel coronary stent in 1985. It was shaped differently than the Gianturco-Roubin Stent and was for several years used by most interventional cardiologists worldwide. Johnson and Johnson bought the stent from Palmaz and Schatz in 1986 and manufactured and marketed it worldwide. In studies the Palmaz-Schatz Stent demonstrated superiority over plain old balloon angioplasty (POBA) and against the Gianturco-Roubin Stent. The development of thinner strut stents as time went by has further reduced post-deployment thrombosis of the stent, as has the use of the dual anticoagulants against platelets, aspirin with either clopidogrel (it replaced ticlopidine in 1999), prasugrel, or ticagrelor, taken for one year with a baby aspirin 81mg. In 1994 the U.S. the FDA finally cleared the Palmaz-Schatz Stent for use on coronary arteries, although they were used since 1987 in Europe and used in 1992 in Europe when I was performing cardiac research in Sweden. The Cook Company Gianturco-Roubin Stent was actually approved earlier by the FDA in May 1993 as the first FDA-approved stent. This stent, meant to be for bailout of abrupt closures and not as a primary device, was quickly overtaken in use by the superior Palmaz-Schatz Stent, which the FDA approved in 1994 for de novo use to reduce restenosis. Ironically the fairly inflexible, immovable Palmaz-Schatz metal stent proved its worth in diseased arteries, even in those that had twists and turns and constantly moved with each heartbeat. Whereas POBA re-narrowing (called "restenosis") was close to 50% at six months, the new bare metal stents brought this down to 20%.

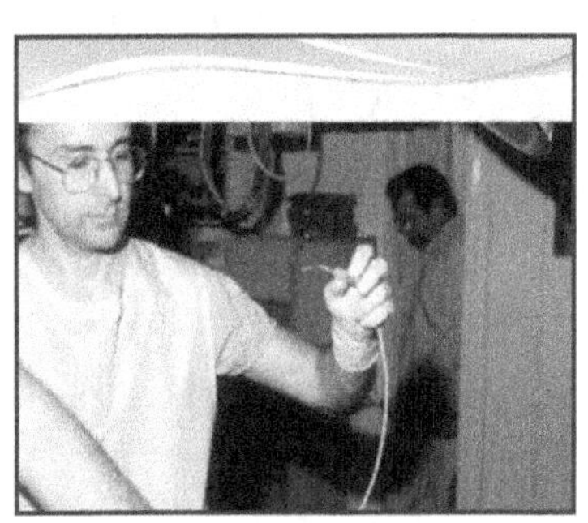

JULIO PALMAZ
by permission of Dr.
Schatz, from his personal
collection

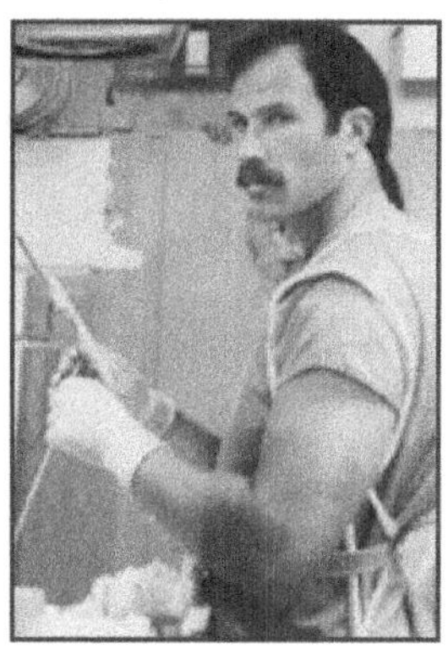

RICHARD
SCHATZ by permis-
sion of Dr. Schatz,
from his personal
collection

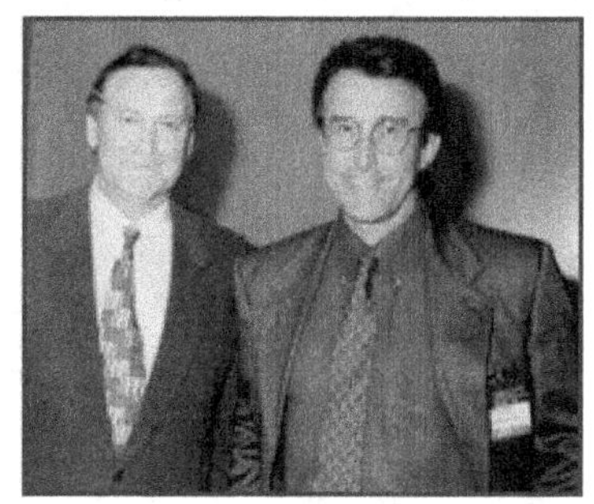

GARY ROUBIN/ JULIO
PALMAZ
Roubin's collection

As the most utilized stent in the world for many years, it was first used in Europe when Dr. Schatz performed the first coronary case with Dr. Raimond Erbel in Mainz, Germany, in February 1987.

Finally, the stent received another improvement. By placing an antiproliferative or an immune-suppressive drug on a polymer, which coats the stent struts, restenosis rates continued to plummet to 5% using Sirolimus (Cordis Cypher stent—first worldwide deployment by Dr. Jose Eduardo Sousa in 1999 in San Paolo, Brazil) or Paclitaxel (Boston Scientific). The drug eluting stents, or DES as they are known (vs. the initial bare metal stents - BMS), elute the drug off the stent over four to eight weeks and prevent the neointimal hyperplasia cells from re-narrowing at the inside layer of the artery that was injured during balloon inflation and where the stent was placed. Subsequently new medications such as Everolimus (Abbott Xience Stent and Boston Scientific Promus Stent) and Zotarolimus (Medtronic Resolute and Endeavor stents) have brought even better results as second-generation drug eluting stents both because of the newer attached medications and thinner stent struts made possible by shifting from stainless-steel to nickel cadmium designs. Now newer polymers have been developed that do not interfere with formation of a more normal lining of the artery under the stent, sometimes remaining "denuded" by the first-generation drug eluting stents. This new normal healing helps prevent thrombosis at stent sites. And recently a study with a bioadaptable stent using cobalt-chromium with the drug sirolimus showed the vessel to have a more normal mobility despite its presence in the artery. With time, other better stents will surely also be developed, including self-absorbing stents.

The field of stenting has expanded its indications because of the work of Geoffrey Hartzler, who pioneered the field of angioplasty for an acute myocardial infarction (heart attack), which is now the accepted gold-standard treatment for a heart attack (angioplasty and stenting).

The Palmaz-Schatz Stent for many years was the most utilized coronary stent in the world. Although not FDA approved in the U.S. until 1994, it was widely used in Europe by 1992, where I was performing research at the time in Gothenburg, Sweden, and had the good fortune of working with the team in at least a dozen stent procedures (Drs. Lars Ekstrom, Hakan Emanuelsson, and Per Albertsson). I was at the Sahlgrenska Institute in Gothenburg, Sweden, in the summer of 1992 when one of my Swedish colleges who had a very thick Swedish accent while speaking English said what at the time I thought was an extremely poetic metaphor about stenting. I thought I heard him say that to complete a successful stent procedure you needed "the right angel." I certainly thought that given the risks of performing stenting, it would be nice to have an angel watching over the operator and the patient. As I reflected upon the episode after the case, I realized my college said what was needed is the right "angle," not "angel." Of course, he said this as the right angle of the x-ray machine was required to prevent blood vessel overlap, which might obscure the proper lesion and stent position. Oh, well, I like my poetic version better.

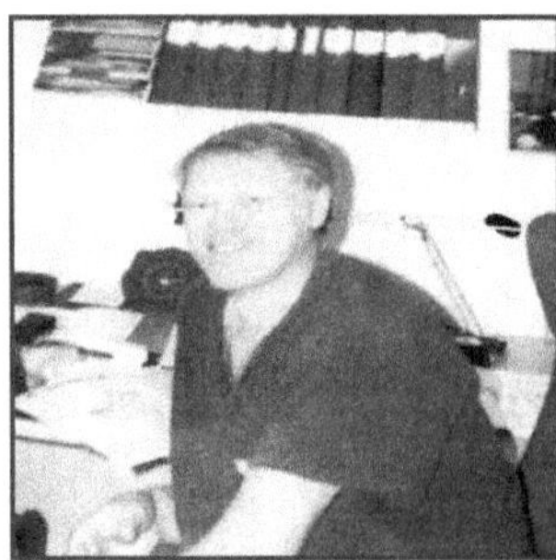

Dr Haakon
Emmanuelson

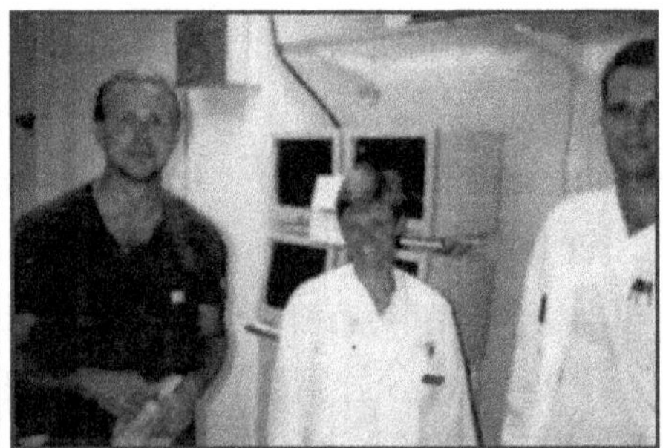

Dr Lars Ekstron, unknown
woman, and Dr Albertson

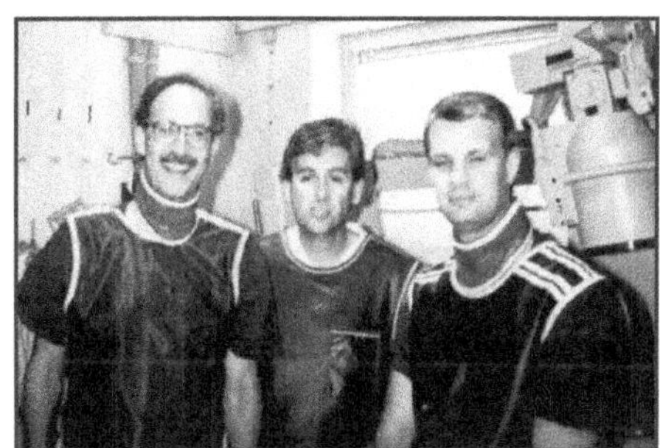

Author, unknown doctor, Dr
Per Albertsson
author' personal collection

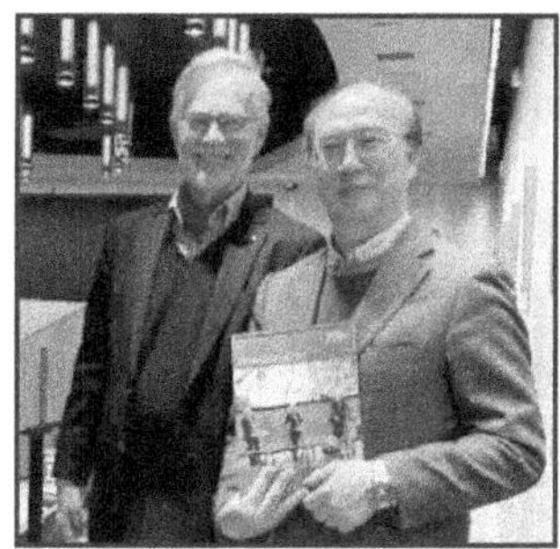

Dr Goran Hansson , Chief of the Lab
at Sahlgrenska Hospital in Gothenburg, Sweden when I was there and
Dr Yong jian Geng, retired head of
cardiovascular research, Texas Heart
Institute
Dr Geng's personal collection

GLOSSARY CHAPTER 7

LAD, or Left Anterior Descending Coronary Artery – the artery down the front of the heart that supplies 40% of the left ventricle muscle, more than the other two arteries

PTA = Percutaneous Transluminal angioplasty – placing a catheter through the skin to open an artery anywhere in the body

Recanalize – reopening a channel

Iliac artery – **connects the aorta at the level of the belly button with the artery** at the groin

Retrograde – pushing the catheter toward the heart

Angina pectoris – a pressure in the chest with exertion when the blood supply to the heart is inadequate for the demand, which goes away with rest

Elastic recoil – like a compressed sponge going back to its original shape

CHAPTER 8

PACEMAKERS, TEMPORARY AND PERMANENT; DEFIBRILLATORS, EXTERNAL AND INTERNAL

When I was a third-year medical student on my general surgery rotation in Boston at the Peter Bent Brigham Hospital, I saw the patients on the wards each morning with Dr. Dwight Harken, a world-renowned cardiac surgeon, and his team (known as "rounding"), who included an engineer from American Optical who was the inventor and designer of the first permanent transvenous pacemaker (placed in a vein), whereas previously permanent pacemakers were placed via an incision into the chest with the pacer wire sewn directly onto the right ventricle muscle from the outside. The designer was Barough Berkovits, whom as a young medical student I found to be very self-assured but clearly very brilliant!!! As we each morning visited the patients who had undergone transvenous pacemaker implantations the day before, I just assumed this was routine and being performed for years. A surgical resident awoke me from my medical student slumber of ignorance and informed me I was witnessing medical history in the making, as such pacemakers had never been implanted previously but in the past required opening the chest to sew the wire onto the heart muscle wall. Wow!! I felt a little ridiculous, but I quickly grasped the importance of what I was observing.

This chapter is about defibrillators and pacemakers. It is difficult to separate them into two topics since they are intertwined from a surgical point of view, and both require a wire inside the heart for the permanent pacemaker and automatic internal defibrillators (AID) and have a control box with software and battery. Most AIDs are coupled with a pacemaker capability so there is only one box. Let's start with the defibrillator story.

Geronimo Mercuriale (1530-1606, born and died Forli, Italy), as a graduate of the famed Bologna and Padua Schools of Medicine, recognized that
people often fainted when the pulse was very slow. Considering he had no
EKG corroboration as the EKG was not yet invented, his problem recognition
was remarkable for the time and his description most likely described patients
with complete heart block. This condition is due to the electrical signal from
the top of the heart, the right atrium, not making it down to the ventricle
(often from scar tissue in the conducting system) to tell the ventricle to contract (i.e. pump).

A Danish physicist, Nicolai Abildgaard (1743-1809, born Copenhagen,
Denmark, and died Frederiksdal, Denmark), stimulated a hen's head electrically,
which made it die (of course). When he electrically stimulated various parts of
the body, nothing happened (of course). However, when he finally stimulated
over the hen's chest, the bird was revived (this was probably the world's first defibrillation...EUREKA!!!).

Even the surgeon John Hunter, in 1776, about whom we read in Chapter 2,
recommended applying electricity to the chest of drowning victims. His friend
John Fothergill (1712-1780, born Wensleydale, England, and died London,
England) invented mouth-to-mouth respiration. The surgeon, Charles Kite (no
photo available), in England in 1788 reported the successful use of a portable
electrostatic generator on a three-year-old girl who had fallen out of a window
and apparently was dead for twenty minutes before Kite's shock brought her
back to life. This may have been the first successful defibrillation of a human,
although there is controversy as to the mechanism of the heart rhythm before
and during the shock.

Without Alessandro Volta (1745-1827, born Como, Duchy, Milan, and died
Como, Lombardy-Venetia, Austrian Empire) we might never have pacemakers
because they require batteries. He published in 1800 his work on placing two
dissimilar metals together to produce electricity—the first battery!! And in 1872
Guillaume Duchenne de Boulogne (1806-1875, born Boulogne, France, and
died Paris, France) resuscitated a drowned child by placing one electrode to a
leg and tapping over the heart with the second live electrode, which caused the
child's heart to restart. It was more probably the first human defibrillation re-

suscitation in history if the Englishman Kite's claims are inaccurate as some have claimed.

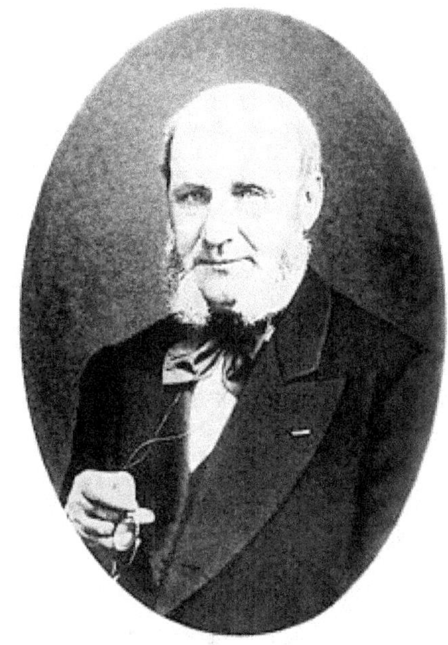

GUILLAUME DUCHENNE
DE BOULOGNE
Creative Commons

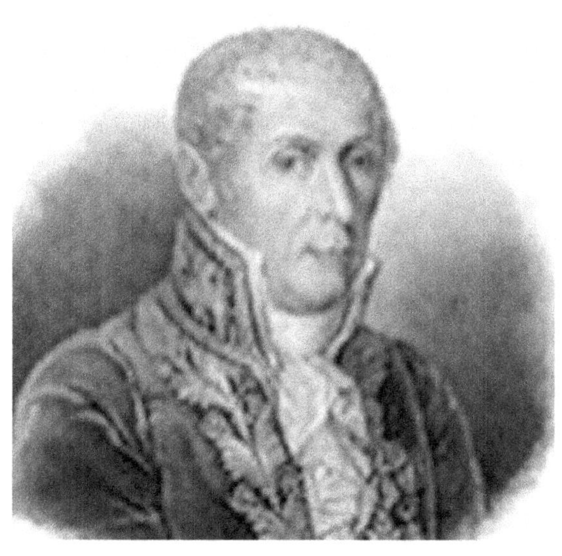

ALESSANDRO VOLTA,
public domain

Carl Ludwig (1816-1895, born Witzenhausen, Germany, and died Leipzig, Germany) (see chapter on the blood pressure machine) in 1850 demonstrated that he could induce ventricular fibrillation in animals by applying an electric current directly to the heart. This German scientist led the way in experimental physiology and taught many of the future scientific leaders of Europe and the British Isles. In the same year, Germany was composed of numerous duchies and principalities. Prussia, the largest and wealthiest and most powerful, agreed to restore the German Confederation in November of 1850, known as the Punctation of Olmutz. Industrial capitalism came to Germany in 1850, and progress ensued. When the Prussian leader, Prince Frederick William IV, in 1857 suffered a series of strokes, his brother succeeded him in 1858. The new prince, William I, was more modern and realized that the old way of doing things was not working. He dismissed his brother's cabinet and announced some modest reforms, winning the approval of the German legislature and ushering in an era of optimism in Germany.

Hugo von Ziemssen (1829-1902, born Greifswald, Germany, and died Munich, Germany), a physician, had performed experiments with electricity for years and with a patient whose heart was exposed due to a chest malignancy. Von Ziemssen demonstrated that applying electricity either directly to the chest or through the chest wall, he could change the rhythm and return it to normal. He was clearly onto something, and an American wrote in 1882, "The therapeutic value of such a means of acting directly and positively on the heart is evident." A British physician had a contrary opinion after performing some experiments himself: "Little is to be expected from electricity as a therapeutic agent in the treatment of disease." This quotation shows how scientists need to bridle their critiques lest mud might be thrown back into their faces. This was the voice of Restrainers.

John Alexander MacWilliam (1857-1937 another Disruptor, born Kiltarlity Inverness-shire, Scotland, UK, and died Edinburgh, Scotland, UK) invented a machine to record the heartbeat and other muscle contractions (pre-EKG machine). He studied under the great Carl Ludwig in Germany. From his studies on animals he surmised that the rapid ineffective heartbeats from the lower chamber, the ventricle, and now known as ventricular fibrillation were the cause of most sudden death. He described basic CPR techniques for keeping his animals alive (but not humans). He determined that his conclusions in cold-blooded animals also pertained to mammals. In 1887 he published "fibrillar contraction…the ventricular muscle is thrown into a state of irregular arhythmic (spelling is correct for its time) contraction, while there is a great fall in the arterial blood pressure. The ventricles become dilated with blood as the rapid quivering movement of their walls is insufficient to expel their contents; the muscular action partakes of the nature of a rapid uncoordinated twitching of the muscular tissue."

In his address to the International Medical Congress in Washington, D.C., in 1887, he reported his own experiments where the heartbeat could be restored in animals by two electrodes when inducing electrical shocks of moderate strength and at a rate of a normal heartbeat (sounds suspiciously like the first pacemaker and/or defibrillator). He also used this technique of cardiac compression and artificial respiration (similar to CPR of today). One electrode was applied to the heart's apex and one on the back of the chest at the vertebra

with the chest opened. Most importantly, he was sure that ventricular fibrillation was most likely the leading cause of sudden death in humans. It is important to remember that MacWilliam's conclusions were based on arterial
wave forms and direct observation of animal hearts without the availability of
an EKG machine, which makes the diagnosis so easy today. He also recognized the association of ventricular fibrillation with "degenerative changes of
a fatty or fibroid nature in the muscular walls" in humans. This is consistent
with previous heart attacks or chronic ischemic damage. But he also recognized that ventricular fibrillation could also occur in humans "apart from gross
structural lesions with no very obvious or extensive alterations of cardiac tissues." At the conclusion of his paper he descriptively wrote, "The cardiac
pump is thrown out of gear, and the last of its vital energy is dissipated in the
violent and prolonged turmoil of fruitless activity in the ventricular walls."
He understood the relationship of ventricular fibrillation to sudden death and
its link to coronary artery disease and heart attacks. He was a Disruptor. His
work was ignored for years for the same reasons that other scientists ignored
the importance of coronary artery disease to heart attacks since they were Restrainers (Chapter 2). It may be that the new field of bacteriology had usurped
the interest and intrigue of the scientific and nonscientific world with its discovery and future promise. Furthermore, sudden death and heart attacks were
not prevalent like today since most people did not live long enough as a rule
to suffer from coronary artery disease. Ironically, as life expectancy was ex-
tended in the twentieth century compared to the three previous centuries,
coronary artery disease became the leading cause of death by 1950. Ironically,
the increased life expectancy may also have been facilitated by the field of bacteriology, which has prolonged life with vaccines, antibiotics, and aseptic techniques. (My oncology colleagues used to say to me that cardiologists are really
good for their business since the cardiological extension of life has produced
more people living long enough to get cancer, which they can then treat.) It
is also said that MacWilliam's modesty prevented him from broadcasting more
loudly and broadly his important scientific conclusions. About all that could
be clinically applied immediately by the work of MacWilliam was the discovery by ALFRED GOODMAN LEVY in 1912 (1866-1954, born Melbourne,
Australia, and died Marlow, England) in dogs and in 1911 with SIR THOMAS

LEWIS in 1881-1945, born Taffs Wells, Cardiff, Wales, UK, and died Hertfordshire, UK, in surgical patients whom they monitored in the operating room. They realized that the sudden death occurring during anesthesia using chloroform (first used in 1847) was due to ventricular fibrillation. Sir Thomas Lewis credits MacWilliam for first thinking that sudden death was often caused by ventricular fibrillation. When the portable EKG became available, it became possible to assess fallen patients out of the hospital during a cardiac arrest rather than only animal subjects in the lab. In fact, Sir Thomas Lewis, the Father of Electrophysiology, also recognized that ventricular fibrillation was seen uncommonly in man at that time because people could not be assessed properly (no EkG available) and most sudden death was sudden and unexpected (an EKG recording would be taken too late and only by the time that asystole had occurred, i.e. the end stage of death). Of note is that the study of ventricular fibrillation, which can be caused by electrocution, owes its early research funding to two large companies, the electrical and telephone companies that were concerned about electrocution of employees and looking for ways to prevent electrocution.

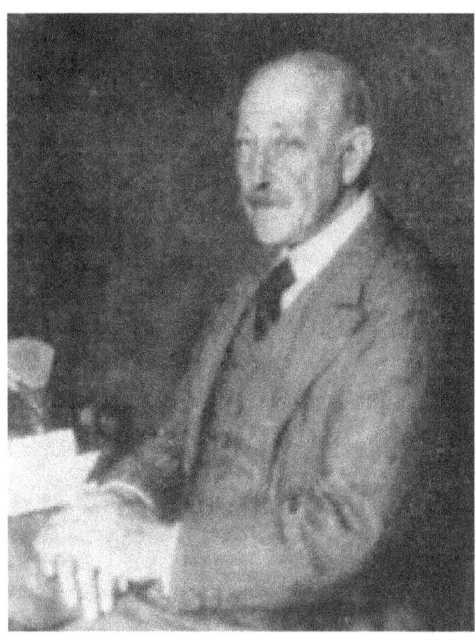

ALFRED GOODMAN LEVY,
public domain

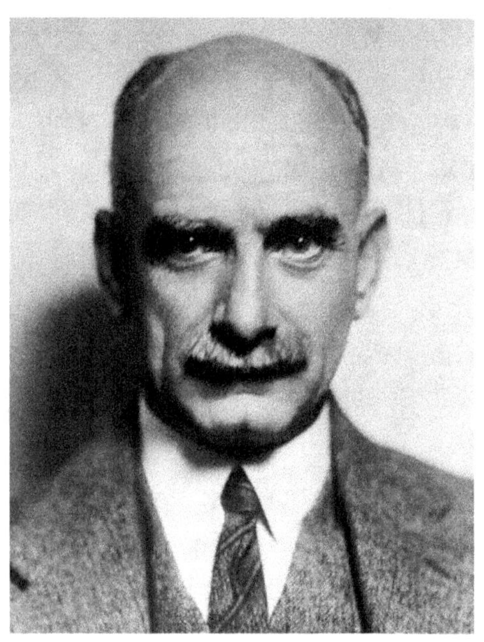

SIR THOMAS LEWIS,
public domain

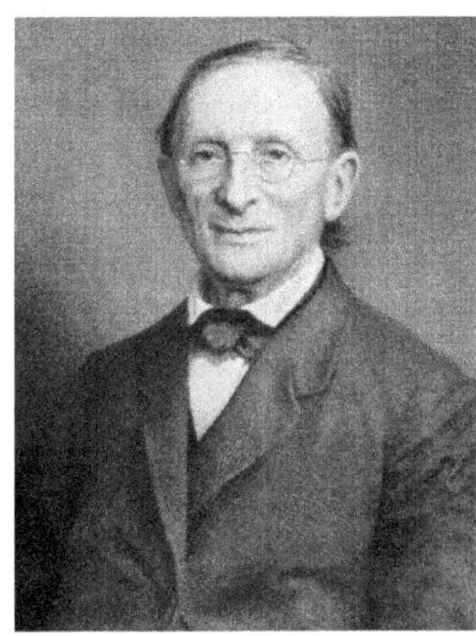
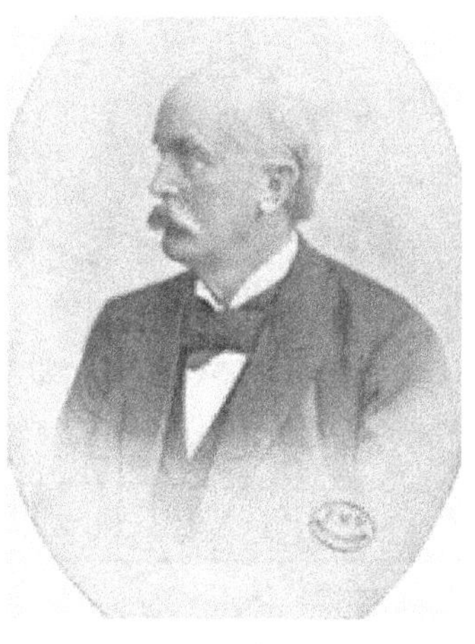
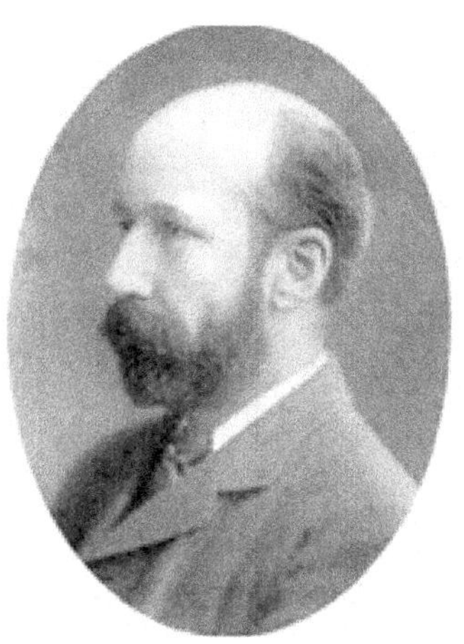

CARL LUDWIG
public domain

HUGO VON ZIEMSSEN
public domain from
Collection Bibliotheque,
public domain interuni-
versitaire de Sante

JOHN A. MACWILLIAM
public domain

In Geneva, Switzerland, Jean Louis Prevost (1838-1927, born Geneva Switzerland and died Geneva, Switzerland) and Frederic Batelli (1867-1941, born Macerata
Feltria, Italy and died Geneva, Switzerland) in 1899 reported both A/C and D/C
voltages could revive their experimental dogs with open chests, thus creating the first
internal defibrillator although not for humans. They found weak shocks could cause
ventricular fibrillation, but they also found that some of their animals when applying
larger current through electrodes in the mouth and small intestine were restored to
normal rhythm. They also used cardiac compression and artificial respiration.

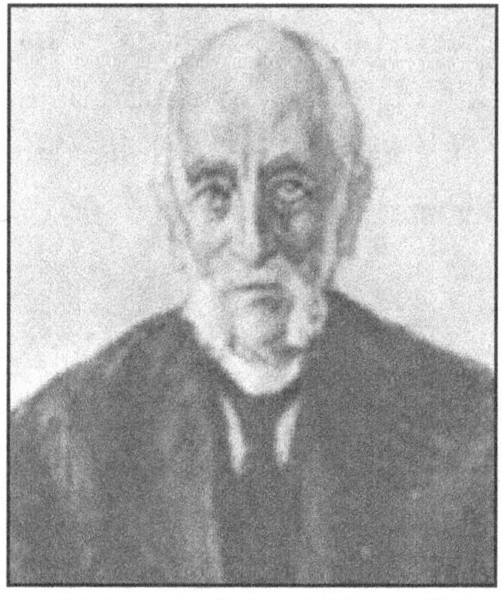

JEAN LOUIS PREVOST,
public domain

An engineer, William Bennett Kouwenhoven (1886-1975, born Brooklyn, NY, U.S., and died Baltimore, Maryland, U.S.), at Johns Hopkins in 1933 used electricity to defibrillate dogs with open chests. He received his funding from Consolidated Edison of NY due to their concern about electrocution from electricity. Despite his findings, the subject was not pursued further at Johns Hopkins. He was an early pioneer in the field and awarded the much prestigious Lasker Prize in 1973.

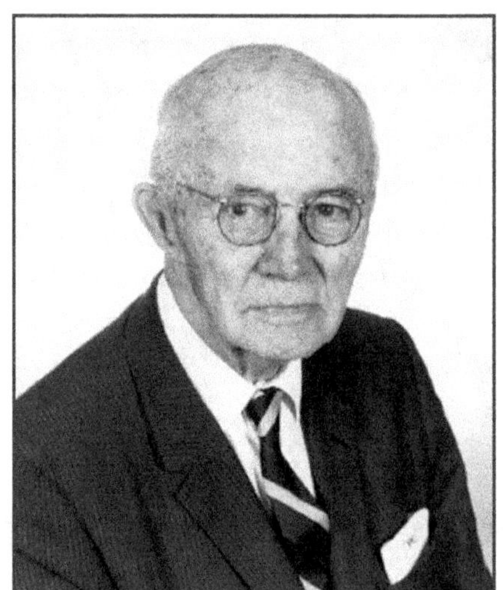

WILLIAM B. KOUWENHOVEN
by permission of the Lasker Foundation

Finally, Dr. PAUL ZOLL (1911-1999, born Boston, Massachusetts, U.S., and died Chestnut Hill, Massachusetts, U.S.), also a Lasker Prize winner in 1973 and a Disruptor, was a cardiologist at the Harvard Beth Israel Hospital in Boston who worked on the first practical external cardiac defibrillator and the first external pacemaker. His pacemaker research came first in 1952. And then in 1956 he published the first transcutaneous approach to treating ventricular fibrillation or ventricular tachycardia (the first is disorganized and the second sometimes more organized but can be ineffective for the circulation and just as lethal) with an A/C shock. Previous work was performed on open-chested animals, usually dogs, although Dr. Claude S. Beck in 1947 used a defibrillator made by his engineer to successfully restart a patient's ventricular fibrillatory heart whose chest was also opened at the time of surgery. Subsequently, and for technical reasons,

D/C electricity has been shown to be more effective and replaced Zoll's original A/C design.

In 1952 Zoll had previously also revolutionized cardiology with the first external pacemaker. Previous pacemakers used a wire surgically attached to the heart muscle of an open chest but attached to an external energy source. Zoll's pacemaker used flat metal leads on the patient's normal closed chest attached to an external box, which housed the controls and battery. Zoll showed that he could control the rate of the heart and pace with an appropriate voltage. Although Zoll's device was revolutionary and sometimes lifesaving (I used it at the Beth Israel Hospital in Boston as a medical resident on rare occasions), it was not very practical for an awake patient. It was quite painful for an awake patient who was electrically paced sixty or more times a minute to feel the 50-150 volts of electricity required to "capture" the heart with each stimulation. However, it paved the way for other inventions, including temporary transvenous pacemaker wires attached to a similar external box as Zoll had made and percutaneous temporary wires placed through the skin during a cardiac arrest, which hooked on to the right ventricle, entering the skin from under the bottom of the breastbone and connected to the external battery box. Interestingly, an external pacemaker similar to Zoll's original device was recycled about fifteen years ago and still is used today for emergency pacing in hospitals until a temporary transvenous (i.e. internal wire) pacemaker can be placed. His research showed the medical profession that asystolic hearts could be stimulated to beat again.

In 1962 Dr. Bernard Lown (1921-2021, born Utena, Lithuania, and died Newton, Massachusetts, U.S.) developed an external direct current (D/C) defibrillator for ventricular tachycardia and ventricular fibrillation cardiac arrests as well as to convert atrial fibrillation back to a normal sinus rhythm. Today Dr. Zoll and Lown's dream have become a reality as small portable battery-operated defibrillators are found in thousands of public spaces due to Zoll and Lown's efforts. Parenthetically, the company Zoll started and bears his name makes a vest, which is worn after a severe heart attack to diagnose and then shock a patient automatically if a dangerous ventricular arrhythmia threatens death.

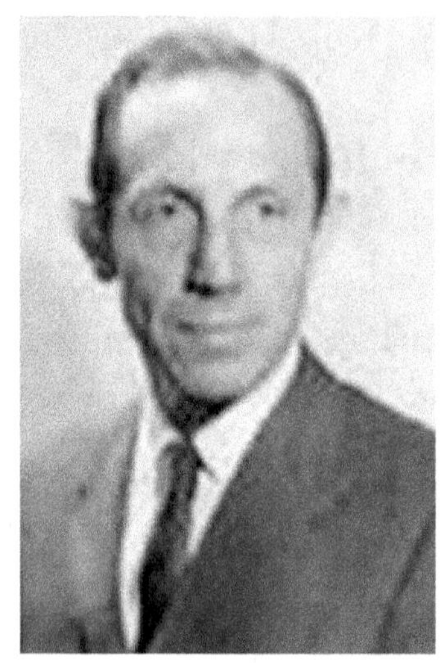 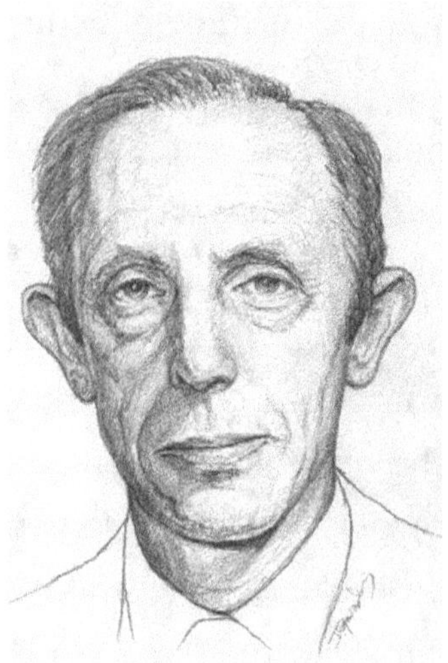 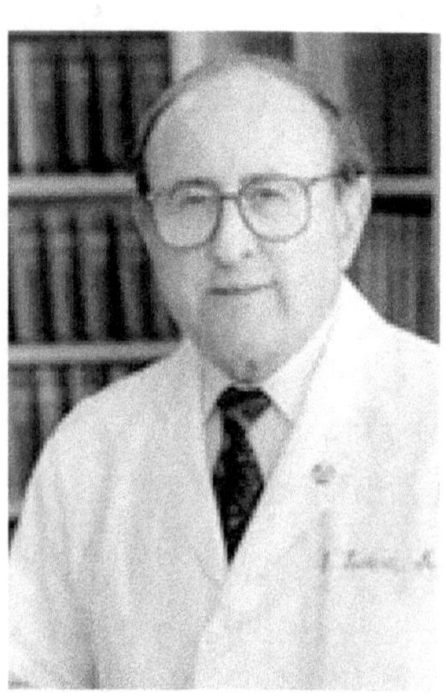

PAUL ZOLL
Public domain
Rhythm

PAUL ZOLL
Public domain
Drawn by D. Gavasheli
From author's personal
collection

BERNARD LOWN
permission from Heart
Rhythm Society

I knew Dr. Paul M. Zoll when I was first a medical student and then an internal medicine intern and resident at the Beth Israel Hospital in Boston between 1966-1970, and I liked him and always got along with him. He was very short and his expression was usually quite severe. I can't remember him smiling, although I am sure he did. He was the attending (i.e. teacher to those of us in training) for one month and met with us every morning to go over the patients under our care. He was a stickler way ahead of his time for not wasting medical resources, and he was correct. I have tried to take this lesson with me over the years. One morning while discussing a patient admitted four days before with pneumonia, he reamed us out for ordering daily white blood counts (he was right) and asked if having this in the chart every day changed our diagnosis, treatment or the patient's outcome (it did not, of course). The next week a patient was admitted the evening before our meeting with Dr. Zoll with a heart attack of the undersurface of the heart (known as an inferior myocardial infarction). Most of the time, and occurring in this patient, it is easy to diagnose on the EKG, and only three of the twelve EKG leads are needed to make the diagnosis. In those days the interns, not technician, took the EKGs. I told my intern to take the usual 12-lead EKG but to give me a second one with only leads two, three and aVF (usually designated II, III, and aVF, showing the heart attack area. Dr. Zoll asked to see the EKG). I presented the abbreviated EKG to Dr. Zoll. He said, "Where is the rest of the ECG?" I answered, "Dr. Zoll, since the patient had an inferior wall infarction, we knew that three leads would give us our diagnosis. You did not want us to waste EKG paper, did you?" If Dr. Zoll thought it was funny, he did not show it on his face or share this with us at the time and gave a very disapproving look to me. Maybe he actually did laugh after being out of sight of us, as no one from administration ever called me to ream me over the coals for the episode, nor was I fired from my residency program.

PACEMAKERS

The theoretical concept of a pacemaker is quite simple yet very complex in engineering design and execution. A box known as a generator or battery (now with software, which can be programmed externally) is placed under the skin near the collarbone by a small incision usually on the left side if the patient is righthanded (righthanded people use this hand most often, so they are less likely to accidently dislodge the lead placed on the opposite side), and a metal wire enclosed within a plasticized outer covering is connected to the generator at one end and is embedded into the tip of the right ventricle (the apex) at the other. After the surgeon pushes it through the subclavian vein (under the collar bone and then into the superior vena cava into the right atrium to the tip of the right ventricle, it can stimulate electrically the right ventricle to make it pump or merely record the electricity of the heart. Normally, if the heart rate, which is recorded from the heart muscle electricity through the wire and into the battery box, is above a certain heart rate, the pacer remains in a quiescent phase, but when the heart rate falls below a preset heart rate, the pacer battery through the electrode wire makes the heart pump at a set higher predetermined rate, which may be anywhere from 40-130, depending upon the needs of the patient's heart. The pacemaker box is about the size of a small cigarette lighter. Although the early pacer patients were implanted for only complete heart block (i.e. the electrical impulse from the upper part of the heart is blocked from reaching the bottom of the heart to tell the heart to pump), as pacemakers became more sophisticated with software and a second lead was placed in the right atrium, many patients with "Sick Sinus Syndrome" underwent pacer implantation as well. Sick Sinus Syndrome is a condition when the starting mechanism at the top of the right atrium does not function properly (like a broken light switch) so heart rates intermittently become exceedingly slow or even stops for a period of time, sometimes causing fainting. The risk of complete heart block was not just temporary fainting but sudden death as well. Although Sick Sinus Syndrome rarely develops permanent cardiac electrical standstill, unlike complete heart block, a long pause with no heartbeat, even one long enough to produce fainting while driving or standing at the top of stairs can be just as lethal, so the condition also requires remediation with a backup pacemaker if the patient's heart rate falls below a preset lower limit. Some pacemakers can also shock or defibrillate a heart that is in ventricular fibrillation (very rapid and poorly organized rhythm from the ventricle leading to death if not aborted) if needed as ventricular fibrillation is otherwise fatal. These are called automatic implantable cardiac defibrillators ((AICD (automatic implantable cardiac defibrillator) or AID (automatic implantable defibrillator) or ICD (implantable cardiac defibrillator)) and is another function added to the other pacemakers sometimes, although uni-purpose AIDs occasionally are implanted. So let's now see how pacemakers evolved historically. It was a long circuitous route, first with defibrillators being invented and then pacemakers. They are interrelated as both require software and a battery source and now usually are coupled both in one unit with a pacemaker using the wire placed in the right ventricle to deliver the shock or to tell the heart to speed up.

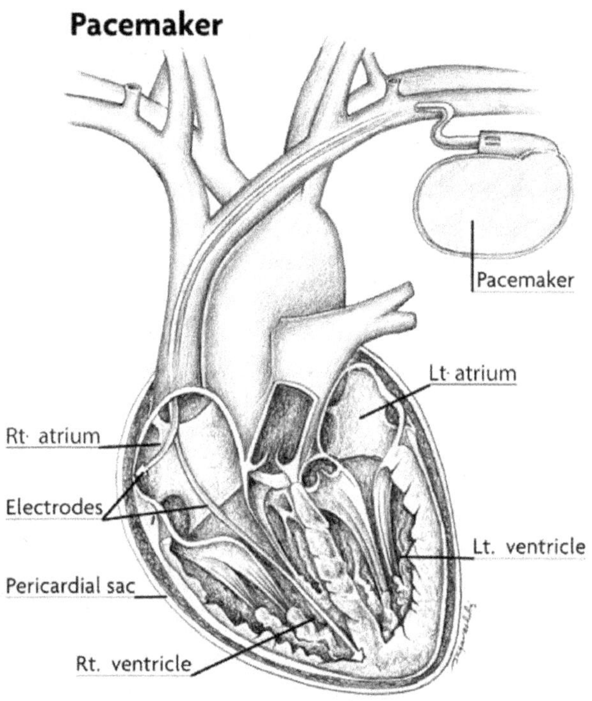

The heart with a right ventricle pacing wire at the tip or apex and a second wire in the right atrium at the outer wall, both connected to the pacemaker battery, which is placed surgically under the skin by the left collarbone, by D. Gavasheli, author's personal collection

The need for pacemakers goes back to those who recognized heart block, where electrical signals from the upper part of the heart get blocked, often from scar tissue formation (other causes also) and prevent these signals from reaching the bottom of the heart either intermittently and for a short period of seconds or much longer, and sometimes so long that the "escape" rhythm of the heart is ventricular fibrillation, which is lethal. Thus, patients may have temporary dizziness, fainting, or even die suddenly unless a pacemaker is placed. It took the EKG machine's invention to lead physicians to be able to diagnose confidently complete heart block (known as third-degree block, although even every other beat blocked of second-degree heart block can degenerate to third-degree heart block). When the diagnosis of complete heart block was finally confirmed as the EKG became available in the early 20th century, the cure for this was a pacemaker.

Before the EKG (now spelled ECG in Canada and the U.S.) machine and long before pacemakers, two men had a fairly good idea that what doctors then called apoplexy, i.e. sudden fainting, was not usually due to the brain but as a result of heart block. The two were William Stokes and Robert Adams.

ROBERT ADAMS (1791-1875, born Dublin, Ireland, then UK, and died in Dublin, Ireland, UK) in 1827 wrote a paper about a patient who had apoplexy (i.e. sudden loss of consciousness or fainting) and a very slow heart rate of thirty beats a minute. Rather than attributing these findings as originating in the brain as most physicians of the time did, he was the first to be convinced that it was a primary cardiac problem ninety years before the EKG was invented. This condition is commonly seen today and is known as complete heart block, usually treated, not cured, by the placement of a pacemaker. He rightfully pointed out that apoplexy was not a specific disease but a symptom. Although others described the same complex of symptoms earlier (Marko Gerbec (Marcus Gerbezius) (1658-1718, born Carniola, Slovenia, Austria, and died Ljubljana, Slovenia, Austria) in 1717 and Morgagni in 1761), earlier descriptions did not consider this a primary cardiac issue but a neurologic problem. Walter Gaskell (1847-14, born in Italy and died Great Shelford, UK) named this "heart block" in 1881 (more to come about Gaskell in the later chapter on EP. He came closest to the true cause but did not have an EKG, which would not be invented for another 24 years. Henri Huchard (1844-1910, born Auxon, France, and died in France) in 1889 named the drop attacks of apoplexy and slow heart rate "Adams-Stokes Attacks" after Robert Adams and William Stokes, who first described this symptom complex. Adams wrote in his "Cases of Diseases of the Heart, Accompanied with Pathological Observations" concerning a patient falling down, sometimes hurting himself, twenty times over a seven-year period. "Heavy breathing loudly stertorous and pulse very slow." He recovered from the attacks with no paralysis but later died within two hours of such an attack. The postmortem showed an enlarged right atrium and thinned wall left ventricle. Had he had access to an EKG (invented by Einthoven in 1901), Adams would have been considered the father of modern cardiac electrophysiology instead of Sir Thomas Lewis.

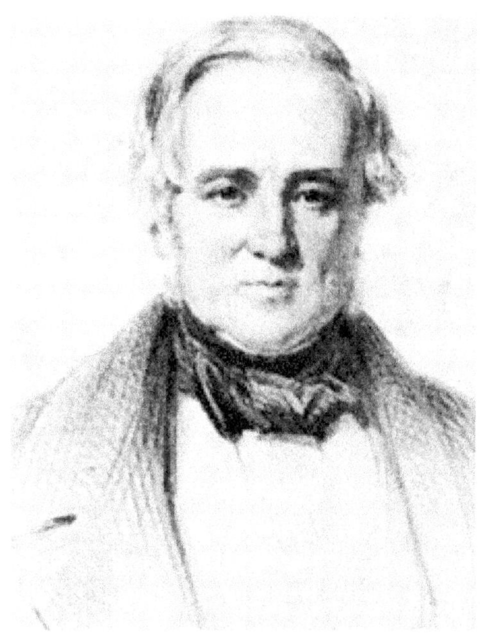

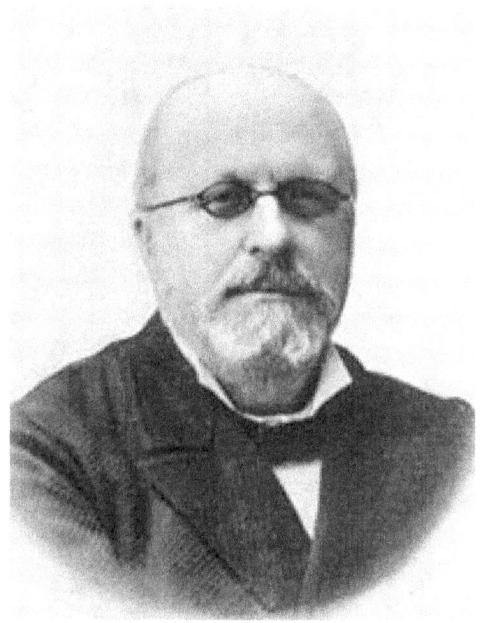

ROBERT ADAMS,
public domain

HENRI HUCHARD,
public domain

The other forerunner in the diagnosis of complete heart block was William Stokes, who we previously learned used mercury to treat congestive heart failure.

WILLIAM STOKES (1804-1878, born Dublin, Ireland, and died Howth near Dublin, Ireland) in 1846 described a patient with a very slow pulse with semi-beating of the heart in between the palpable beats. He was most likely seeing in the neck veins the cannon waves of the right atrium contracting against a closed tricuspid valve, which occurs in complete heart block when electrical signals from the upper heart do not get through to the bottom of the heart. Thus, he was associated as the second name on the Adams-Stokes Attacks of losing consciousness with a very slow pulse, usually due to complete heart block.

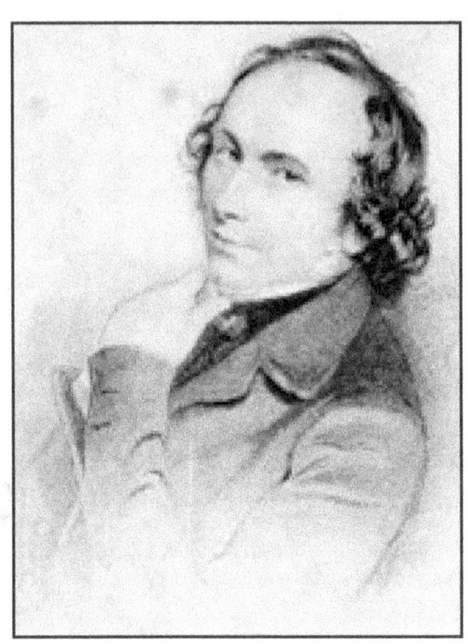

WILLIAM STOKES, public domain

Although Zoll developed the first external pacemaker in 1952, the first internal permanent pacemaker procedure in 1958 was performed by Dr. AKE SENNING (1915-2000, born Rattvik, Sweden, and died Zurich, Switzerland). The device placed the leads on the outside surface of the heart (epicardium) with the battery external to the body. Despite the fact that this first device lasted only a few hours and its successor in the same patient for six weeks, it was a historical first and heralded what was to come. Kirk Jeffrey and VICTOR PARSONNET (1924-, born Newark, NJ), in their classic review article of pacemakers from 1960-1985 (Circulation 1998:1978-1991), went on to write that this first patient was still living as of the publication of their article in 1998 after 26 battery changes at age 83. Coincidently, Dr. Senning also performed the first cardiac transplant procedure in Switzerland in 1969 and promoted coronary artery bypass in Europe. He also stood by in case emergency bypass was needed when his colleague Dr. Andreas Greuntzig performed his first angioplasty procedure in 1977. He was also the first to use elective defibrillation in heart surgery.

In 1960 WILLIAM CHARDACK (1917-2006) of the VA Hospital in Buffalo, NY, and head of thoracic surgery collaborated with WILSON GREATBATCH (1919-2011, born West Seneca, NY, U.S.A., and died Williamsville, NY, U.S.A.), an engineer, and surgeon William Gage implanted the first fully internal pacemaker in 1960, although with epicardial leads (on the heart surface requiring opening the chest leads rather than current transvenous leads) in the U.S. in a patient with multiple faints from Adams-Stokes disease (the electrical signal from the upper part of the heart is blocked midway before reaching the ventricle so that no contraction occurs (known as complete heart block)). These attacks, according to Jeffrey and Parsonnet, required the patient to wear a football helmet to protect his head. They ceased after his pacemaker was implanted, and he lived another two and a half years of normal life. Chardack developed this pacemaker with William Greatbatch first while working on dogs. A few weeks later in 1960 at the Beth Israel Hospital in Boston, the surgeon (Dr. Howard Frank, 1914-2004, born Manhattan, NYC, NY, and died Brookline, Mass., U.S.) working with Dr. Paul Zoll implanted a similar epicardial permanent fully internal pacemaker. As Dr. Victor Parsonnet has written, "Clearly, the idea for the implantable pacemaker was not the exclusive property of any one group but was in the air."

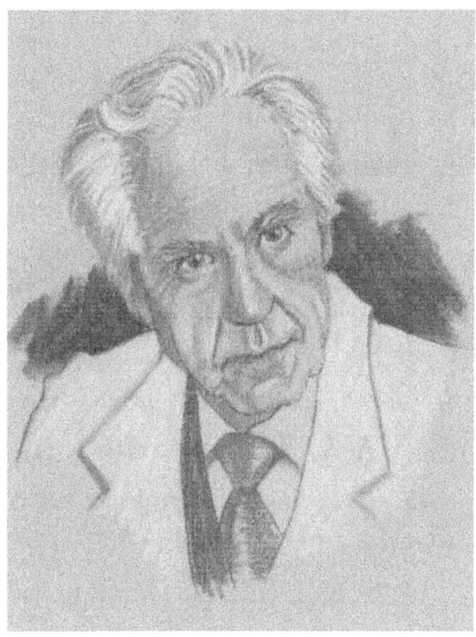

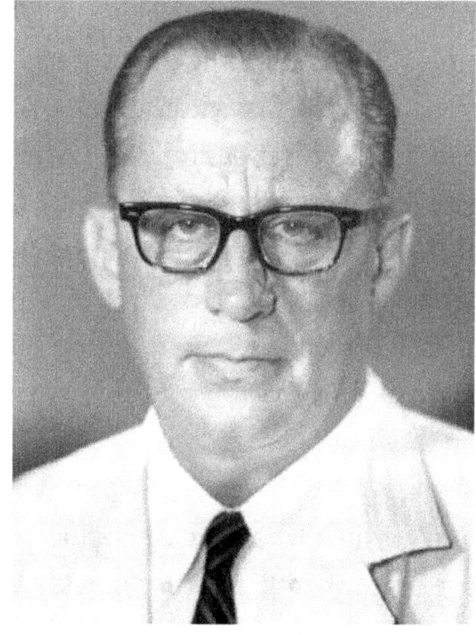

AKE SENNING   WILLIAM CHARDACK

drawing and photo by permission Heart Rhythm Society

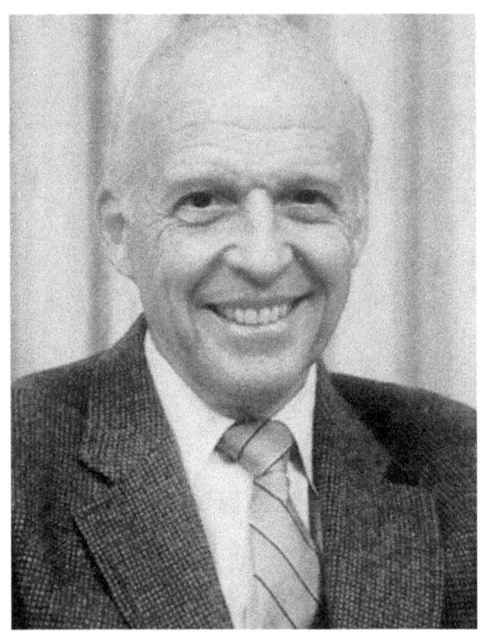

VICTOR PARSONNET
permission of Heart Rhythm Society

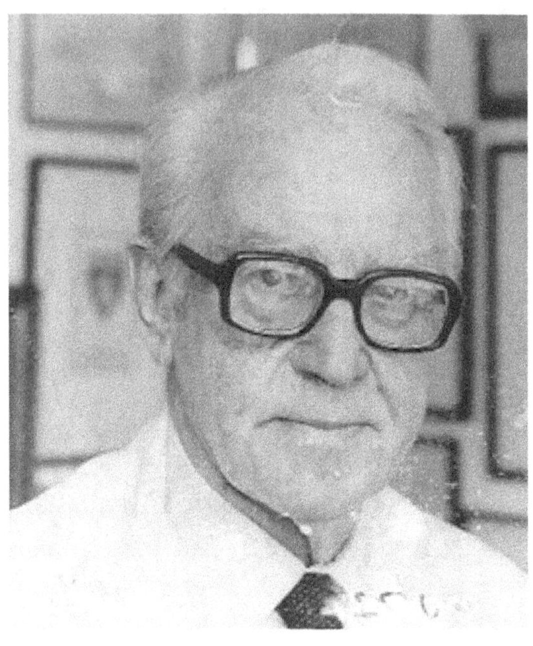

DWIGHT HARKEN
From private collection of his son Dr.
Alden Harken

Early pacemaker batteries were quite large and ran out of charge much earlier than the promised five years, usually less than two years. Broken wires (lead fractures) were frequent. Mercury zinc batteries were not well hermetically sealed and hydrogen gas leaked out and body fluids leaked in. Nuclear-powered batteries were a good answer to the problem of battery life and first suggested and then tested and implanted by Dr. Victor Paronnet, age 98 at the time of this writing. The battery could last forever, which was their advantage but also their disadvantage. They became impractical as new and continuously changing and upgraded software and wiring were being designed but could not easily be added for nuclear pacemakers. Such modifications for the nuclear battery pack was more difficult, and they quickly became obsolete. The nuclear battery was eventually replaced by lithium batteries. Newer methods were no longer made by researchers but by the pacemaker companies and their engineers. Moreover, physicians were the first to find other issues and problems with new pacemakers and worked with the company engineers to solve them. Originally the pacemaker paced a fixed rate set by the surgeon. Competition with intrinsic beats that might still be present could cause physiologic adverse consequences. Engineers with proper circuitry design determined how to overcome this competition so that pacers would not fire when the patient had his or her own beats. These were called "demand pacemakers," and Dwight Harken of the Peter Bent Brigham Hospital implanted the first one in 1966 in conjunction with the American Optical engineer Barough Berkovits.

Temporary epicardial (heart muscle surface) pacer wires placed by thoracotomies (opening the chest) were replaced in 1966 by endocardial leads placed via small cutdowns on the antecubital vein by the elbow and later from the groin femoral vein or jugular or subclavian (under the collarbone) percutaneously, which were connected externally to a pacer battery box and used for temporary pacing until a permanent pacemaker could be implanted. This venous wire was carefully pushed through the vein to the right ventricle apex inside the heart with the aid of a fluoroscope. All venous pacing wire techniques (either permanent or temporary) were able to be performed with low-voltage pacing. The temporary pacemaker was much quicker than preparing for thoracic surgery of even for permanent endocardial pacemakers with wires placed in the vein under the collarbone and threaded to the right ventricle. Seymour Furman (1932-2006, born Bronx, NY, and died Bronx, NY, U.S.A.) used a transvenous approach in 1958 for a temporary pacemaker with a fluoroscope for guidance (i.e. real-time x-ray visualization) and an external pacemaker battery box prior to his patient having lung cancer surgery at Montefiore Medical Center, Bronx, NY. A second patient had the pacing wire remain in him for 96 days with no complications. Furman a Disruptor was the first to use a temporary transvenous endocardial (inside surface of the heart muscle, whereas previous pacer wires placed on the heart were epicardial, or on the outside surface of the heart and required opening the chest) pacemaker.

By 1964 Vogel demonstrated the use of flexible wires with no fluoroscope needed for guiding the wire into the right ventricle for temporary pacing. Thomas Killip did the same in 1965 at the bedside with no fluoroscope.

By the mid-1970s permanent pacemakers were externally programmable with multiple possible settings required by the individual patient, and the only epicardial leads were used when open heart surgery was being performed for other reasons. By 1980 permanent dual chamber pacing (atrium and ventricle on right side) was added.

Finally, a built-in defibrillator function (ICD or AID or AICD) was first invented and implanted through the efforts of Michel Mirowski (1924-1990, born Warsaw, Poland, and died Baltimore, Maryland) a Disruptor at

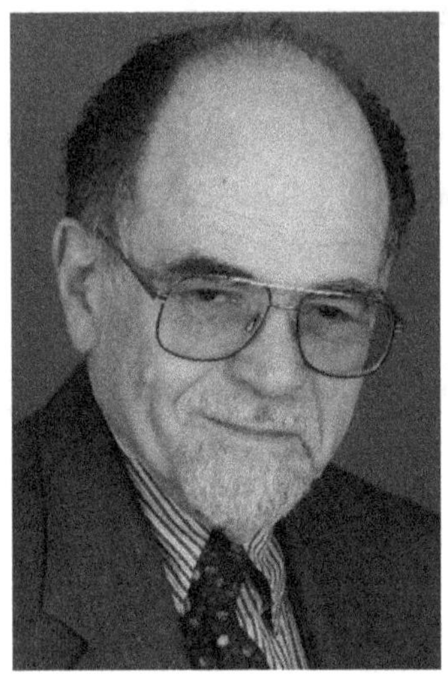 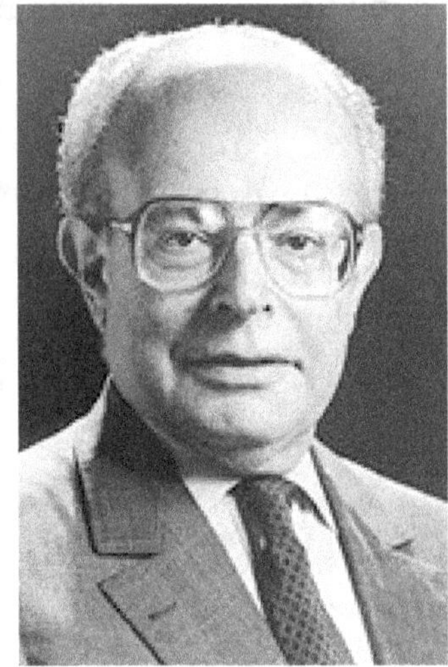 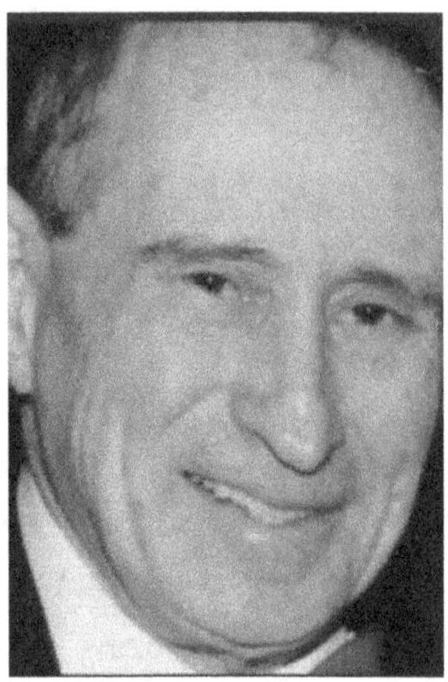

SEYMOUR FURMAN   MICHEL MIROWSKI   MARTIN MOWER

all three permission from Heart Rhythm Society

Sinai Hospital in Baltimore in 1980 (size of a deck of cards and weighed nine ounces) that he had been working on since 1968 using a single right ventricular wire. Subsequently, this function was added to many dual chamber pacemakers units when clinically indicated. Mirowski worked with Dr. Martin Mower (1933-2022, born Baltimore, Maryland, and died Denver, Colorado, U.S.A.) at first and then showed his concept to Stephen Heilman, with whom he cooperated in the research. Heilman later founded the Medrad medical device company. A prototype ICD was place in a dog in 1975 with the first human implant in 1980 by thoracotomy and in 1988 transvenously. I was interviewed in 1974 by Mirowski for my first job after training for the Mt. Sinai Hospital in Baltimore, Maryland, which I decided was not for me, although I may not have been hired if I decided otherwise. I was impressed by Dr. Mirowski's dedication and determination, which eventually bore fruit. I was not certain of this outcome in 1974 when I interviewed. Today's ICDs are smaller in volume and weight and may last nine years using lithium-silver-vanadium batteries compared to the two-year life expectancy of earlier models.

I personally knew Victor Parsonnet, who became a leader in pacemakers. He was tall, elegant, brilliant, innovative, and a gentleman to the nth degree. I remember when I was a young practitioner having a minor disagreement with him about a patient's ejection fraction calculation, which I am certain now that I was wrong and he was correct.

I also knew Paul Zoll, as he was one of my instructors as a medical student and internal medicine resident in Boston. He was the researcher and clinician and inspiration for his group but was not a surgeon so he did not physically implant the pacemaker, but I am certain he was in the OR and scrubbed during the procedure, which Dr. Howard Frank performed. I still remember as an intern at the Beth Israel Hospital in Boston in 1967 transporting a patient from the CCU with complete heart block and multiple fainting episodes emergently to the operating room for a permanent pacemaker, as there were no good temporary pacemakers at the time. Along the way, despite an intravenous drip of isoproterenol to speed up his intrinsic heartbeat (only partially and intermittently successful), I had to perform cardiac massage. It was a harrowing few minutes, but the patient survived the procedure and was discharged home.

I was told of a patient who died at the Massachusetts General Hospital in Boston with a nuclear pacemaker long after my training days. Whether the story is true or made up, I cannot verify. In those days the U.S. government kept strict records on these batteries and insisted on removal of them upon death. A family had a loved one hospitalized who had a nuclear pacemaker. Unfortunately with his age, severe diabetes, and congestive heart failure, he died in the hospital. When the cardiologist after pronouncing him dead went to console a very emotional family and explain that the pacemaker by law must be returned, the family said that they needed to see their beloved and discuss it among themselves before they would agree, although the doctors knew he was dead and had pronounced him so. They came out of the room and a family representative said that "my father (the deceased) told them that he refused to have his body cut to remove the device." After the cardiologist explained that this would be a Federal offense with some of the family going to jail as well as a hefty monetary fine, the family went back to their dead father a second time. When they returned, they said their father changed his mind and now agreed to have the pacemaker box removed. I guess occasionally cardiologists can be smarter than a dead patient.

Arrhythmia – any heart beat not from the normal source in the upper-right atrium, the SA node. It may be one beat or continuous.

EKG – electrocardiogram, now called ECG in the U.S.and Canada, as the original was European Dutch and German with a K

CHAPTER 9
THE BIRTH OF HEART SURGERY

My father and mother from Omaha were visiting my wife and me in New Jersey when he was 72 years old. He casually asked me to make an appointment for him with the senior cardiologist of my group. I asked him if he was feeling well and briefly questioned him about chest discomfort with effort such as during his morning walk. He reassuringly answered, "None, I am fine." The appointment was three days later, and my partner afterwards came into my office and said, "Do you know that your father has angina pectoris?" I said, "He does?" We quickly scheduled him for a nuclear stress test, and it was abnormal (positive). The next step was for another of my partners to perform a coronary angiogram (x-ray with contrast invasively) to look at his coronary arteries for cholesterol buildup, and it showed two vessel diseases (there are three coronary arteries). Four days later he was on the operating table for double bypass performed by my friend Dr. Grant Parr. As he was being wheeled into surgery and holding my mother's hand, my mother said to him, "Don't you dare die or I'll kill you." He died six weeks short of age ninety, eighteen years after his surgery, not from his heart.

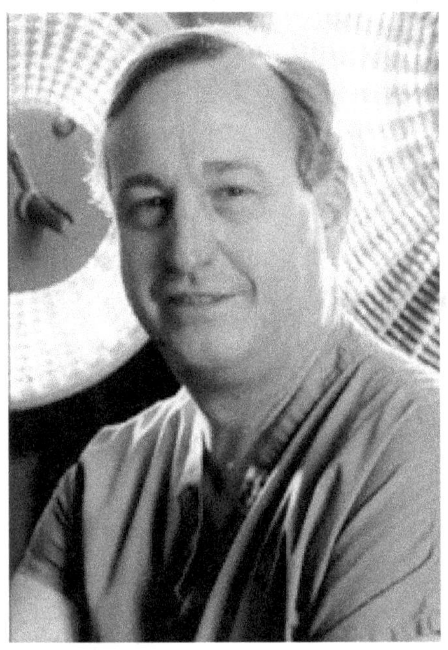

permission: Dr. Parr's personal
collection

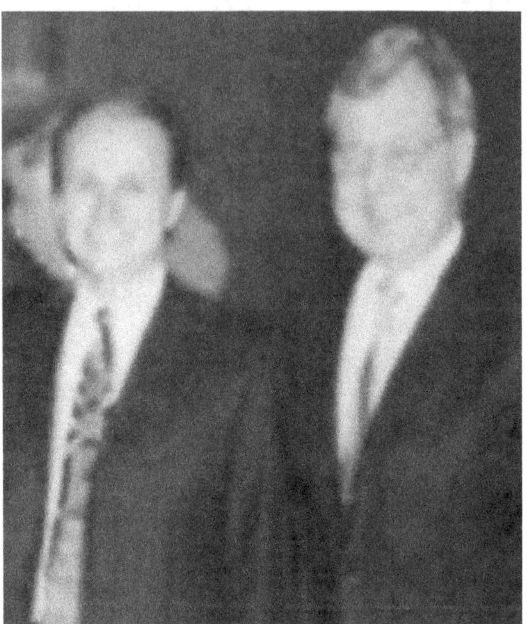

Dr Karel Raska and Dr Lawrence
Lubow managing partners of MCA
Dr Lubow was cardiologist to aurthor's
father

EARLY SURGERY

Physicians for generations thought that no one could survive if the heart was
even manipulated. let alone operated upon. The famous German surgeon Bill-
roth said that any surgeon operating on the heart would lose the esteem of his
colleagues.

Industrialization in Norway precipitated a mass migration to North America
occurring in the 1860s. In 1884 the Norwegian king appointed a new prime
minister, Johan Sverdrup, which began the era of parliamentary government in
Norway. For a long period of time Norway and Sweden had been one country,
but in 1905 this union was dissolved, which had been created in 1814.

A Norwegian surgeon, AXEL CAPPELEN (1858-1919, born Selje, Norway), performed the first heart surgery known in the world in this era and certainly in the western world in 1895 on a bleeding coronary artery caused by a
stabbing. Although the patient seemed fine for 24 hours after surgery, he succumbed to infection a day later but may have survived if antibiotics had been
available during that era.

However, in 1891 DANIEL HALE WILLIAMS (1856-1926, born Hollidaysburg, Pennsylvania, and died in Idlewild, Michigan, U.S.A.), an African-American surgeon from Chicago's Provident Hospital, came pretty close to being the first surgeon to operate on the heart muscle. His patient, James Cornish, suffered a severe stab wound, but it evidently did not penetrate the heart, only the outside layer, the pericardium, which is a membrane of two layers but can lead to death if bleeding occurs into it after a gunshot or knife wound. It was a success, and his patient survived many years. However, without the benefit of blood or antibiotics it was a miracle, and it is not clear how deeply the wound penetrated. Williams helped open Provident Hospital, the first interracial hospital on Chicago's South Side, which also established a nursing and a medical intern program because African-American doctors were being refused admitting privileges to other hospitals. He had served as an apprentice to a surgeon but then completed further training at Chicago Medical College and became a charter member of the American College of Surgeons in 1913. Technically Dr. Hale's operation was not fully cardiac since the wound did not reach the heart muscle, but it was very, very close.

In 1896, one year after Cappelen's operation, a German surgeon named LUDWIG REHN (1849-1930, born Bad Sooden-Allendorf, Germany, and died Frankfurt, Germany) sutured a cardiac laceration in a 22-year-old gardener's right ventricle, which he suffered from a knife wound. Lo and behold, the patient survived! These were the first known successful heart surgeries in the world and opened the possibility of heart surgery previously thought impossible. These surgeons may also have been the first people to see and describe a living, beating human heart. By 1907 Rehn had gathered 124 cases of heart suturing with a 60% mortality (terrible results by today's standards but excellent for his time). Cappelin, Williams, Rehn were all Disruptors.

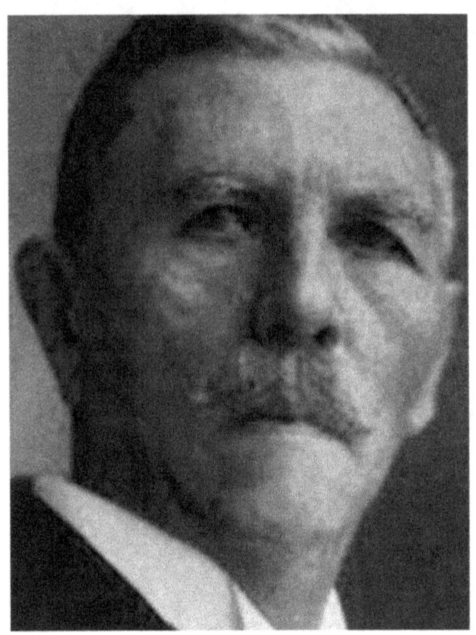
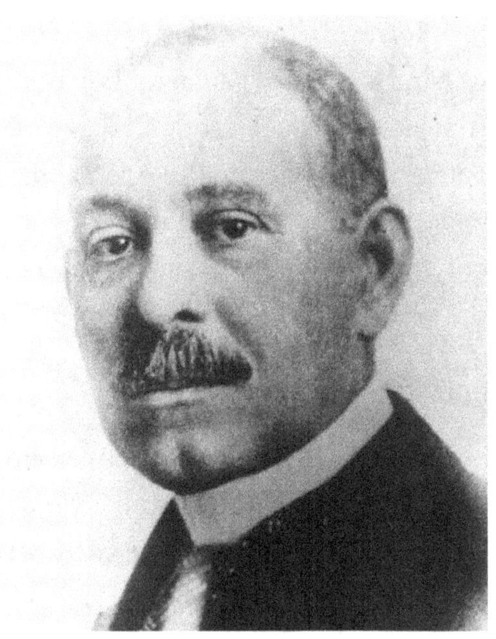

LUDWIG REHN
public domain

DANIEL HALE WILLIAMS
public domain

Although there are four valves within the heart, two on the right and two on the left, the aortic valve, which allows blood out of the heart from the left ventricle to supply the body, arguably is the most important. The first valvular heart surgery was performed by THEODORE TUFFIER (1857-1929, born Belleme, Orne, France, and died Paris, France) in 1914 with his fingers (no metal instruments) to digitally improve the opening of the aortic valve, which would not open properly (known as aortic stenosis). Of note is that he worked with the "to be" Nobel winner, Alexis Carrel, who pioneered vascular surgery techniques.

In 1923 Dr. ELLIOT CUTLER (1888-1947, born Bangor, Maine, U.S.A., and died Brookline, Massachusetts, U.S.) of the Peter Bent Brigham Hospital in Boston and Harvard Medical School performed the world's first intra-heart surgery in 1923 (inside the heart—Rehn, Hale, Cappelen, and Tuffier operated on or from the outside and Tuffier on the aortic valve from outside the heart) on a twelve-year-old patient with rheumatic heart disease and mitral stenosis, a condition where tissue leaflets (the mitral valve has two, one in front and one behind), which open and close to allow blood to enter the left ventricle from the left atrium above, are thickened and fused and cannot open properly to allow blood to pass through it easily, usually due to rheumatic heart disease and remote streptococcus throat infection. Although at the time Dr. Cutler received worldwide acclaim, including by the *British Medical Journal* as "a milestone," the procedure was abandoned by Cutler in 1928 due to a 90% mortality. It took twenty more years before American heart surgeons again operated on a valve.

The next year, in 1929, the U.S. Stock Market crash occurred.

Dr. Henry Souttar (1875-1964, born Birkenhead, UK, and died London, UK) performed a similar operation two years after Cutler in 1925 on the mitral valve as an intra-cardiac heart surgical manipulation on a fifteen-year-old female also with severe mitral stenosis. Like Tuffier and Cutler before him, he performed this without modern anesthesia techniques, before the heart lung machine was invented and before antibiotics. He performed his procedure blindly only using his tactile senses, as did Cutler and Tuffier. His patient survived, but the operation would not be repeated for another 22 years. Ironically, his colleagues would not allow him to perform the operation again (was this professional jealousy that impeded cardiac surgical progress?). The early surgical pioneers were all Disruptors, but Suttar's work was a victim of the Restrainers

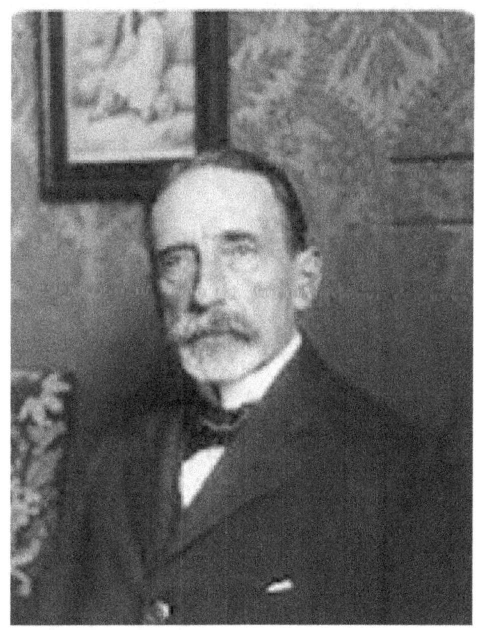

THEODORE TUFFIER,
Alamy License

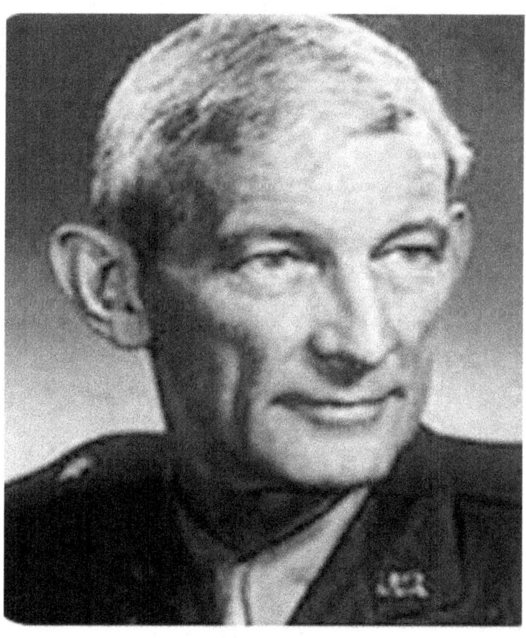

ELLIOT CUTLER,
public domain

In 1943 and 1944, DWIGHT HARKEN (1910-1993, born Osceola, Iowa, U.S., and died Cambridge, Massachusetts, U.S.) removed fragments from in and around the myocardium (heart muscle) in over one hundred soldiers' hearts, saving many American lives during WWII. This was the next big step in heart surgery and was published in 1946 in the journal *Surgery, Gynecology and Obstetrics*. It clearly was a milestone in surgical success as Harken was a Disruptor.

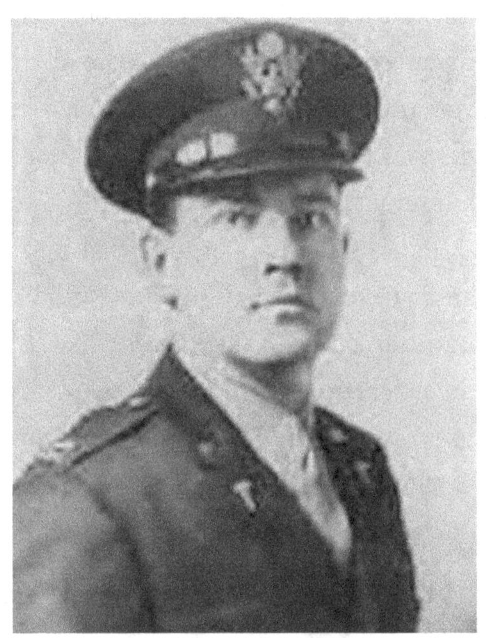

DWIGHT HARKEN
public domain

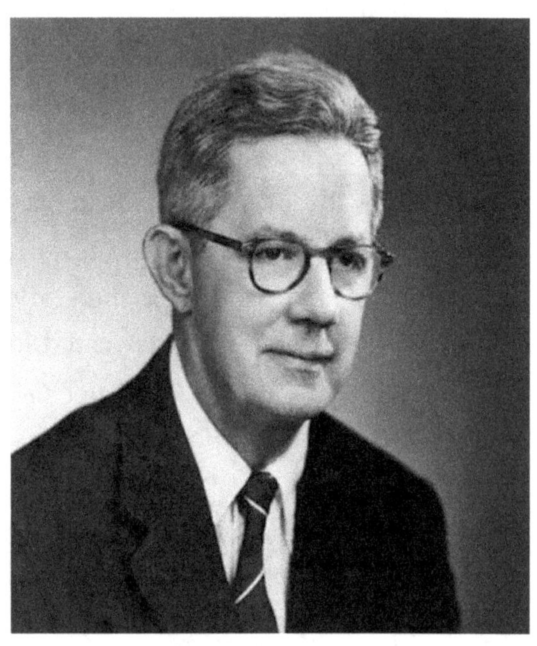

ALFRED BLALOCK
permission: Lasker Foundation

A major cardiac surgical breakthrough occurred in 1944 by ALFRED BLALOCK (1899-1954, born Culloden, Georgia, U.S., and died Baltimore, Maryland, U.S.) of Johns Hopkins (the Blalock-Taussig Shunt, it was called) on a blue baby (cyanotic, inadequate oxygen to the tissues) with a congenital heart defect called Tetralogy of Fallot. His operation increased the flow of blood through the pulmonary vascular circulation. Unfortunately, the early surgeons were hampered by a major factor: time. They had a limited amount of time in which the heart would tolerate manipulation without an artificial circulation, which at this time did not exist. This was soon to change and change the entire field of heart surgery forever when the heart lung machine was developed and finally perfected.

Development of the heart lung machine for open heart surgery (also known as pump oxygenator or bypass pump)

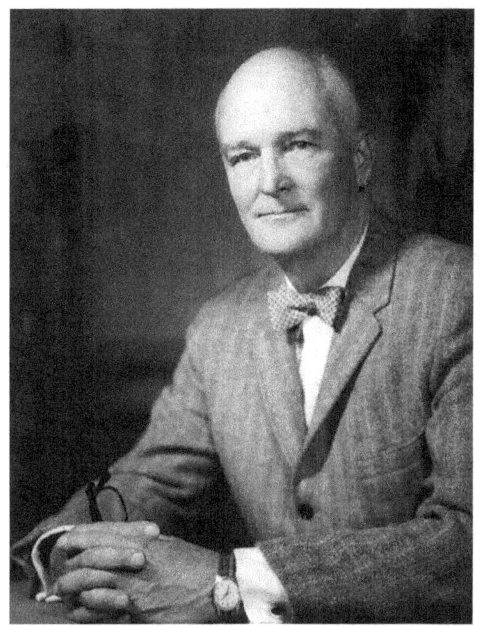

JOHN H. GIBBON
permission: Lasker Foundation

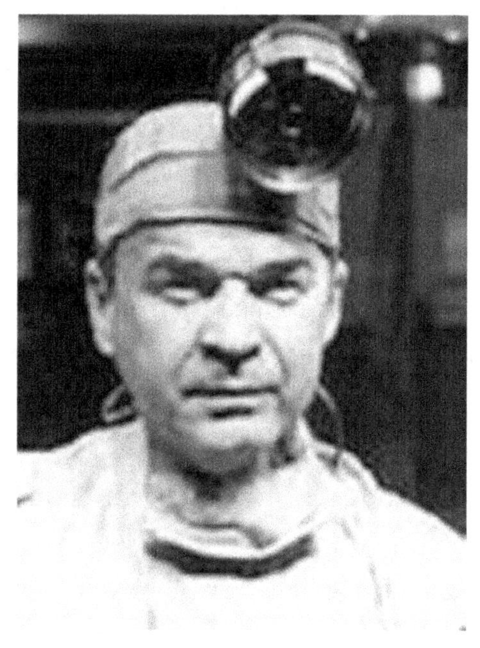

C. WALTON LILLEHEI
Permission of the U of Minnesota Archives

CLARENCE WALTON LILLEHEI of the University of Minnesota (1918-1999, born Minneapolis, Minnesota, U.S., and died St. Paul, Minnesota, U.S.) pioneered early open heart surgery and was called "The Father of Open Heart Surgery" by the famous Texan surgeon Denton Cooley. He was a major Disruptor in the field. In his first operations Lillehei used a cross circulation with the mother's (or father's) blood as the oxygenator for the patient child. This connection of circulations allowed an hour's time to perform his procedures, longer than for previous procedures, usually to correct a hole between the right and left ventricles occurring at birth known as a ventricular septal defect. He joked that his "technique was the only one he knew with a potential 200% mortality," as both parent and child could potentially die. Fortunately, only one complication, a stroke, was suffered by a parent during his operations.

Although Lillehei's technique was a huge step forward, the most important development was to come and invented by Dr. JOHN H. GIBBON (1903-1973, born Philadelphia, Pennsylvania, U.S., and died Media, Pennsylvania, U.S.), who developed the first heart lung machine (also called pump oxygenator or membrane oxygenator). He had worked for years (1937-1953) on his invention, which revolutionized heart surgery, making him one of the most important Disruptors in the history and cardiac surgery. His invention made today's complicated and lengthy open heart surgeries possible. Although Dr. John Lewis of the University of Minnesota had previously experimented with deep hypothermia (cooling the body) during surgery to arrest the heart, this technique was also limited in time to about an hour, whereas most modern cardiac surgical cases require several or even more hours of operative time to accomplish their goal. Dr. Gibbon's machine was able to take over the function of the heart and lungs by circulating or pumping the blood around and oxygenating it. His work started at the Massachusetts Hospital in Boston and continued at Jefferson Medical College in Philadelphia. His first machine was made in collaboration with the IBM Corporation but was not able to pump large enough volumes of blood for humans. The first operation using his new model (called Model II) was in February 1952 on a fifteen-month-old baby who was thought to have a hole in its atrium, although the diagnosis was inaccurate due to cardiac catheterization techniques still in their infancy and often not able to provide a precise diagnosis. Unfortunately, the baby died. But on May 6, 1953, the first successful open heart surgery was performed using Gibbon's machine on an eighteen-year-old patient who did have a hole in her atrium (atrial septal defect). She made an uneventful recovery, and the hole at repeat catheterization at six months post-op showed the atrial septal defect to be closed. The case was hailed by the press for its success. However, the next two patients died at surgery, and Dr. Gibbon was so concerned about his failures that he declared a moratorium on the procedure using his bypass machine. However, without his creative pioneering thought, hard work, and courage, open heart surgery of today would not be possible.

In 1953 Ake Senning of pacemaker history fame, after using his own pump oxygenator on dogs in 1951, successfully used it on a young woman in 1953 to remove her left atrial myxoma (a benign but symptomatic tumor of the heart, which can cause severe symptoms), and according to Dr. Denton Cooley in a paper in memoriam to Senning written in 2000, that the patient "is still alive today."

It would take others to subsequently come along to successfully complete Gibbon's early and pioneering work. (Dr. John Kirklin (1917-2004, born Muncie, Indiana, U.S., and died Birmingham, Alabama, U.S.) finally refined and perfected Gibbon's machine at the Mayo Clinic in 1955, and it has become the standard for open heart surgery with some modifications.

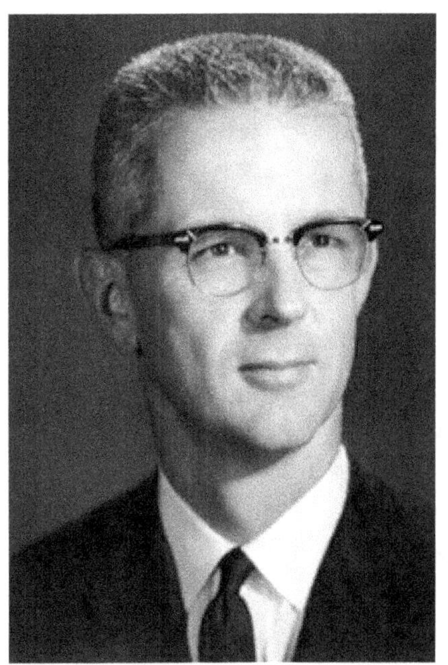

JOHN KIRLIN
permission: Mayo Clinic

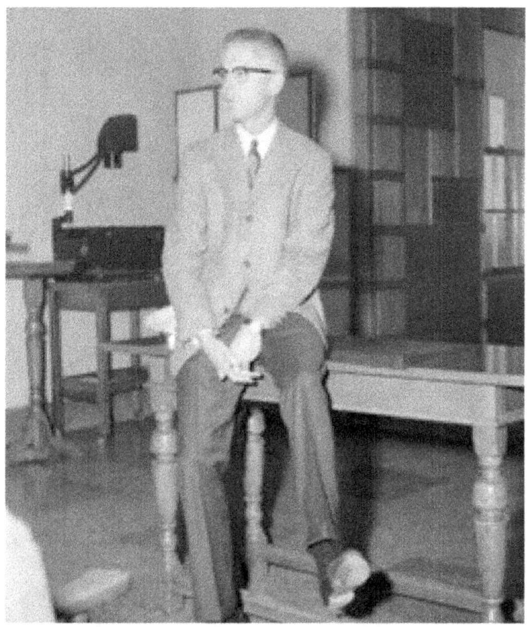

JOHN KIRKLIN
permission: Mayo Clinic

I recently attended a high school 60ᵗʰ reunion in Omaha, Nebraska, delayed two years due to the pandemic. A woman I had not seen since high school and I were talking when she asked what I had done for a living. When I responded that I was a cardiologist, she told me that her husband was in the first group of seven patients to undergo heart surgery at the Mayo Clinic using their new heart lung machine developed by Dr. John Kirklin. What a small world!

GLOSSARY CHAPTER 9

Aortic stenosis – fusion of the aortic valve leaflets to restrict blood out of the heart

Mitral stenosis – fusion of the double leaflet valve separating the upper-left atrium from the lower-left ventricle. When this occurs, usually from rheumatic fever, shortness of breath with effort occurs.

Pulmonary vascular circulation – **pulmonary arteries leaving the right ventricle** bring deoxygenated blood from the body organs to get oxygenated blood from the lungs, which is then brought to the left atrium by pulmonary veins

CHAPTER 10
DEVELOPMENT OF CORONARY ARTERY BYPASS SURGERY

One of the other most important developments in cardiology and cardiac surgery in the 20th century was the invention and success of coronary artery bypass graft surgery, known as CABG. Although I have been an interventional cardiologist who performed thousands of angioplasty and stent procedures in my career, I am able to easily concede that CABG was even more important than the field I spent my career in for angioplasty and stenting. Coronary angioplasty would have probably never been invented had CABG not been perfected. CABG was and continues to be the "bailout" procedure if we interventionalists get into severe trouble during our cases.

To demonstrate this concern, early angioplasty always required an open heart surgical team "on standby" with an open operating room "just in case." As we became more adept and equipment evolved and improved, no longer was a surgical team kept on standby in most hospitals, and the backup became the "first available operating room" and surgeon. Most of the time this system has worked well, as angioplasty techniques have improved and have become more reliable with only on rare occasion requiring a surgeon's rescue, but it is always reassuring to know that our surgical colleagues are available to save the day if necessary.

Having given my surgical colleagues their due, let me describe the history leading up to today's very refined CABG. First, CABG as we know it would not be possible if Mason Sones had not stumbled into coronary angiography in 1958, which provided the surgeons (and now interventional cardiologists) with a roadmap for operating on the diseased coronary arteries and a precise localization of the areas of narrowing. Without coronary angiography, the surgeons would have to operate without knowing where the blockage was and we cardiologists would not know what area needed opening with a balloon and stent. I wrote the previous chapter (Chapter 5) about coronary angiography and coronary angioplasty and stenting before this chapter because both were the direct outgrowths of coronary angiography and require a coronary angiogram to be taken frequently during the procedure. But CABG actually preceded coronary angioplasty historically and was also the beneficiary of the Sones procedure of coronary angiography. Coronary artery bypass needed to precede coronary angioplasty and stenting because of the need for a backup, although rarely needed for angioplasty or stenting anymore, but in the early days of angioplasty required emergency bypass heart surgery in approximately 1% of cases. The coronary artery bypass (affectionately known as a CABG – "cabbage") procedure takes a piece of artery (usually from the chest wall or even the wrist) or vein from the lower leg and connects one end to the aorta not far above the aortic valve and the other end beyond where the coronary artery is narrowed, which is why the surgeon requires a precise location of the coronary artery narrowing (stenosis) for his procedure given to the surgeon by coronary angiography. As time went by the left internal and/or right, internal mammary arteries were left in place under the chest wall, where they originated with the most downstream segment attached beyond the narrowing in the coronary artery. However, even now occasionally the internal mammary artery is detached at its origin and connected as a free tube to the aorta just above the aortic valve, similar to when a vein is used. But this road took many years and many surgeons to make it one of most frequent surgical procedure today. Although there has been a downward trend in CABG procedures due to coronary artery angioplasty and, subsequently, stenting, between 240,000-350,000, coronary artery bypass procedures are still performed each year in just the U.S.

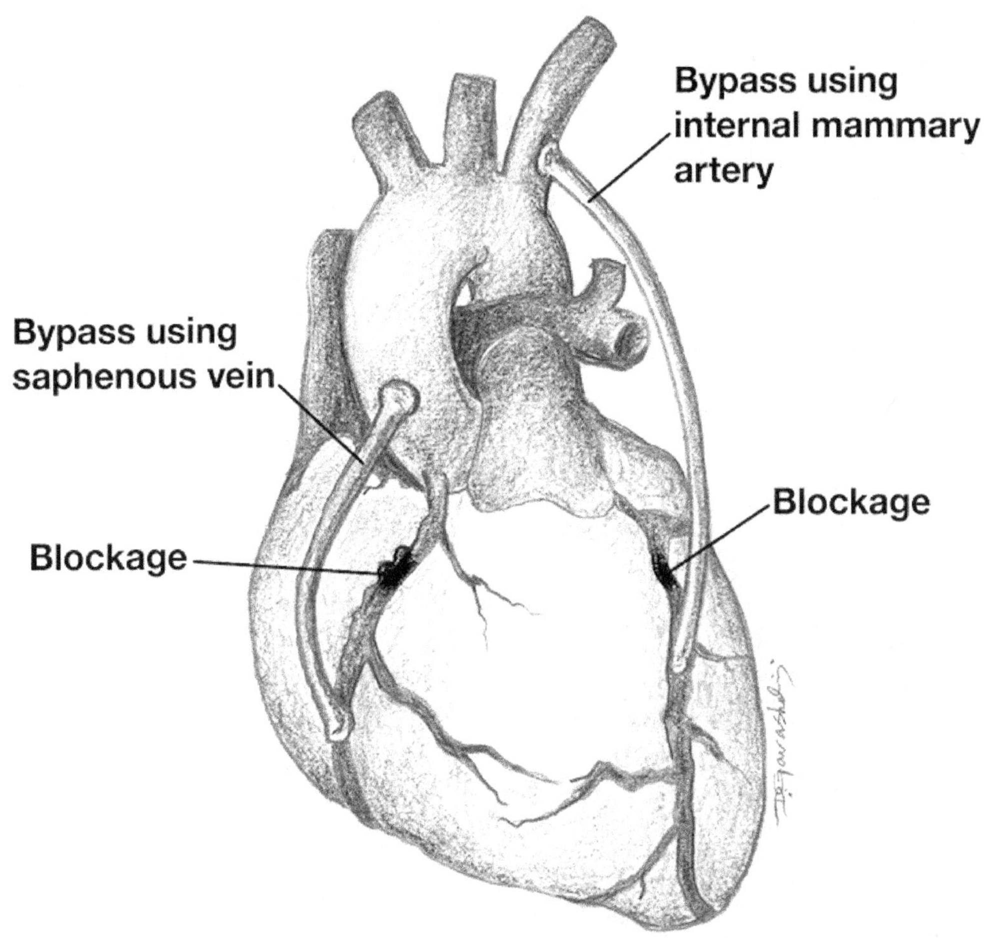

Double bypass with vein to right coronary artery and internal mammary graft to left anterior descending artery by D. Gavasheli, author's personal collection

In 1910 ALEXIS CARREL (1873-1944, born Sainte-Foy-les-Lyon, France, and died Paris, France) performed aortic to coronary artery anastomoses (connections) in dogs. He was the first to develop the technique of connecting blood vessels end to end (i.e. connecting the open end of one vessel to the open end of another) or end to side to another blood vessel (the open end of one vessel is connected to a second vessel by making a round or elliptical hole in the receiving blood vessel). In addition he demonstrated that blood vessels could be kept for long jhnnk,.periods of time in cold storage for later use. His research was paramount in leading others to be able to perform CABG and organ transplantations. For his contributions Carrell received the Nobel Prize in 1912 with his collaborator, Dr. Guthrie.

CLAUDE BECK (1894-1971, born Shamokin, Pennsylvania, U.S., and died Cleveland, Ohio, U.S.) in 1935 placed chest wall muscles inside the heart's covering, the pericardium, to enhance blood flow. In 1946 a Canadian surgeon, ARTHUR VINEBERG (1903-1988, born Montreal, Canada, and died Montreal, Canada), used the left internal mammary artery and placed it on the front wall of the heart for added circulation and collateral development without any downstream attachment but with the hope that small vessels would find their way to connect with the in-place coronary artery segments. Clinical results were inconsistent so the procedure's benefit remained debated throughout years, but the actual improvement in flow was actually proved after coronary arteriography (angiography) was developed.

However, an even better procedure soon supplanted and replaced the Vineberg Procedure, the coronary artery bypass graft procedure, or CABG.

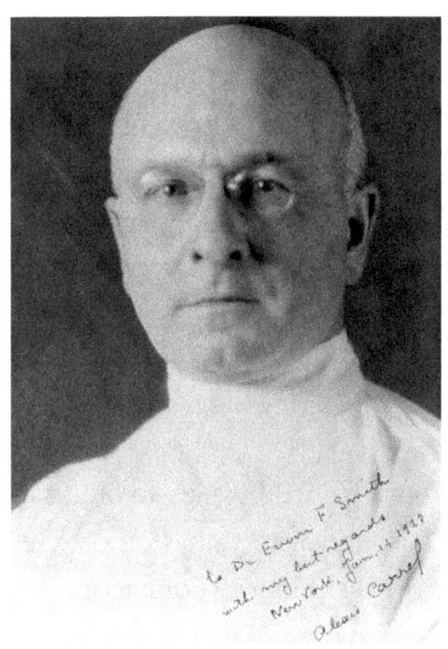

ALEXIS CARREL
Smithsonian Institution/
public domain

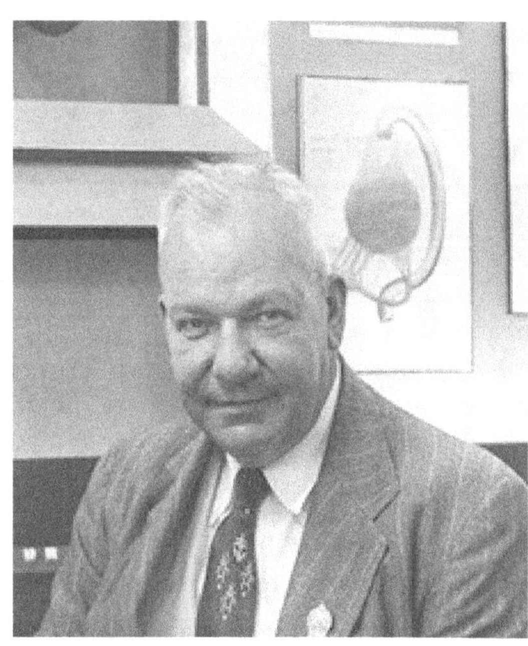

CLAUDE BECK
Courtesy of the Stanley A. Ferguson
Archives, U Hospitals of Cleveland

In 1956 CHARLES BAILEY (1910-1993, born Asbury Park, New Jersey, U.S., and died Marietta, Georgia, U.S.) was the first to perform a procedure to open the diseased part of a coronary artery and clean it out (the term is coronary endarterectomy). At the time coronary arteriography was not yet invented, so his procedure was limited to very few patients where the anatomy inside could be surmised before making an incision on the outside of the coronary artery, usually by feeling the area first but not knowing for sure if the artery segment was the culprit. Thus, he was the first to operate on a coronary artery to allow increased blood flow through it.

Five years later, in 1961, AKE SENNING (1915-2000, born Rattvik, Sweden, and died Zurich, Switzerland) used a piece of pericardium as a patch to enlarge a narrowed "widow maker" left anterior descending artery, and a few months later at the Cleveland Clinic DONALD EFFLER (1915-2004, born Roosevelt Island, New York, NYC, U.S., and died Jamesville, New York, U.S.) performed the same procedure. These were the early efforts to improve blood flow to the heart muscle and were the forerunner operations to today's Coronary Artery Bypass Surgery.

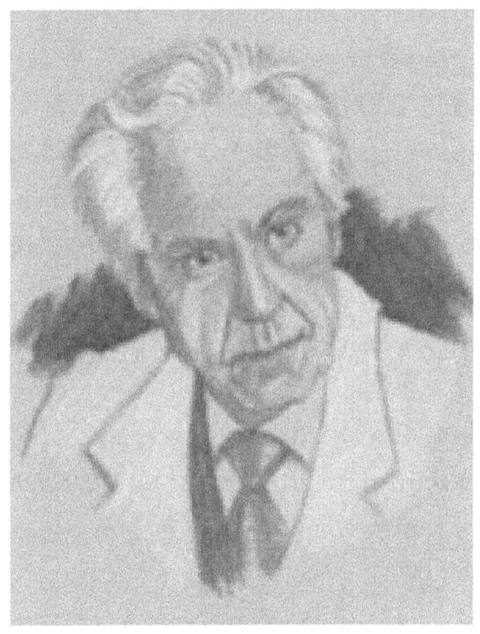

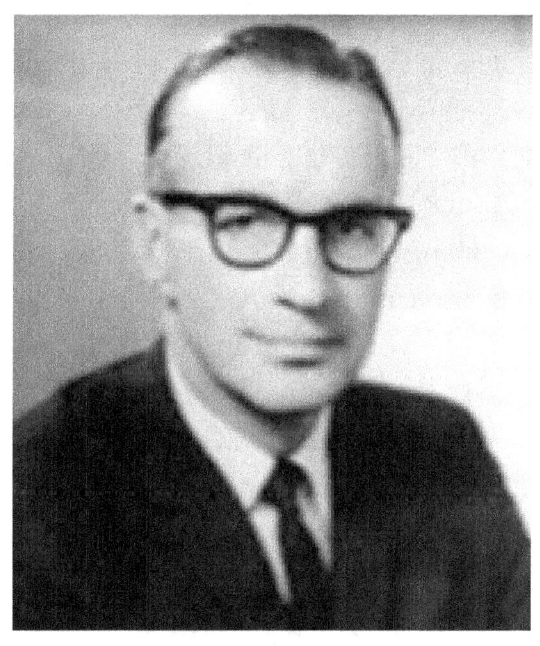

AKE SENNING
permission: Heart Rhythm Society
(drawing)

DONALD EFFLER
permission: Cleveland Clinic

But after coronary angiography spread throughout the world, many surgeons now had an anatomical map and could attempt more complicated coronary artery procedures and experiment on various types of bypass connections since the precision of where the problem was could be seen long before opening a chest.

Dr. ROBERT GOETZ (1910-2000, born Frankfurt, Germany, and died Scarsdale, New York, U.S.), on May 2, 1960, at the Albert Einstein Bronx Municipal Hospital Center in NY, performed the world's first coronary bypass procedure by connecting a right internal mammary artery (supplying the chest muscles in the front to the right of the breastbone) to the right coronary artery. Despite his success and being the first of hundreds of thousands of future successful bypass procedures, Goetz's colleagues demonstrated resentment, and no further cases were performed by him or his team, a supreme example of a Disruptor against the Restrainers holding back progress. This would not be the first time that professional resentment or jealousy stopped medical progress. Goetz's team placed their piece of blood vessel in tantalum rings attached to the downstream artery and made a small hole in the downstream artery to connect the two.

The first handsewn connection for a bypass graft anastomosis using the vein not attached to a ring became the surgical gold standard for the CABG. It was performed by Dr. DAVID SABISTON (1924-2009, born Jacksonville, North Carolina, U.S., and died Durham, North Carolina, U.S.) in April of 1962 while at Johns Hopkins University Hospital. He attached a piece of leg vein on the ascending aorta at one end and to the right coronary artery at the other beyond the coronary narrowing (stenosis). He did not report his success until 1974 because he was so disheartened by his patient's death from an unrelated stroke three days after surgery.

MICHAEL DEBAKEY (1908-2008, born Lake Charles, Louisiana, U.S., and died Houston, Texas, U.S.) and H. Edward Garret in November 1964 performed coronary bypass surgery but did not report the outcome of their twelve coronary bypass procedures performed until 1973.

In 1968 Dr. GEORGE GREEN (born 1932-, Brooklyn, New York) performed the first left internal mammary artery to left anterior descending artery bypass in 1968, and this procedure has become the standard for bypassing the LAD even though leg vein grafts are most commonly used for the circumflex and right coronary arteries, making him a major Disruptor.

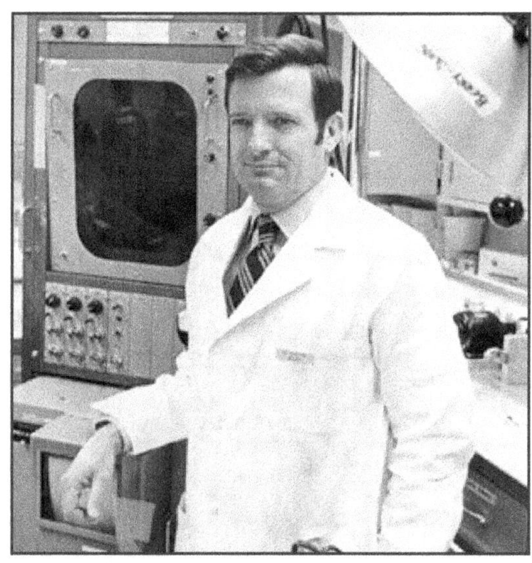

DAVID SABISTON,
permission of Duke U Archives

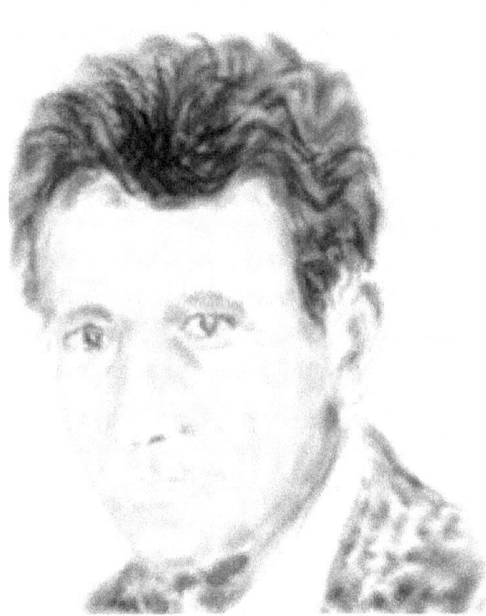

GEORGE GREEN, original
drawing by Dr. Roy Nuzzo

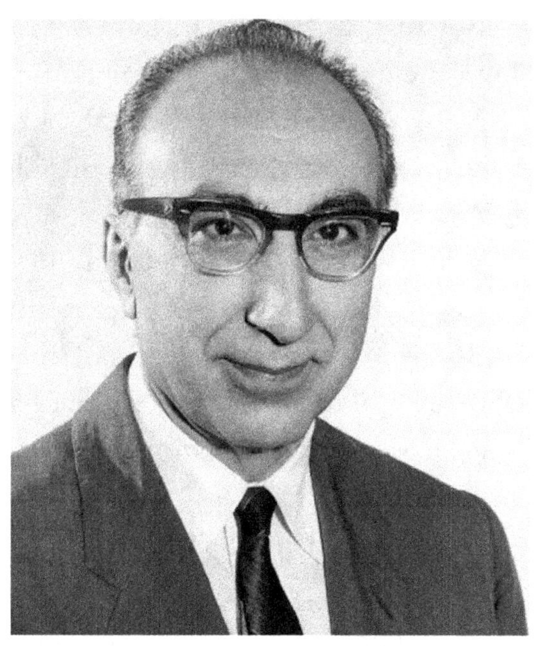

MICHAEL DEBAKEY, permission:
Lasker Foundation

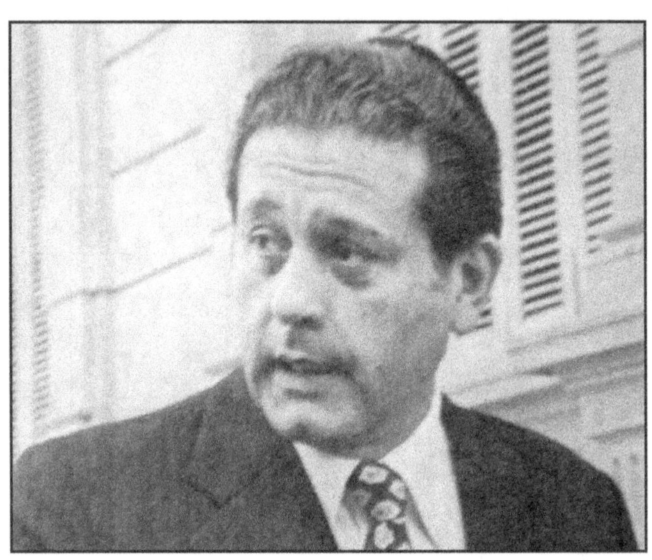

RENE FAVALORO,
Alamy License

But just as it took Dr. James Herrick to convince the medical world about the link between blocked coronary arteries and heart attacks, it took RENE FAVALORO (1923-2000, born Plata, Argentina, and died Buenos Aires, Argentina), who came to the Cleveland Clinic with his expertise and in May 1967 and performed his first procedure in Cleveland and then convinced the surgical world of the importance of coronary bypass surgery with his large number of cases and excellent results. He became the salesman for CABG by his numbers, success of his patients, and lectures. A year later he reported 150 cases and by 1970 he had performed one thousand cases!!!!! This Disruptor changed treatment of symptomatic cardiac patients around the world.

Subsequently, in the mid-1980, Floyd Loop (1936-2015, born Lafayette, Indiana, and died Lynhurst, Ohio), also from the Cleveland Clinic, published a ten-year comparison of saphenous vein grafts versus right and left internal mammary artery grafts. The internal mammary grafts, first performed by George Green, were the clear winners, including survival, less revascularization (i.e. second operations), and fewer subsequent heart attacks.

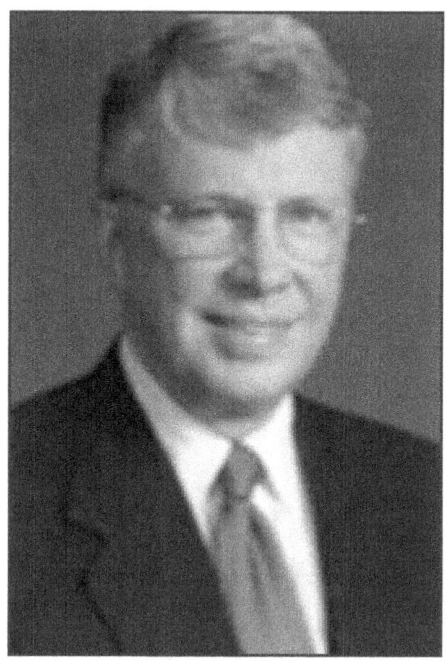

FLOYD LOOP,
permission: Cleveland Clinic

GLOSSARY CHAPTER 10

Anastomosis – connection

End-to-side anastomosis – connecting end of artery or vein tube into the side of another artery or vein

Endarterectomy – scooping out of arterial plaque or "cleaning it out"

Revascularization – fixing the blood supply to an organ

CHAPTER 11
HEART VALVE SURGERY AND THE TAVR PROCEDURE

None other than the great Leonardo DaVinci first described the aortic valve in the 1500s and understood its function was to prevent backflow, known as regurgitation, of blood from the main artery, the aorta, back into the left ventricle after blood was pumped out of the left ventricle. The valve can either not open properly, a condition known as aortic stenosis, or not close properly, allowing blood backflow, known as aortic regurgitation or insufficiency, or even have a combination of both. Most cases are of the three leaflet aortic valves that with aging (usually age 60-90s) acquire aortic stenosis, although 10-15% are from congenitally bicuspid aortic valves (two leaflets). Bicuspid aortic valves were first described by the British surgeon James Hope based on autopsy studies in 1832.

The two earliest descriptions of the pathology of aortic stenosis were by the Frenchman LAZARE RIVIERE (1589-1655) in 1663 and by the father of pathologic anatomy, Giovanni Battista Morgagni (see Chapter 2). In the same century, Corvisart (who first described thickening of the left ventricle wall (Chapter 2)) also published that he saw an aortic valve so fused that even the little finger could not be introduced. The first description of the stethoscope's auscultatory findings was in 1832 by JAMES HOPE (1801-1841, born Stockport, Cheshire, UK, and died Hampstead, UK).

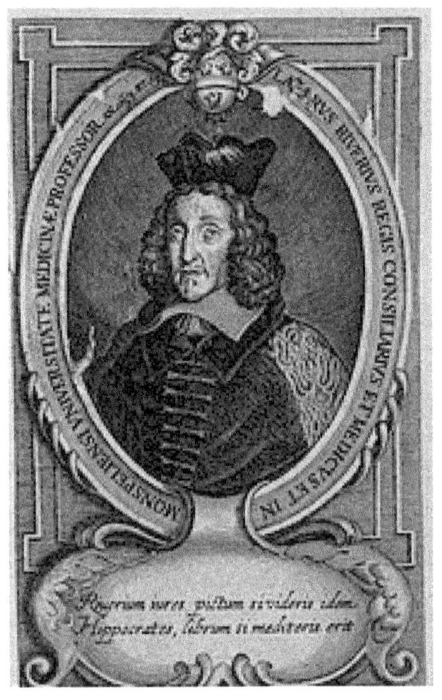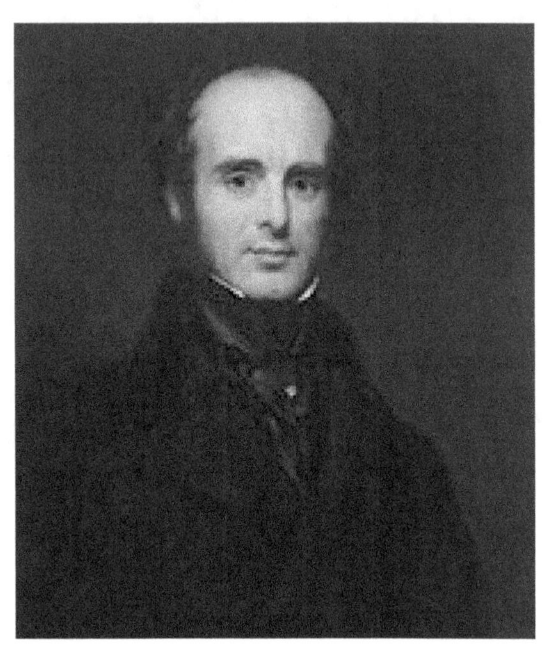

LAZARE RIVIERE Creative Commons via Wellcome Foundation

JAMES HOPE, public domain

A leaky aortic valve allows blood meant for the body to inappropriately and harmfully flow backward from the main artery to the left ventricle, from whence it originated, This was first described by DOMINIC CORRIGAN (1802-1880, born Dublin, Ireland, UK, and died Ireland, UK). He was known for his observations on heart disease and described the rapidly collapsing pulse felt in severely leaking aortic valves (aortic insufficiency, also called aortic regurgitation) to which his name is associated (Corrigan's Pulse) to this day. He explained the nature of this pulse and the rumbling sensation felt over the chest (known as a thrill) and the heart murmur associated with this condition more thoroughly than any predecessor. His conclusions were discovered from his experimental studies of 1836. To this day very little has been added to the physical diagnostic description made by Corrigan.

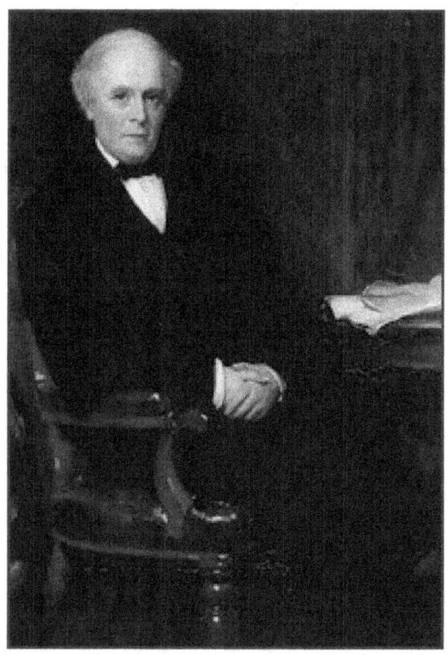

DOMINIC CORRIGAN, public domain

AUSTIN FLINT (1812-1886, born Petersham, Massachusetts, U.S. and died Brooklyn, NY, U.S.) in 1862, using the stethoscope, described the association of aortic insufficiency with a diastolic murmur (in the resting phase) not associated as it usually was with a sticky mitral valve (mitral stenosis) but with aortic regurgitation. To this day cardiologists listen for and still use the term "Austin Flint murmur," associated with severe aortic insufficiency.

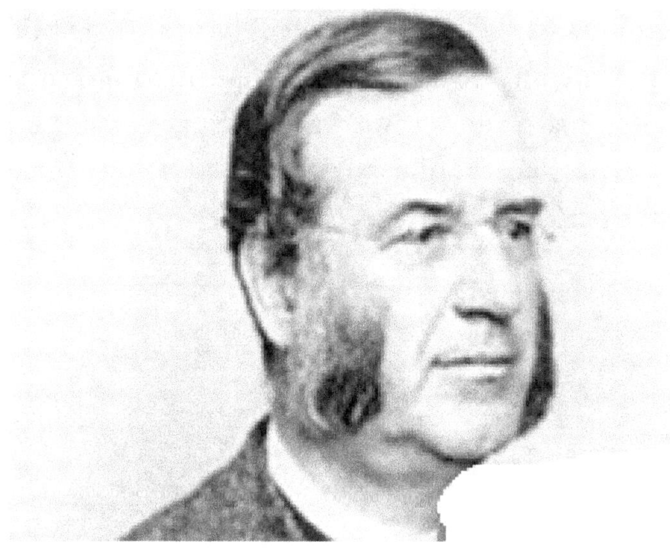

AUSTIN FLINT, public domain

HEART VALVE SURGERY

The early work of Souttar, Tuffier, Blalock, and Cutler is discussed above as runups to how heart surgery was performed before the development of the cardiopulmonary bypass machine. Once surgeons could operate more leisurely with a better visual field, and aided by the cardiopulmonary bypass machine and newer techniques, more complex internal operations of the heart became possible.

The early history of operating on these sticky, fused stenosed aortic valves was suboptimal for most patients until artificial valves were developed. Even to this day, no adequate operation exists to repair a diseased aortic valve without replacing it.

THEODORE TUFFIER (1857-1929) performed dilatation in 1912 with his finger with some relief, but it took the development of artificial aortic valves for the field finally to take off. The first aortic valve surgery performed by an the American surgeon was by ROBERT GLOVER (1914-1961) from the Mayo Clinic, who developed a dilating instrument, which he used in 1950 instead of a manual dilatation. As he wrote in his 1958 paper on seven years of experience with the aortic valve, "Anatomically, the valve is the least accessible to exploration, for it lies centrally placed within the confines of the heart." The first step to using artificial valves was by Dr. CHARLES HUFNAGEL (1916-1989, born Louisville, Kentucky, U.S., and died Washington, D.C., U.S.) who, in 1952, placed an acrylic ball in a cage prosthesis not in the upstream aortic valve position but in the descending aorta in the abdominal aorta far away from the native valve for aortic regurgitation, thus bypassing the diseased valve itself. Two hundred of these procedures were performed.

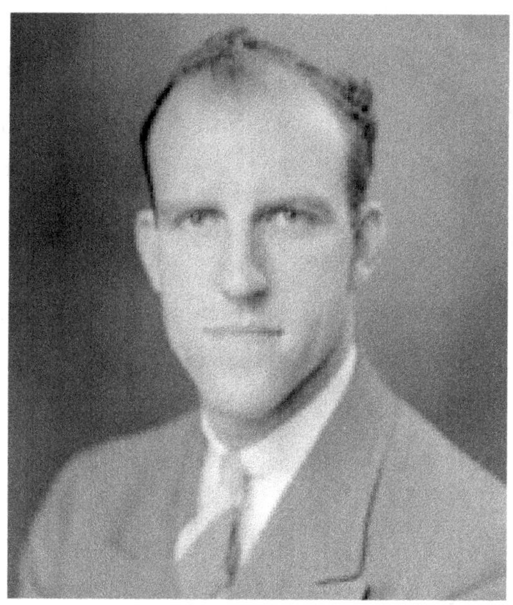

ROBERT GLOVER
permission: *Mayo Clinic*

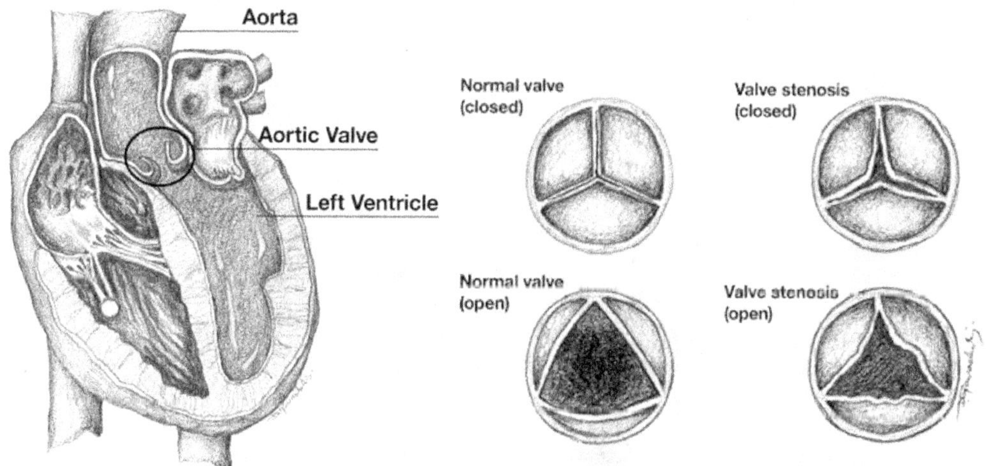

Left: Heart with normal AORTIC VALVE.
Right: Top two aortic valves in cross section by D. Gavisheli from the author's personal collection.

Once the heart lung machine was developed, surgeons could perform valve replacement with an artificial valve, as they now had more time to operate and no longer were racing against the clock before the patient's brain met disaster. The first such operation was performed by Dr. WALTON LILLEHEI, whom many consider the Father of Open Heart Surgery, in 1957 with a plastic valve in a cage for the aortic valve. Then Dr. DWIGHT HARKEN in 1960 at the

Peter Bent Brigham Hospital (who has been mentioned in this book previously) developed a double-caged ball, which moved forward to allow blood out of the heart and then back to a closed position in the resting diastolic phase. In the same year Dr. ALBERT STARR (1926-, born NY, NY, U.S.A.) worked with an engineer, Lowell Edwards who, at age 65, according to Starr, "in 1958 stepped out of his Cadillac and into my office with an ambitious plan to build an artificial valve." Within two years, in 1960 they implanted a ball in a cage aortic valve, which became a standard until bi-leaflet prostheses came along. The Starr-Edwards valve was superseded by the Medtronic Hall and St. Jude bi-leaflet valves, which became the dominant valves used by surgeons until tissue valves were finally perfected (1962) and have mainly replaced mechanical aortic valves except for certain specific but limited indications. Yet despite innovations and replacements, the original Starr-Edwards valve has remained predictably reliable for years and years, with some of the original valves still in place and working well. Unlike tissue valves, mechanical valves require strong anticoagulation with Coumadin and monthly or even more frequent blood checks of the anticoagulation with a test known as a prothrombin time, or PT for short.

As the famous surgeon from Houston, Denton Cooley, pointed out, heart valve innovation was driven by the philosophy "Apply, Simplify, and Modify."

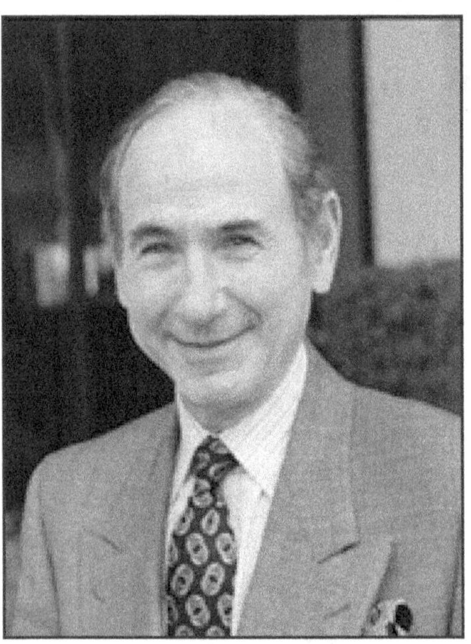

ALBERT STARR
permission: Edwards Lifesciences Co.

Not long after the artificial aortic valve was developed, a total mitral valve replacement was developed and implanted by Dr. NINA BRAUNWALD (1928-1992, born Brooklyn, New York, U.S.A), who was among the first women to become a cardiothoracic surgeon. Her mitral valve design was implanted by her in 1960 with her team. Her Braunwald-Cutter cloth-covered valve was implanted into thousands. Braunwald's colleagues described this surgeon and mother of three as "pioneering, determined, yet gentle."

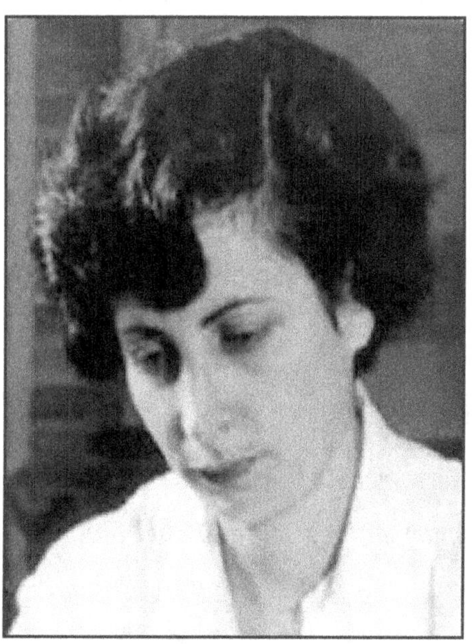

NINA BRAUNWALD,
public domain

THE TAVR PROCEDURE

I still remember my group performing the first balloon valvuloplasty at Morristown Medical Center long before the TAVR was approved. Dr. Alain Cribier from France had been the pioneer and leader of the balloon valvuloplasty and later the TAVR procedure as well. The procedure used a very large balloon on a fairly large- diameter catheter inserted in the groin to cross the narrowed aortic valve. One then would inflate the balloon sitting inside the valve, and hope the valve opened enough and was not damaged. I had a patient in his early eighties with severe aortic stenosis and congestive heart failure who statistically was going to die within a month or two without surgery. However, his risk of surgery was extremely great, and he was turned down by our surgeons for valve replacement. I called my friend Igor Palacios at the Massachusetts General Hospital, who trained with me and was now a world leader in balloon valvuloplasty of the mitral valve and aortic valve. I asked him if he could come down to help us perform our first procedure. He could not come due to other obligations but sent his #2. What stands out in my memory are three things. First, the procedure was a success and the patient had six more months of useful life before his readmission for restenosis and congestive heart failure and a second balloon valvuloplasty, as he was not still a surgical candidate and would have died on the OR table. Second, Igor's stand-in, along with two of my partners who would assist at the procedure, and I first went to lunch at a local Indian restaurant, which was spicier than we had anticipated. This was not a good idea since the four of us around the catheterization table all intermittently were suffering from heartburn. Third, when I returned home later in the day, I was literally jumping up and down with excitement. My wonderful wife Toni was already outside at the front door removing cobwebs under the eaves with a long stick with a cloth attached. There were areas too high for her to reach, so she asked me for some help. Normally I would jump in to give her a hand, but I was still distracted by the excitement of our team's success and absentmindedly answered her with "You know, I just performed the first successful balloon aortic valvuloplasty in NJ." She responded, "I know, and I am so proud of you, but please don't forget the area in the corner." Toni has always kept my feet on the ground.

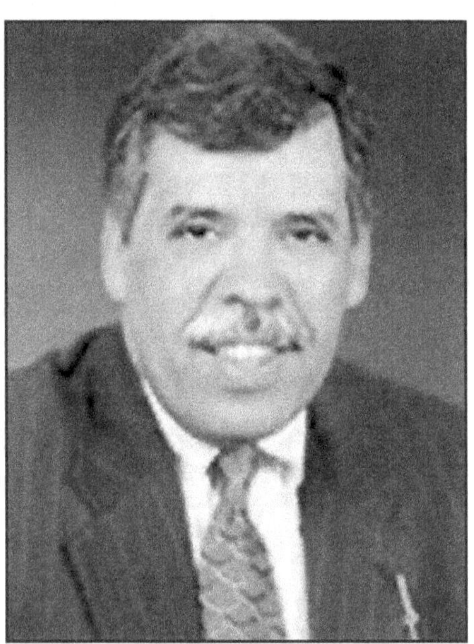

Dr. IGOR PALACIOS
permission Dr Palacios' personal collection

As of today's writing, the TAVR (transcutaneous aortic valve replacement) or TAVI nonsurgical procedure (see below) has outnumbered surgically replaced aortic valves (SAVR) for patients with severe isolated aortic stenosis. In the elderly over age eighty, TAVR is now the preferred procedure for aortic stenosis valve replacement if other cardiac surgical procedures such as coronary bypass are not also required. In addition, patients with previously placed aortic valves, if lucky enough to have been given tissue rather than mechanical valves, are able to have a TAVR placed inside the original surgical tissue valve without reopening the chest but now placed via a catheter. On the other hand, if the original valve was one of the mechanical valves, a repeat open chest operation is necessary if valve malfunction occurs in order to replace the aortic valve, as the metal and hard leaflets will not allow placement inside them of a TAVR valve.

So what is a TAVR, sometimes called TAVI (transcutaneous aortic valve implantation)? The TAVR is a non-surgical procedure to give a patient a new aortic valve without opening up the chest by a surgeon. Human beings are always trying to go one step further and advance progress. Part of this ingenuity was manifested by attempts by both cardiologists and surgeons to spare the patient a painful and prolonged convalescence and increased risk of open heart surgery. To avoid open heart surgery, percutaneous procedures were designed, implemented, and perfected. Early attempts to repair the aortic valve but avoid open surgery were developed by the French surgeon named ALAIN CRIBIER (1945-2024, born Paris, France and died Rouen, France), who had also trained at Cedars Sinai in Los Angeles. He was already known as the inventor of aortic balloon valvuloplasty, which he first performed in Rouen, France, in 1985. A very large balloon is wrapped around the end of a catheter after it is inserted into the groin artery, known as the femoral artery, and then inflated to crack open the fused aortic leaflets. This is fairly safe and results are often immediately successful. However, re-narrowing (known as restenosis) almost always occurs within six months, and the patient is back to square one. Although I personally have performed these in the pre-TAVR days, even twice on several of the same patients, the expected results were only short term (lasting six months the first time and three months the second time until restenosis occurred). This procedure by and large became abandoned even before the perfection of the TAVR and remains used only occasionally as a bridge for future open heart surgery. The hope is that the patient and his condition will improve enough to make the patient a better surgical risk once his valve is relieved of its stenosis using the balloon. And the hope has been that surgery can be performed before the valve re-stenoses. The TAVR procedure procedurally is similar to the aortic balloon valvuloplasty, but like coronary angioplasty and subsequently coronary artery stenting, in the TAVR a tissue aortic valve is placed onto a metal stent, and crimped onto a large balloon , and positioned across the diseased aortic valve. The balloon is then inflated, leaving the new valve inside the old thickened valve which had been literally "pushed to the outside rim" where the aortic valve normally sits. The ballon and catheter is then removed with the new valve in place inside the old valve . This describes the Sapien Edwards valve which is known as a balloon expandable valve. The Medtronic Core Valve is similar but self-expands into place when a long covering tube known as a sheath is withdrawn and removed from the body due to the properties of nitinol which is used instead of steel. Once the valve expands, the catheter on which it was placed is also removed from the body leaving the new valve inside the old aortic valve. Both Sapien and Core valves have three cow pericardial tissue pieces much like a normal aortic valve which open and close as the heart pushes blood into the aorta. There are certain anatomic or clinical indications dictating whether the operator chooses the Sapien valve or the Core valve.

Henning Rud Andersen (1951-, born Himmerland, Denmark) invented and fabricated the first TAVR in 1989, placing it in an adult pig, but could not find a company to work with him to perfect and manufacture it. He presented his research in 1990 at the Danish Society of Cardiology. Ironically his paper was rejected by the two major U.S. cardiology journals, the first *Journal of the American College of Cardiology and Circulation*, where his research was called "gimmicky." Once again original thinking was rejected by the establishment Restrainers.

Andersen was a Disruptor, and the academic American cardiology world of research journals the Restrainers. Henning Rud Andersen from Aarhus University in Denmark had the original idea of an aortic valve placed on a metal frame and delivered with a catheter percutaneously. He said he formed the idea while at an international meeting in Scottsdale, Arizona, and listening to a lecture by Dr. Palmaz from the Palmaz-Schatz coronary stent. Although placing stents in pigs, he was not able to raise the money he needed to pursue his great idea. His patent was eventually purchased by Edward Life Sciences and became the basis for the second TAVR Sapien valve, the Sapien XT valve. The first Sapien valve which was by the FDA in 2011 although studies using this valve date back to 2006.. The Sapien valve has a metal frame of cobalt chromium whereas the other major TAVR valve, the Medtronic Core Valve, has a frame of flexible self-expandable nitinol which is why no balloon is required to deploy it.

Although not the inventor or manufacturer, Dr. Cribier implanted the first artificial aortic valve into a human being on April 16, 2002, and his leadership, teaching, and clinical research really is the reason its use has surpassed open heart valve replacement worldwide. As written in the American Journal of Cardiology for his "In Memorium" on February 17, 2024, Dr. Cribier was quoted in 2022 , "When you decide to innovate in medicine, you have a number of people against you. The biggest lesson is to make sure you are right, then persevere and try to jump all obstacles in your way. Never be discouraged." Dr. Alain Cribier was already the world renown pioneer for the balloon valvuloplasty, performing the world's first aortic valvuloplasty in 1985. By 1990 he realized that the valvuloplasty was not the right road, and he started research on the TAVR. . Evidently nearly deciding to become a concert pianist, the world is eternally grateful that he chose cardiac surgery as his calling instead. He spent his professional career in Rouen, France where he died slightly under a month on February 16, 2024 at the age of 79, slightly under a month before I reviewed the first draft of this book for editing.

The first human procedure of this TAVR was performed in Rouen, France, in 2002 by Dr. Cribier after first working on his device implanted in sheep. This is known as a story of "Disruptive Technology," and Dr. Cribier may be one of the most important Disruptors in the history of cardiology and cardiac surgery to this day. The U.S. FDA approved the Edwards Sapien aortic valve for human use in 2011. Given the number of TAVRs performed each year, it is fair to say that Dr. Cribier, a heart surgeon, started a revolution in cardiology. The lifespan of the TAVR valve is thought to be ten to twenty years, not bad since most patients are in their 80s when it is deployed.

In 2019, 72,991 TAVRs were performed in the U.S. compared to open heart aortic valve replacements (SAVR – surgical aortic valve replacement), 57,626. Around the world since 2002, more than four hundred thousand TAVRs have been performed. In the U.S. alone, in 2019 there were 716 centers performing this procedure, not possible without the work of Cribier. A randomized prospective study in 45 centers of 795 patients showed a one year mortality of

14.2% for the Core Valve versus 19.15 for open heart aortic valve surgery. Other studies have shown a 2.8% stroke rate and requirement for a permanent pacemaker of 28.7% with a 93% early survival and one year mortality of 17.1%. Comparing the two valves has shown no real difference in operative and follow up mortality. The Core valve due to its design required more pacemakers at 22% vs 5% for the Edwards Sapien valve. The leakage rates were similar.

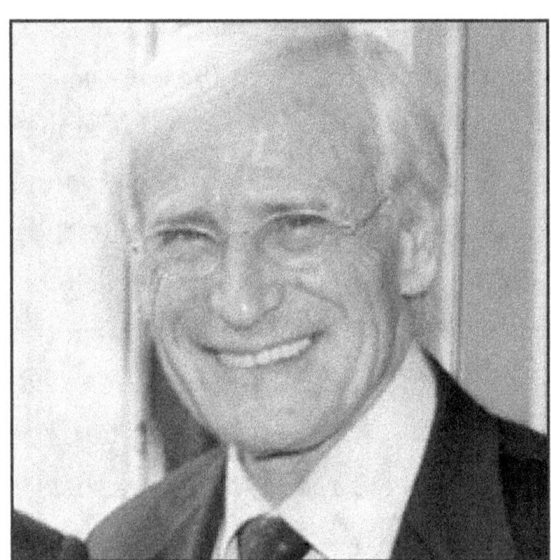

ALAIN CRIBIER
permission: American College of Cardiology

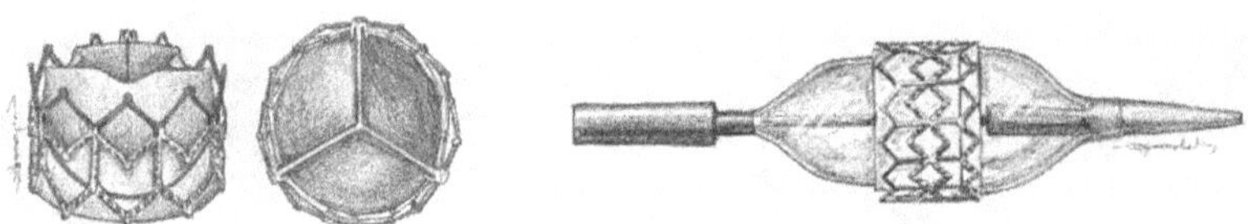

the TAVR Valve

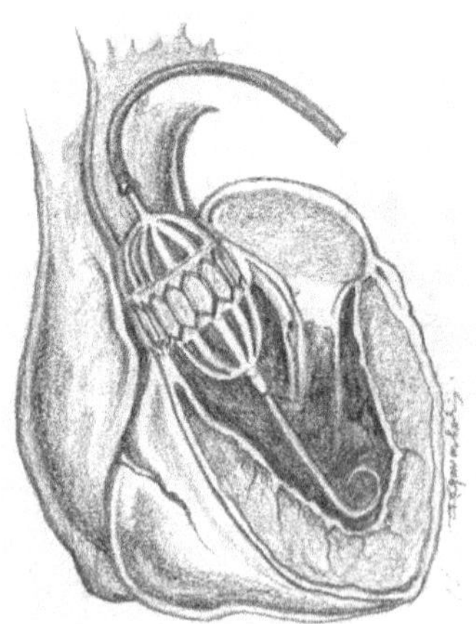

Balloon inflated to expand TAVR, inflating the balloon in place

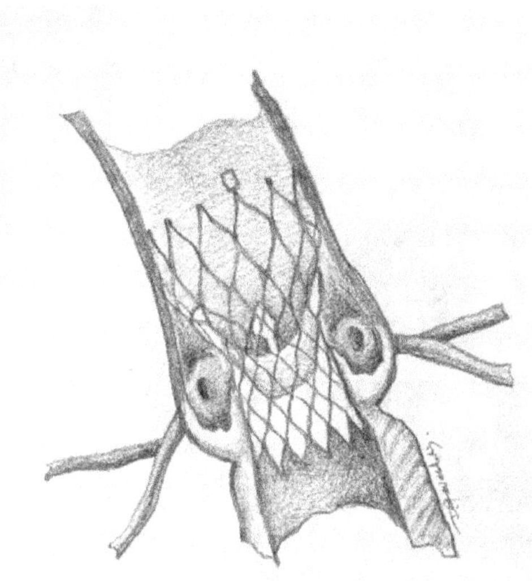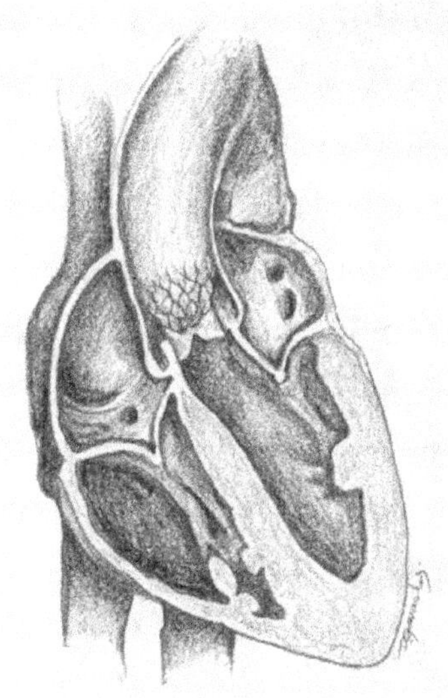

TAVR is deployed, procedure completed
Drawing by D. Gavasheli, from author's personal collection

The TAVR (transcutaneous aortic valve replacement and sometimes called TAVI for transcutaneous aortic valve implantation) uses a catheter usually placed from one of the two groin femoral arteries to gain access to the arterial tree and a route back to the heart. The catheter is then directed to the aortic valve, where a very thin wire is literally and sometimes with difficulty fished across the minimal opening of the valve through the larger tube (catheter). Then a smaller catheter with the stent-mounted aortic valve is placed on a balloon, which is on the tip of the catheter, then pushed into proper position through the first larger catheter but also over the wire. The balloon is then inflated. At the tip of the catheter on the balloon is a wire metal mesh scaffold called a stent in which a cow or pig aortic valve is attached. The balloon is similar to what was previously used to expand the valve during the older valvuloplasty procedure, then is inflated under the compressed metal stent mesh, pushing the scaffolded stent into position against the aorta wall (there is also a type with a self-expanding valve) and the valve, which rests in the scaffold, into place just outside the left ventricle with its circular scaffold resting circumferentially against the aorta. The catheter is withdrawn and removed from the body. The self-expanding variety is released by withdrawing its covering sheath, which sits on top of the stented tissue valve, allowing the valve to expand by virtue of the expansive nitinol material used for the scaffold. Since untreated, severe aortic stenosis leads to premature death, and valve replacement becomes mandatory in severe cases since surgical repair attempts have been suboptimal. Most eligible patients are over age eighty. As of this writing, there are two types of TAVR devices, one, which is expanded when in place by a balloon inside it, and the other, which self-expands. Although a boon to patients, especially the elderly and sicker with congestive heart failure, this procedure is not without its complications. The mortality is still about 2%, with a third of deaths occurring after discharge in the first thirty days. However, strokes, artery injury, need for a permanent pacemaker placement, and infection can also occur as complications despite the success and popularity of the procedure.

The job is not completed. Artificial valves have now been implanted or being developed for the pulmonic, tricuspid, and mitral valves, as well as the FDA-approved aortic valve. The pulmonic valve for children was actually the first percutaneously approved valve. The FDA has approved recently a tricuspid percutaneous valve, and multiple mitral valves are now in clinical trials. In addition, stitching procedures to repair leaking mitral and tricuspid valves are now being used by interventional cardiologists to alleviate the need for open heart surgery.

GLOSSARY CHAPTER 11

Thrill – rumbling sensation felt on the chest by the examiner and caused by a very loud heart murmur, which is audible, and due to severe blood flow turbulence

CHAPTER 12
HEART TRANSPLANTATION

At the end of my third year in medical school in the summer of 1967, I had a rotation on general surgery and its subspecialties at the Peter Bent Brigham Hospital in Boston. We were on call every other night, which usually meant being up most of the night as a surgical assistant usually holding the retractor for the surgeon and trying not to fall asleep and falling into the sterile open surgical field. I distinctly remember doing whatever medical students did on a triple valve (there are four heart valves) replacement being performed by Dr. Dwight Harken and his cardiothoracic surgical fellow, who later became well known at Cedars Sinai in California, Dr. Jack Matloff. Dr. Harken was nice but all business and no nonsense. I still remember that even to me, at 6'2.5" in height, Dr. Matloff seemed like a giant with hands the size of Yogi Berra's catcher's glove and fingers to fit. I never could understand how he performed flawlessly such intricate and delicate surgery with those hands, but he did and for years to come. I was at this stage of my career fairly naive and clueless, but what was about to be discussed by Dr. Harken and Dr. Matloff I clearly understood. There was in the intensive care unit at the Peter Bent Brigham Hospital a young man in his twenties who was braindead from a motor cycle accident (from that day I have resisted ever getting onto a motorcycle). Dr. Harken and Matloff could not get their patient, a female, off the bypass machine no matter how hard they tried, and she was certain to die. This was in August of 1967, with Dr. Christiaan Barnard of South Africa (more to come) not performing the world's first cardiac transplant until December 3, 1967. I distinctly remember the following and immediately understood the implications of a possible historical moment. I have no idea what preparation Dr. Harken and Matloff had for this moment, and I have always been sorry that I did not ask either of them at the time (medical students would never do that in that day) or subsequently. I even recently called Dr. Harken's

When one thinks of heart transplantation, two names immediately pop into the head of a cardiologist and cardiac surgeons—Dr. Christiaan Barnard and Dr. Norman Shumway, two important Disruptors. Dr. Barnard is remembered as performing the world's first successful human heart transplant. Dr. Shumway was known for performing basic transplantation research for years and performed the world's fourth human cardiac transplant, but his work and his team are most remembered as working out what was required not only to perform the procedure but to make sure the follow-up and survival were enduring, especially in terms of preventing rejection of the foreign transplanted heart by the receiving patient. Without the research of Dr. Norman Shumway and his team, there would be no heart transplantation today.

However, before either of them came onto the scene, others prepared the ground. As far back as 1905, the first cardiac transplantation was performed at the University of Chicago by Dr. ALEXIS CARREL (1873-1944, born Lyon, France, and died Paris, France) with Dr. CHARLES GUTHRIE (1880-1963, born Gilmore, Missouri, and died Columbia, Missouri, U.S.), not in a human being but from one dog to another dog (both surgeons were working together at the University of Chicago). Their interest was not really in heart transplantation per se but in perfecting connections between arteries, and they were mainly interested in limb re-implantations and, to a lesser extent, the kidney and heart for transplantation. Carrel's dog died two hours later, possibly because aseptic technique (and with bilateral ventricular clots) was not utilized, and the flow was not physiological. Carrel subsequently transplanted a dog's head into another dog, giving that recipient two heads. This was the beginning of organ transplantation. Carrell and Guthrie, two Disruptors, received the Nobel Prize in Physiology in 1912 for their work in blood vessel transplantation and connections. FRANK C. MANN (1887-1962, born Adams County, Indiana, U.S., and died Rochester, Minnesota, U.S.) and his colleagues in 1933 at the Mayo Clinic performed the world's second heart transplant using another canine model and placing the transplanted heart into the neck of the recipient dog. The longest-surviving animal was eight days with the average of four days' survival. Mann was head of vascular research at the Mayo Clinic. His team studied the mechanism of rejection, noting that not the surgical technique but the body's inflammatory response caused the failure of the procedure. Of course, little was really known about immunology in 1933.

The Russian VLADIMIR P. DEMIKHOV (1916-1998, born Volgograd farm region, Russia, and died Moscow, Soviet Union) published in 1962 extensive research he began on transplantation back in 1940. He was the first to establish (in the dog) that total circulation could be established. His dog survived fifteen hours. In 1946 his transplanted dog survived 32 days. His experiments kept the recipient heart just where it was but isolated from the donor heart.

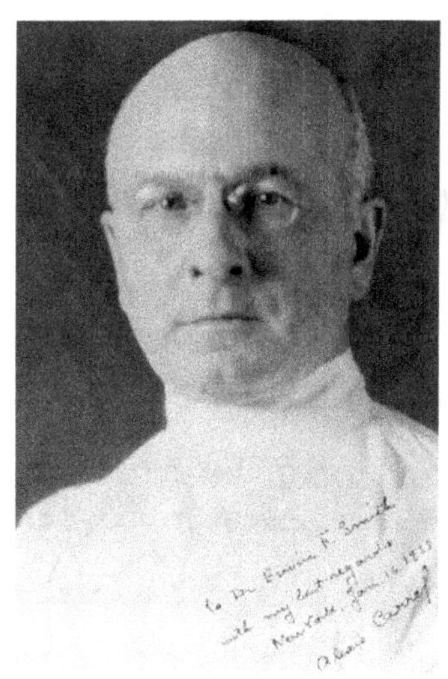

ALEXIS CARREL
Smithsonian
Inst./Copyright Status
unknown/Science
Photo, Library License

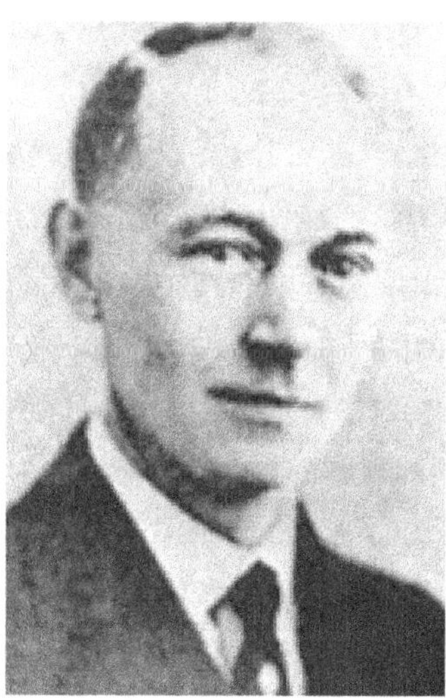

CHARLES GUTHRIE
National Library of
Medicine,
public domain

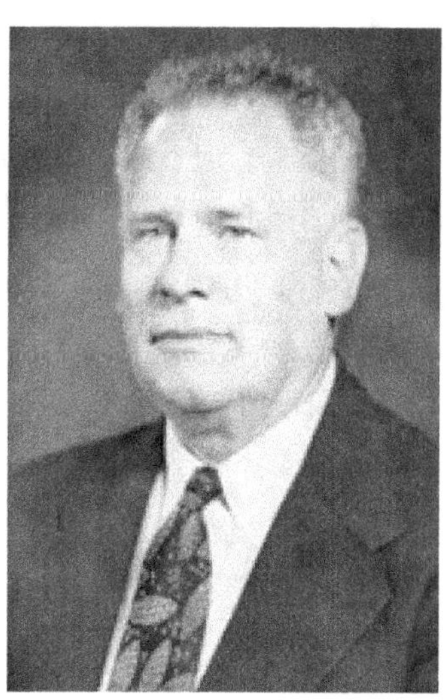

FRANK C. MANN
permission: Mayo Clinic

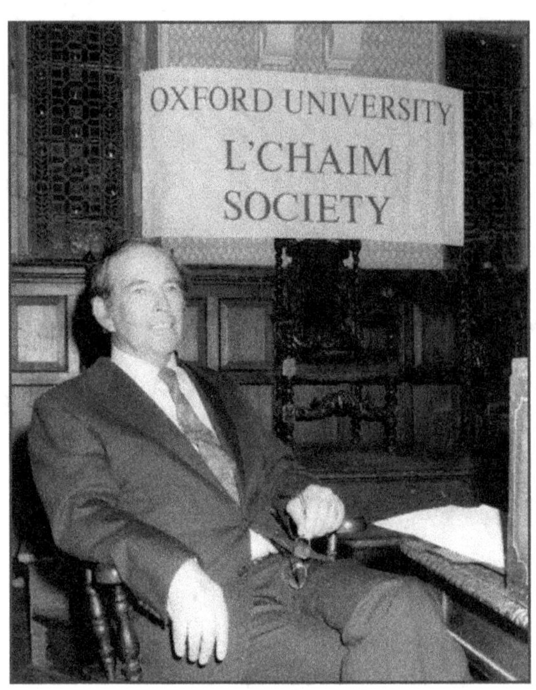

CHRISTIAAN BARNARD
Jewish Chronicle Archive Heritage Images/Science Photo Library License

RICHARD LOWER (1929-2008, born Detroit, Michigan, and died Twin Bridges, Montana, U.S.) (no relation, I believe, to Richard Lower, discussed in Chapter 2) and NORMAN SHUMWAY (1923-2006, born Kalamazoo, Michigan, and died Palo Alto, California) of Stanford University in 1960 published their experience of dog transplantation without immunosuppression with dogs surviving up to 21 days. During their research they discovered an ominous portent of rejection. They noticed the EKG voltage was reduced in size from baseline when rejection occurred and returned to normal when the rejection process was suppressed using azathioprine (immunosuppressive agent) and methyl prednisolone (a steroid), allowing animals to survive over eight months. PHILIP CAVES (1940-1978, born Belfast, Northern Ireland, and died Glasgow, Scotland) worked with Dr. Shumway both in the OR and in the lab. He is credited with inventing the cardiac surgical bioptome, allowing small samples to be taken easily and repeatedly if required from the right ventricle of the wall shared with the left ventricle. His instrument was inserted in the internal jugular vein through the skin. This technique has been indispensable in diagnosing early transplant rejection, which requires more aggressive medication treatment. He so impressed Dr. Shumway that he was made his chief cardiac surgical resident in 1972 and a staff surgeon in charge of the transplant program in 1973. In 1965 Caves was made professor of cardiac surgery in Glasgow, Scotland. His untimely death due to a heart attack while playing squash in 1978 at age 38 certainly deprived the cardiac transplant field of more innovations by this surgeon.

Once the technical and rejection problems were solved in the animal laboratory, soon the procedure was performed on a humans. On January 23, 1964, Dr. JAMES HARDY (1955-1987, born Newala, Alabama, and died Jackson, Mississippi), at the University Hospital in Jackson, Mississippi, performed the world's first human transplant, but he used a large heart from a chimpanzee into a human rather than human to human. Unfortunately the circulation failed, and the patient died one hour later. Hardy was ridiculed by his colleagues, probably for using a donor chimpanzee. I would conclude he was cautious and a Disruptor with mocking from Restrainers.

But on December 3, 1967, the world was impressed and shocked when in Cape Town, South Africa, Dr. CHRISTIAAN BARNARD (1922-2001, born Beufort West, South Africa, and died Paphos, Cyprus), who assisted by his brother, MARIUS BARNARD, also a heart surgeon, performed the first human-to-human successful cardiac transplant at Groote Schur Hospital in Cape Town, South Africa. His patient, Louis Washkansky, a 54-year-old grocer, had a five-hour operative procedure that December day. Some criticized Barnard for quoting his family an 80% chance of success, but Barnard subsequently wrote: "For a dying man it is not a difficult decision to make because he knows he is at the end. If a lion chases you to the bank of a river filled with crocodiles, you will leap into the water, convinced that you have a chance to swim to the other side."

Barnard had previously worked under Dr. Shumway in California and used the techniques Shumway and Lower developed. Despite the initial hurrah, the patient died on the 18th day. Barnard performed his second transplant on a local dentist on January 2, 1968

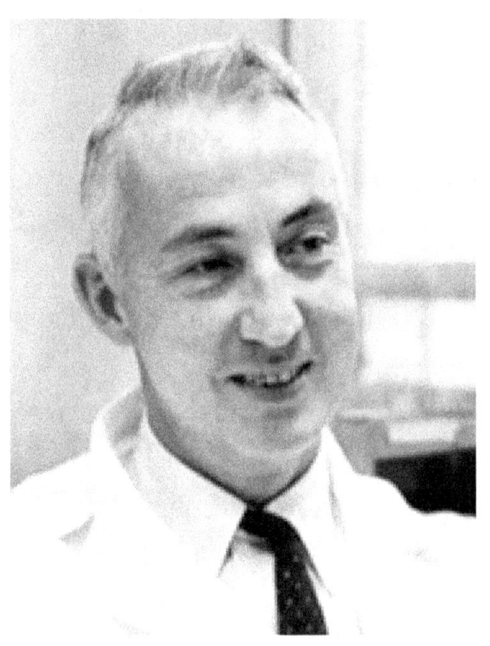
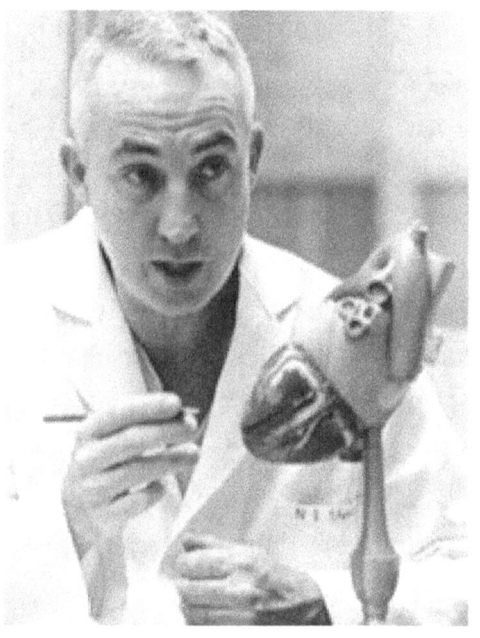

NORMAN SHUMWAY   NORMAN SHUMWAY

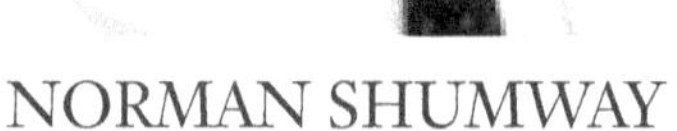

permission: Stanford University Medical History Center

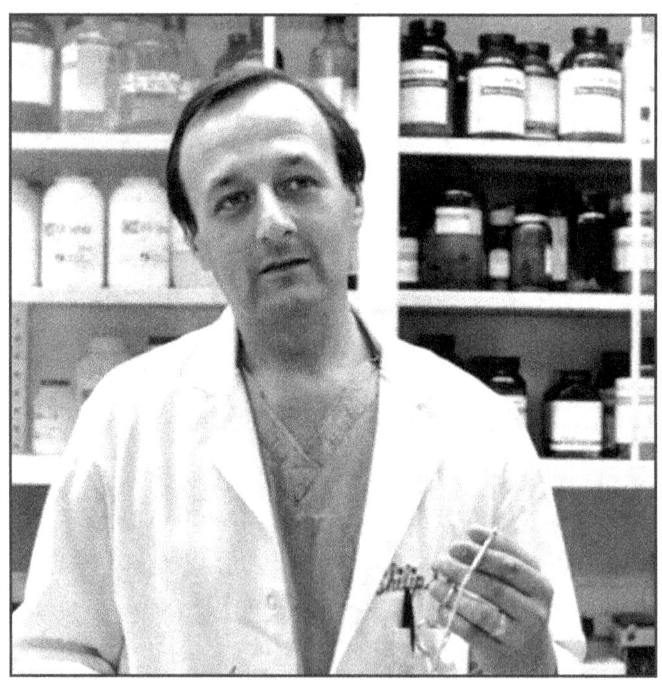

PHILLIP CAVES
permission: Stanford University Medical History Center

On December 6, 1967, Dr. Adrian Kantrowitz (1918-2008, born New York City, NY, and died Ann Arbor, Michigan), a pediatric heart surgeon from Maimonides Hospital in Brooklyn, NY, U.S, performed the world's second human transplant from a patient born with no brain (anencephalic) into an eighteen-day-old child with congenital heart disease. The baby survived six hours.

Barnard performed the world's third human transplant on January 3, 1968, and the patient survived 19 months.

Shumway's team finally was able to perform the second U.S. and fourth world's human adult transplant on January 6, 1968 at Stanford University Hospital on a 54 year old man who lived 15 days before dying of several complications.

An interesting sidelight is that several public publications from Texas give Denton Cooley credit for performing the first "successful" U.S. cardiac transplant, but he did not perform his procedure until May 2, 1968, nearly four months after Shumway's heart transplant. Cooley's patient was a 47-year-old man who survived 204 days. This may be considered the first successful U.S. heart transplant since Cooley's patients lived over six months rather than fifteen days, the survival of Shumway's first transplant. Cooley also performed 22 transplants the next year, including three in a single day.

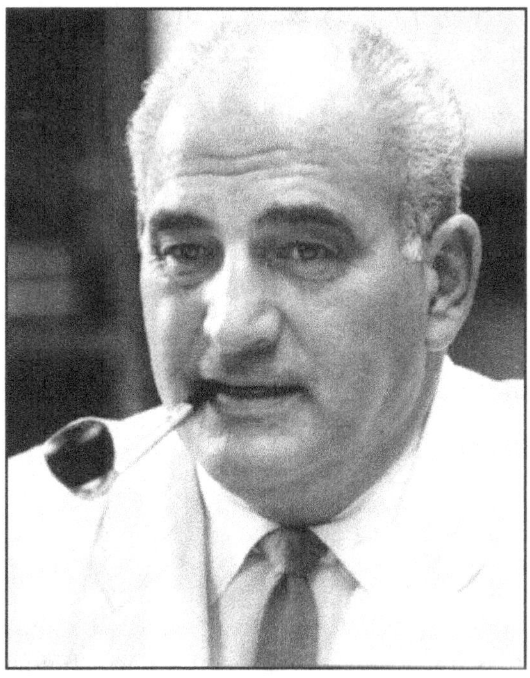

ADRIAN KANTROWITZ,
Alamy License

Surgeons were "off and running" with 107 heart transplantations being performed in 52 centers in seventeen countries by the end of 1968. What an incredible, contagious beginning from multiple Disruptors. The next year only fifty patients worldwide underwent cardiac transplantation, and in 1970 fewer than twenty patients underwent the procedure. In 1971 only ten. After an international meeting concerning cardiac transplantation, the centers dwindled to four performing the procedure, Marius Barnard (Christiaan's brother) in South Africa; Richard Lower in Richmond, Virginia, having left Stanford; Norman Shumway and his group at Stanford University; and Christian Cabrol-La Pitie Salpetrieri in Paris. The technique for monitoring the immunosuppressive regimen of azathioprine and steroids was developed by Shumway and Philip Caves (1940-1978, born Belfast, North Ireland, UK, and died Glasgow, Scotland, UK), who was working with Norman Shumway's group when he developed a biopsy device to take small pieces of the inside of the heart to look for inflammation under the microscope, which is a sign of rejection of the transplanted heart. This changed the entire picture and outlook for the field of heart transplantation, making the prognosis improved with this knowledge so treatment for rejection could be started early, before a cardiac catastrophe occurred.. In 1980 an even better antirejection drug than azathioprine was introduced. The drug was cyclosporine, having shown to be successful in kidney transplantation since 1978. It was originally discovered in 1969 by Dr. Hans Peter Frey from a soil sample. While he was working for Sandoz Pharmaceuticals, he had collected his sample in Norway while looking for antifungal agents. His company encouraged employees to do so in hopes of discovering new pharmaceuticals. Cyclosporine was isolated from his samples of fungi taken on that trip. For legal scholars, I found a paper asking the question if international law allowed taking for commercial purposes soil samples from another country. I am not an expert, but apparently it is.

Dr. Jean F. Borel (1933-, born Antwerp, Belgium), also of Sandoz, in 1973 recognized cyclosporine's antirejection properties and its ability to antagonize T cell lymphocytes. A pure form was then synthesized. It is said that Borel even tested it on himself. Despite early findings of side-effects and an incidence of lymphoma in humans, in 1980 it was given to eleven liver transplant recipients and finally was FDA approved in 1983. At first it was used mainly for kidney transplants. Its long-term nephrotoxic effects are still an issue. But the Stanford group under Shumway led the way for successful human heart transplant using it. Although even newer methods and techniques are now being used, the credit must go to Dr. Norman Shumway and his group for their impressive research, including using cyclosporine to prevent heart rejection. In 2021, worldwide 3817 heart transplants were performed (24,669 kidney transplants and 9236 liver transplants). More hearts have recently become available for use due to newer guidelines for withdrawing life support, whereas previously surgeons waited for brain death before removing donor hearts. This change has helped to preserve heart function. In addition, due to the availability recently of oral drugs to cure Hepatitis C, even more and older patients have become potential candidates, whereas previously age seventy was the upper limit of age eligibility.

A patient and friend of mine for years developed irreversible heart failure over a period of several years and had less than six months to live were it not for the heart transplant he received in NYC. At age 73$^{1/2}$ he was not a candidate for the usual heart donation for cardiac transplantation, as the cutoff was age seventy. After agreeing to accept a heart of a patient with Hepatitis C, he became a candidate. He received the heart of a 35-year-old, and after several months of medication given orally the Hepatitis C was cured. He is fully functional now, and I joke with him that at age 77 he does not look like the age of the heart that keeps him alive. We also still joke about the day I visited him in the hospital after his transplant and brought him a real New York pastrami sandwich (his surgeon gave permission). He is grateful to be alive and living a good life, even practicing law again until last year, when he decided finally to retire.

GLOSSARY CHAPTER 12

Heart transplant – removing a heart from a dead patient and operatively placing it into a live patient with a very diseased, poorly pumping heart

Immunosuppressive drug – a drug used to block the body's effort to prevent foreign tissue from being rejected by the body

CHAPTER 13
RESEARCH ON THE TOTAL ARTIFICIAL HEART

In discussing cardiac transplantation, some discussion of artificial hearts must also be written. Early on there was great promise, and they have been perfected over time. Rather than replace transplantation, artificial hearts have primarily become a bridge in patients whose lives hang in the balance and have long waiting times 'til a donor heart is available or ineligible for a heart transplant, usually due to age over seventy years.

Physicians thought about artificial hearts over two hundred years ago. Julien Jean Cesasr LeGallois, a Frenchman, had a theory of a mechanical circulatory support in 1812, but of course this was only a theory. Two unlikely people worked together on such a project. Alexis Carrel of vascular transplantation and a Nobel Laureate, and Charles Lindbergh, the celebrity aviator but also an inventor and a pro-Nazi Germany under Hitler supporter, worked together on a heart pump for a time. A pump was made but mainly for organ perfusion, not as a substitute for the diseased heart. Subsequently, their animals survived thirty days post-op. Carrel also performed a coronary artery bypass on his dogs. Carrel was a pioneer in many cardiac fields, clearly a Disruptor.

The first artificial heart placed in an alive animal was made in 1937 by the Russian physician Valdimir P. Demikhov (1916-1998, born, Russia, and died Moscow, Russia), who developed a total artificial heart and placed it into a dog's chest. The dog lived for five and a half hours. In 1957 Dr. Willem Kolff (1911-2009, born Leiden, Netherlands, and died Newtown Square, Pennsylvania, U.S.) of the Cleveland Clinic developed a total artificial heart, which he placed into an animal that lived an hour and a half after implantation. The technical details of the artificial heart are beyond the scope of this book but can be looked up in multiple references for those who care about such details.

Sufficed to say, a total mechanical heart finally was developed. Dr. DOM-INGO LIATTA (1924-2022, born Diamante, Entre Rios, Argentina, and died Buenos Aires, Argentina), an Argentine surgeon, created some new designs and he went to work for Dr. Michael DeBakey of Baylor University in Houston, Texas, at Methodist Hospital. When Dr. Liatta felt that Dr. DeBakey was not appreciating his work and ignoring what he had developed, he sought out Dr. Denton Cooley (1920-2016, born and died Houston, Texas, U.S.), who no longer was collaborating with Dr. DeBakey and had moved to St. Luke's Epis-copal Hospital in Houston and later established the Texas Heart Institute. Then Dr. Denton Cooley also began working with Domingo Liotta, who had left Dr. DeBakey's lab. Cooley and Liatta implanted the first artificial heart into a 47-year-old male in 1969 (the Liotta-Cooley Artificial Heart). The patient had suf-fered multiple heart attacks in the past, but unfortunately the new artificial heart also failed. Cooley's patient lived with his artificial heart for 64 hours until re-ceiving a heart transplant at hour number 64. Unfortunately, he still died 32 hours later of heart rejection of the transplanted heart and possibly infection. It would take another fifteen years before cyclosporine as an antirejection drug was discovered, which might have saved him.

Dr. Cooley and Dr. DeBakey subsequently developed what was to become the Hatfield and McCoy feud of medicine. Dr. Cooley and Dr. DeBakey were physically and temperamentally opposites. Dr. Cooley was from a well-known Texas family and did his training at Johns Hopkins on the East Coast. Dr. De-Bakey was a son of Lebanese immigrants to Louisiana and had established an amazing reputation already in Texas. The move of Dr. Liatta to Cooley, who was bringing his (and what Dr. DeBakey claimed was his) artificial heart to Coo-ley, was looked upon as treason by DeBakey, the mentor and twelve years Coo-ley's senior (in his autobiography Cooley denied that the device was stolen from DeBakey). They were enemies for forty years until they reconciled when De-Bakey was 99 and Cooley 87 years old in 2007. Their feud is reminiscent of the John Adams-Thomas Jefferson feud with a reconciliation at the end of their lives (incidentally, Adams and Jefferson both died on July 4th, 1826) or Yogi Berra and George Steinbrenner, the NY Yankees manager (they finally recon-ciled fourteen years later).

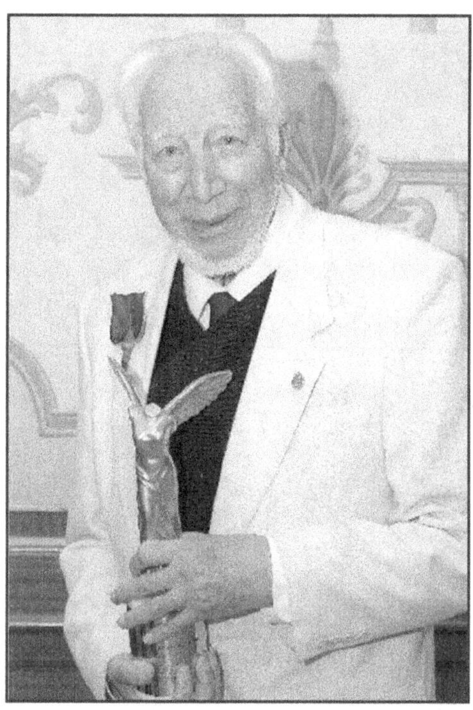

Willem Kolff permission: Lasker Society

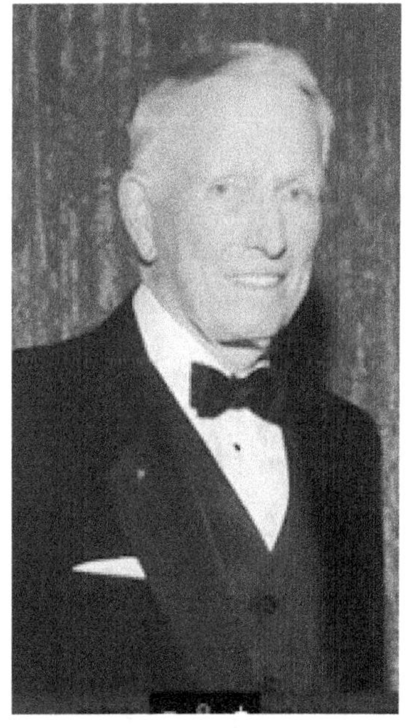

DENTON COOLEY
permission of Dr.
Yong-Jian Geng's
personal collection

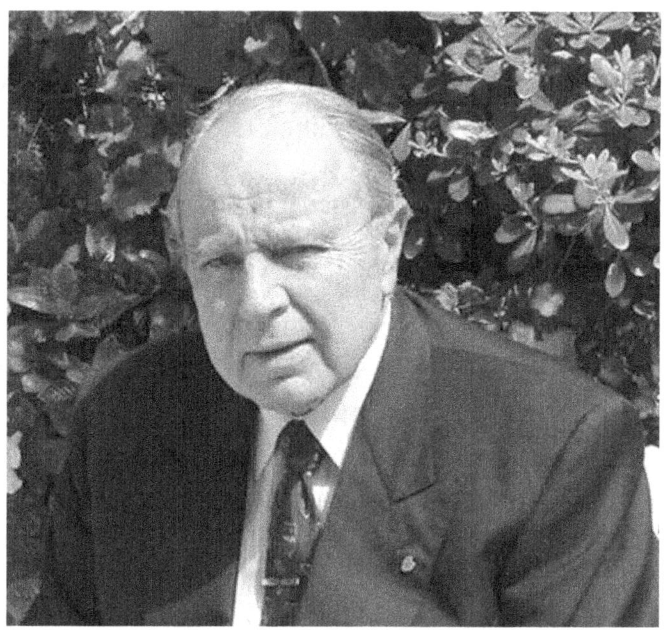

DOMINGO LIOTTA
permission: creative Commons Wikimedia

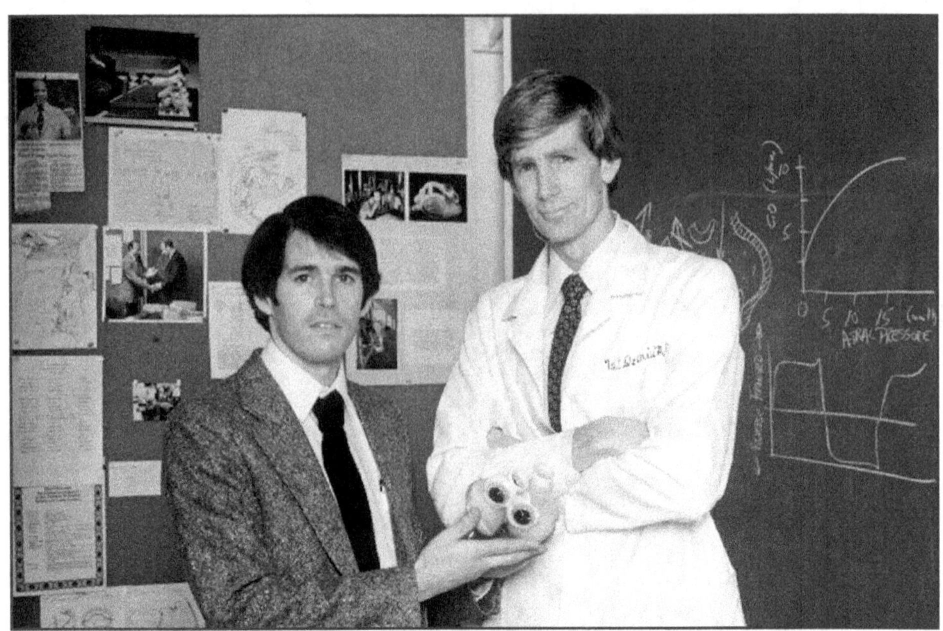

ROBERT JARVIK and WLLIAM DEVRIES
Hank Morgan/License by Science Photo Library

Dr. Robert Jarvik (1946-, born Midland, Michigan, U.S.) is known for inventing, along with Williem Kolff, the first total artificial heart that was successful in humans after working with calves. He worked on the invention with Dr. Willem Kolff who, in the meantime, left the Cleveland Clinic for the University of Utah (it is said that Dr. Kolff always wanted the name of the device to go to the person with whom he was working). The Jarvik 7 (aluminum and polyurethane device connected to a 400-pound air compressor outside the patient) was first implanted in 1982 into a patient.

The patient was Barney Clark, who lived 112 days after his procedure performed by the heart surgeon by William DeVries (1943-, born Brooklyn, NY, U.S.) from the University of Utah and who was working with Jarvik and Kolff. Subsequently patients were living up to fourteen months with the air-powered Jarvik 7 pump. In 2004 the FDA approved the Jarvik as a bridge to transplant. Remember that these early artificial hearts had the pumps externally and were replacements for both ventricles internally. The first totally self-contained internal artificial heart by AbioCor, weighing two pounds, was implanted in 2001 with FDA approval in 2006. The totally internal heart was made possible due to miniaturization, biosensors, plastics and rechargeable energy sources.

Only fifteen patients received this device, including one after FDA approval. The SynCardia replaced the AbioCor. Clots within the artificial heart continued to plague the inventors, surgeons, and receiving patients. Over six hundred patients have received the SynCardia Total Artificial Heart but also with an external energy source known as a driver. The longest living recipient of an artificial heart, Jarvik 7, implanted in a hospital in Louisville, Kentucky, lived 620 days with it.

What has become more common and as a bridge to transplantation are implantations of the LVAD (left ventricular assist devices) to take over the work of a very diseased left ventricle until a transplant can be found and performed and occasionally a RVAD (right ventricular assist device) when the right ventricle fails.

An elderly patient of mine, who was 85 years of age and had been my patient for over thirty years, had severe heart failure and was not a candidate for cardiac transplantation based on age nor was he a candidate for coronary artery bypass based on the anatomy at heart catheterization. He was offered by our cardiac surgeons an LVAD for life prolongation. The pump was outside the body and required recharging regularly. After two months, he was found on the floor dead with the connection from his LVAD to the external pump disconnected, a finding that we confirmed was impossible to occur accidentally. He clearly had decided that even his extra life given by the pump was not tolerable and worth it.

GLOSSARY CHAPTER 13

Artificial heart – device to assume the heart's function. Most have external to the body energy sources

CHAPTER 14
ELECTROPHYSIOLOGY (EP)

When I was a medical resident rotating in the CCU at the Beth Israel Hospital in 1969, the field of electrophysiology was in its infancy. Available then were pacemakers with leads placed on the chest wall externally but used only when a patient was unconscious, for the electrical stimulus would be quite painful. One day I had a patient in a potentially fatal rhythm known as ventricular tachycardia (a rapid and potentially fatal rapid heart rate from the bottom of the heart, i.e. from the right or left ventricle). I wondered if I could pace him out of it with electrical stimuli to restore the rhythm, but it worked for only a few seconds. I turned on the external pacemaker and applied the leads to the unconscious patient's chest and was able to "capture" his heart (i.e. pace his heart) if the pacer set rate was higher than his own, which was already quite fast. The ventricular tachycardia stopped but each time I turned down the rate of the pacemaker, his ventricular tachycardia was seen again and not aborted by pacing. I gave up and felt this technique would not work. Unfortunately, I was not persistent enough or had an unusual patient, as subsequently electrophysiologists have used this technique to terminate ventricular tachycardia. I was close to the solution but not able to cross the finish line. Furthermore, I was unaware that Dr. Paul Zoll, only seven years earlier, in 1960, had demonstrated and published that by increasing the rate of an external pacemaker, he could terminate ventricular tachycardia. Ironically, I was in the very same hospital where Dr. Paul Zoll practiced and trying my technique with Dr. Zoll's own designed external pacemaker. It has subsequently become an accepted technique and is programmed into pacemaker and internal defibrillator software design before delivering an electrical shock.

Electrophysiology (also known as EP) is probably the most complicated of all cardiology specialties. To simplify this complex field, let me try to explain what it is.

Electrophysiology is the study of irregular rhythms of the heart and understanding their mechanisms and treatments. The treatment is sometimes medication and sometimes a procedure burning out the focus of the irregular heartbeat or arrhythmia, called ablation. Many practitioners of this field, i.e. electrophysiologists, also place pacemakers and automatic defibrillators. Because the father of electrophysiology started his studies with atrial fibrillation, a brief discussion of atrial fibrillation will follow. But the reader should understand that atrial fibrillation is only one of many irregular rhythms of the heart (known as arrhythmias). Unlike the coronary artery tree and coronary artery disease, where many nonphysicians have some idea about blood flow and its relationship to heart attacks, electrophysiology, also known as EP for short, is much more complicated and less well known to the public than the field of heart attacks and blocked coronary arteries.

Being very complex, electrophysiology even today is still in its infancy despite over one hundred years of study and research. I like to say that electrophysiology is at the stage interventional cardiology (angioplasty, coronary artery stents, TAVR, repair and replacement of heart valves without surgery) was fifteen to twenty years ago, but electrophysiology is quickly catching up.

The heart is basically a pump, with the heart muscle receiving blood and pushing it around the entire body to each organ. It should be remembered that the heart requires an energy source that is an electrical stimulus as its signal to pump mechanically. This is the function of the electrical system of the heart, which has tissue wires analogous to the electrical wires connected to my laptop, allowing me to type this book. The electrical stimulus starts at the top right of the heart, the right atrium, in the sinoatrial node (SA node for short) and spreads to the other atrium (left) and down the right atrium to the interventricular septum, the muscle separating the right and left ventricles. There is a way station at the top of the interventricular septum that divides the right and left ventricles, and this station is a web or node of fibers called the atrial ventricular node (AV node for short). The AV node's job is to slow down the speed of conduction so that the heart will not beat too rapidly in order to maintain a normal blood pressure, which would fall if the heartbeat was too fast. It takes under two-tenths of a second for the electricity to travel from the sinoatrial node through the AV node (150-160 milliseconds) and then 45-60 milliseconds to traverse down the interventricular septum through what is known as the bundle of HIS and finally reach the heart muscle, where it branches into a right-sided branch (the right bundle) and a left side (the left bundle). Finally these nerves branch into multiple small fibers known as the Purkinje fibers, which tell the heart muscle to contract when their electricity finally reaches the heart muscle. Whew!

Arrhythmias are irregularities of the electrical heartbeat. Sometimes only a single irregular beat occurs, sometimes for short periods of time and sometimes continuously. As a rule of thumb, arrhythmias from the upper part of the heart (the atria) may be bothersome but rarely fatal. Conversely, arrhythmias from the lower part of the heart (ventricles) may be catastrophic, leading to either fainting or death. Some ventricular arrhythmias are short-lasting and benign and may even be asymptomatic. The EKG is required to distinguish the location and sometimes the danger!

What is the story about the electricity of the heart, and who were the scientists who made the great discoveries? We must start with the basis of the heart's electrical signal, the electrical conducting system.

ELECTRICAL CONDUCTING SYSTEM

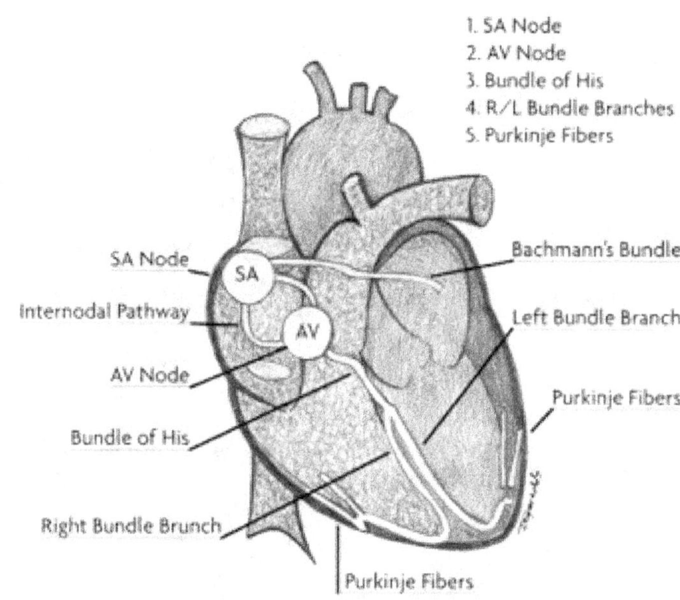

Drawing by D. Gavasheli, from author's personal collection

First it took multiple scientists to determine that the heart produced electricity. But the real coup was from five anatomists who dissected and identified each fiber component separately. The initial scientists included, in 1842, Dr.

Carlo Matteucci (1811-1868, born Forli, Italy, and died Ardenza, near Livorno, Italy), working at the University of Pisa in Italy. He discovered that each heartbeat in the frog produced an electrical current. This was an inspirational groundbreaker in the electrical understanding of the heartbeat.

The British physician and physiologist Augustus Desire Waller (1856-1922, born Paris, France, and died London, England) recorded the first human electrocardiogram in 1887, and even Einthoven (inventor of the EKG) acknowledged his important contribution. Waller used an instrument known as a capillary electrometer with leads on the front and back of a patient. Waller showed that electrical activity preceded each mechanical contraction of the ventricle. He could not record atrial activity unlike the EKGs of today because his instrument was neither sensitive enough nor free of background noise. But he did coin the term "electrocardiogram," which Einthoven picked up and is still used today. Waller also noted that the heart muscle started its contraction at the apex (the tip) and ended its motion at the base (closer to the head) of the ventricles, a finding long forgotten until recently. It should be noted that Einthoven called his machine the "electrocardiogram" or "EKG" for short The term in recent years in Canada and in he U.S. has been changed to "ECG," but I shall stay with EKG for historical reasons and because it is still the term of preference in most of Europe.

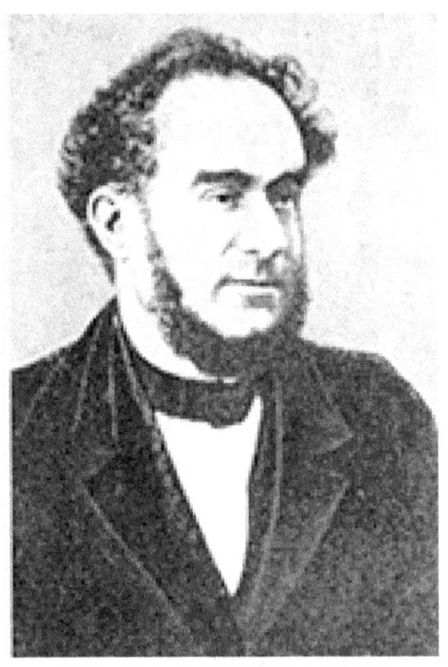

CARLO MATTEUCCI
public domain

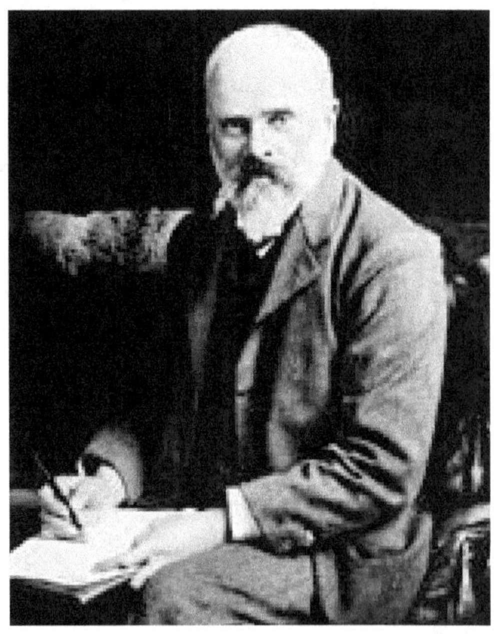

AUGUSTUS D. WALLER
National Library of Medicine

It took scientists seventy years to determine how the heart's electricity traveled down to the ventricles. The consensus came from five anatomists who dissected and identified each component separately.

The earliest description of a segment of the conduction system was by Johannes Purkyne (a.k.a. Purkinje) (1787-1869, born Libochovice, Czechoslovakia, and died Prague, Czechoslovakia). Examining sheep hearts in 1839, he discovered the anatomic fibers of large neurons, which carried electricity to the ventricles to excite mechanical contraction and its many branches. These are now known by his name as Purkinje fibers. They are the end of the line of the heart's wired electrical system.

He lived in the Austro-Hungarian empire. When he discovered his finding in 1839, the first opium war broke out between China and Britain. The new Republic of Texas in the new world started a war with the Cherokee Indians when the president of Texas, Mirabeau B. Lamar, announced that it was time to exterminate the Cherokees, also in 1839. The Brits were fighting in Afghanistan in 1839, and the first photograph of the moon was taken by the French photographer Louis Daguerre in January of 1839. Not long after this the Crimean War between Russia and the United Kingdom allied with France, Sardinia-Piedmont (part of Italy) and Turkey against Russia was fought in 1853. Russia lost territory at the war's conclusion. Triggering the Crimean War was a dispute between Czar Nicholas I and the Ottoman emperor in present-day Turkey, Abdulmejid, who had authority over Christians living under the Ottomans. The famous Charge of the Light Brigade occurred during this war.

Next came along a Swiss scientist, Willhelm His (1863-1934, born Basel, Switzerland, and died Lorrach, Germany), who discovered in 1893 a muscle bundle in the interventricular septum connecting to the Purkinje system below, which also helped transmit electrical impulses. His father was a well-known and respected anatomist.

Willhelm His was convinced and one of the earliest to realize that the heartbeat had its origin in the individual cells of heart muscle. Besides being an excellent scientist, he was also a proficient violinist and painter. Despite being Swiss by birth, he became a German citizen and served in the medical corps of the German army in World War I.

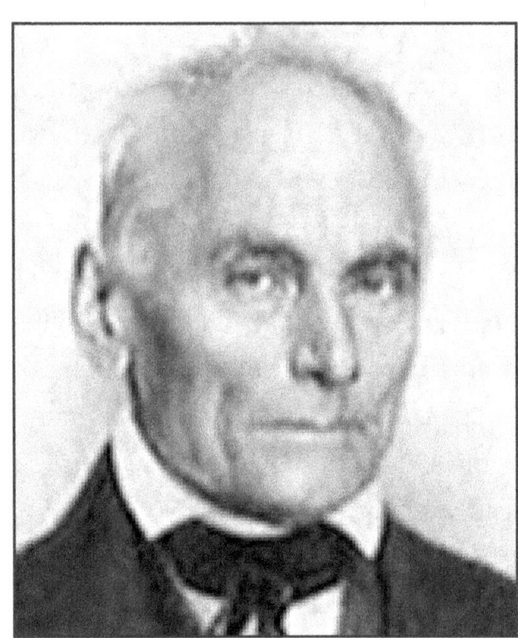

JOHANNES PURKINJE,
National Library of Congress, public domain

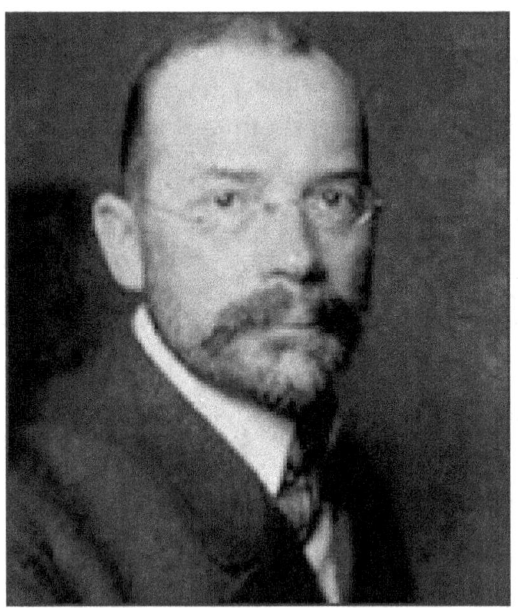

WILHELM HIS, public domain

The search for the origin of the heartbeat was partially discovered by Walter Gaskell (1847-1914, born Naples, Italy, and died Great Shelford, UK), who found during his research from 1874 to 1899 that the initial trigger for the heartbeat was electrical from somewhere in the upper-right atrium, although it took another researcher to find the precise location in the sinoatrial node (SA node). Gaskell found that the electrical current went from the atrium down to the ventricles and concluded that the autonomic nervous system (fight-or-flight center) had strong control over the heart rate. He made zigzag incisions in the heart's electrical conducting system, causing a discontinuity of the upper and lower heartbeat, which he named "heart block," a term still used today when the atria beat independently and not sequentially with the ventricles (often this requires a pacemaker for treatment).

Gaskell lived in the Victorian era of England, when the empire continued to grow and enrich itself. England became the first global industrial power. It also produced most of the world's coal, iron, steel and textiles.

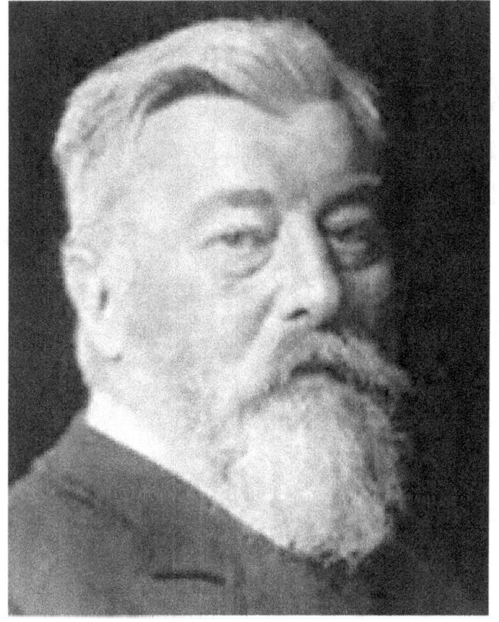

WALTER GASKELL,
Alamy License

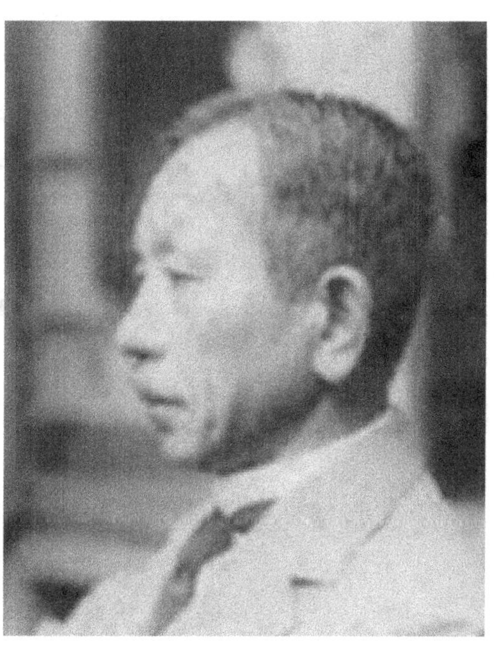

SUNAO TAWARA,
public domain

Sunao Tawara (1873-1952, born Oita Prefecture, Japan, and died Oita Prefecture, Japan) was a Japanese pathologist who discovered the atrioventricular node (AV node), which sits at the top of the interventricular septum and slows electrical conduction time, preventing the heart under normal circumstances from beating too rapidly. He discovered the treelike structure of the AV node, which is contiguous with the HIS bundle system below it. Tawara studied in Marburg, Germany, but went back to his native Japan in 1906, a year after making his historic AV node discovery in 1905 while still in Germany.

When Tawara made his discovery, the Russo-Japanese War had just been fought over the Manchurian Peninsula for control over resources by Russia against Japan. It started in 1904, when Japan attacked the Russians at Port Arthur on the Manchurian coast. This was a surprise attack without provocation or a declaration of war. A first Russian revolution in 1905 occurred after Russia lost to the Japanese. Some temporary democratic reforms occurred after the war in Russia, which were all nullified when the communists took over in the 1917 revolution. In 1917 the Russian communists deposed and killed Czar Nicholas II and his family. The Russo-Japanese War was the first war to unleash a brutality not previously seen in battle, according to experts. U.S. President Theodore Roosevelt helped craft a treaty to end the war in 1905, which Japan won due to its naval superiority.

Finally, the Scotsman Arthur Keith, along with his Oxford medical student Martin Flack, discovered the "wonderful structure in the right atrium" in the small animal the mole in 1907. They named it the sino atrial node (SA node), which is at the high-right atrium near the outside wall.

This occurred during the time of the suffragette movement in England, with a large rally occurring in 1908. In 1907 Russia and England signed a treaty to ally them together. Many think this treaty helped determine the origins of World War I, as these two nations allied themselves along with Serbia, France and Italy before the entry of the U.S. to fight the Germany, Austria-Hungary, Bulgaria, and the Ottoman Empire alliance.

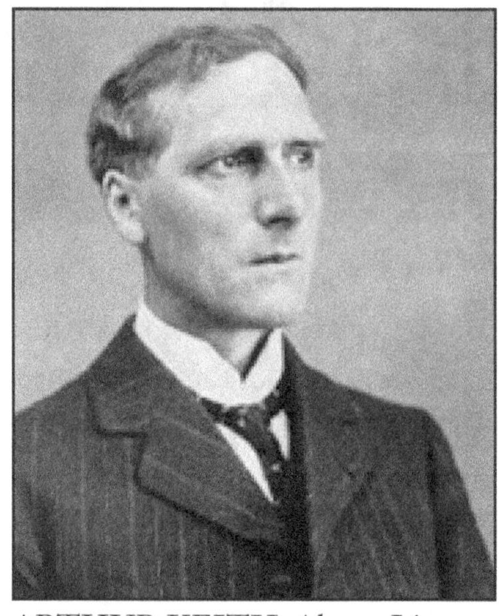

ARTHUR KEITH, Alamy License

The various components of the heart's electrical system, as you have already noted, were discovered from bottom up or the reverse of the actual direction of electrical depolarization, which starts at the top of the heart and travels down to the bottom. The SA node was discovered in 1907, AV node in 1905, Bundle of HIS in 1893 and the Purkinje network in 1839. The SA node is the dominant determinant of the heart rate or, as Anthony Gomes says in his textbook *Heart Rhythm Disorders*, the "Maestro of the conducting system."

Lastly, Jean George Bachmann (1877-1959, born Mulhouse, Alsace, France, and died Atlanta, Georgia) in 1916 discovered the last component of the cellular electrical pathway later named for him. The "Bachman's Bundle" goes from the upper-right atrium to the left atrium.

He was a talented and interesting man. After running away from home in France, he joined the Merchant Marines but settled in the U.S. and went to medical school at Jefferson Medical College in Philadelphia, graduating in 1907 at the top of his class, and then served in the U.S. Army in WWI. He became the first professor of physiology in 1915 at Emory University in Atlanta, Georgia. He was known for his wit, art, cooking, and humor, as well as his intelligence.

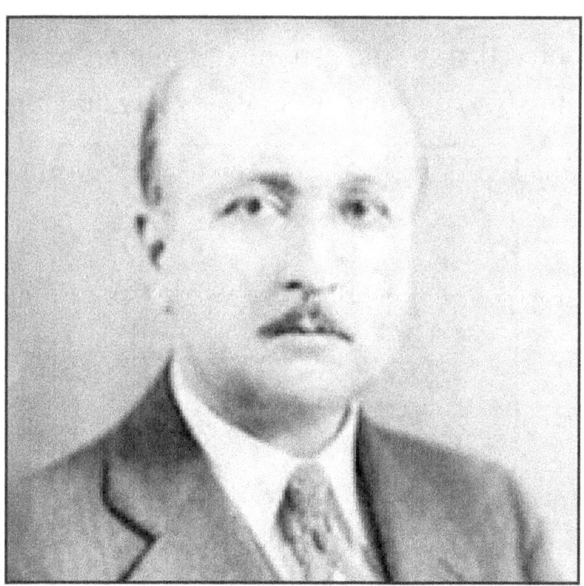

JEAN GEORGE BACHMANN
permission of Atlanta History Photograph collection, Kenan Research Library

Without Einthoven's invention of the EKG (also known as ECG) machine, there would be no field of electrophysiology. The EKG opened the first door to understanding arrhythmias in ways impossible for physicians who came before this invention. The title of Father of Electrophysiology goes to Sir Thomas Lewis (1881-1945, born Cardiff, Wales, UK, and died Breconshire, Wales, UK). He used the first EKG machine that was available in England in 1908 and had his own machine brought from Germany in 1909. One of his great contributions to cardiology was teaching his profession the value clinically of the EKG in diagnosing heart disease. The early tracings taken by Lewis in 1909 showed an irregular rhythm with normal-looking QRS complexes, which is atrial fibrillation, but the fibrillatory waves from the atrial fibrillation were not apparent until several years later on an improved version of the EKG machine. This allowed Lewis to prove that atrial fibrillation arose in the upper part of the heart, although it would take a Frenchman, Michel Haissaguerre (1955-, born Bayonne, France) in Bordeaux nearly ninety years later to show that most atrial fibrillation actually started from extra heartbeats in the pulmonary veins leading into the left atrium.

The pulmonary vein origin of these beats then becomes quite rapid, producing atrial fibrillation. This occurs due to left atrial muscle extending into the pulmonary veins, which empty oxygenated blood into the left atrium. A discussion of atrial fibrillation and its treatment is beyond the scope of this book, but it should be noted that it is an extremely common condition occurring in young and old, with 30% of people over age seventy developing it.

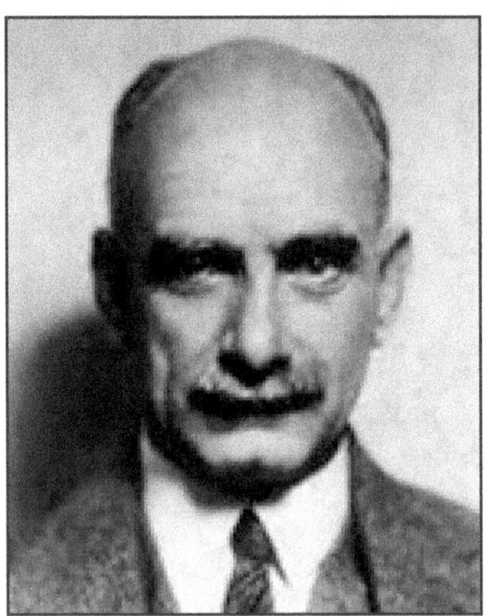

THOMAS LEWIS
public domain

Over 50% of stroke patients have strokes caused by atrial fibrillation, so prolonged use of blood thinners is required to prevent a stroke once atrial fibrillation is diagnosed, even if it converts back to normal rhythm since reoccurrence
is so common. Medications such as quinidine, procainamide, disopyramide, beta
blockers (such as carvedilol or metoprolol), propafenone, flecainide, droneda-
rone, digoxin, verapamil, diltiazem, sotalol, dofetilide, and amiodarone are
among the medications used by themselves or in combination to maintain a normal rhythm (sinus rhythm). To convert atrial fibrillation to sinus rhythm electrical cardioversion (electrical "zapping is a commonly used procedure to return
the rhythm to normal. The patient is asleep via IV propofol sedation, and the
operator pushes a button set to a certain electrical wattage connected by wires
from the control unit to two leads attached to the patient's chest. The leads are
near the right shoulder and at the left nipple area or in the middle of the front
of the chest and directly behind on the spine at the same level. However, when
recurrent atrial fibrillation becomes a clinical nuisance, a surgical procedure
known as a Cox-Maze procedure was developed in the late 1980s and performed
using surgical slicing inside the heart to isolate the part of the heart causing
atrial fibrillation. Today, most attempts to rid the heart of atrial fibrillation are
performed with a catheter and a procedure known as ablation. It basically is cau-
terizing electrically by radiofrequency, burning out the initiating focus around
the four pulmonary veins as they enter the left atrium. The radiofrequency ablation of each pulmonary vein is performed with as small wire-coated catheter
with a magnet at its tip to create a 3D map showing the origin and path of the
arrhythmia to ablate. Then the radiofrequency catheter with a small loop like a
lasso on the end is used to deliver the cautery where each pulmonary vein enters
the left atrium. The first ablation attempt to prevent recurrence of atrial fibrillation was performed by Dr. Melvin Scheinman(1935-, born NY City, NY) in
1983 using D/C electrical shocks. But the procedure really did not take off until
Dr. Haissaguerre showed in 1998 that a circular-tipped radiofrequency catheter
(like a lasso) in the mouth of each pulmonary vein for ablation was more effective in preventing recurrent atrial fibrillation than Scheinman's approach. Improvements continue even today with a new method known as pulsed field
ablation recently becoming more and more popular in the EP field and advertised as being safer.

Once the conduction pathway map was developed and understood, invasive electrophysiology awaited to be born. With the invention of Einthoven's EKG machine, many of the abnormal rhythms of the heart could be identified, understood, and their origins located within this electrical map.

A major contribution to this understanding was first due to the invention of the ambulatory EKG machine to record heart rhythms for days or longer and invented by Norman "Jeff" Holter (1914-1983, born Helena, Montana, U.S., and died Helena, Montana, U.S.) in 1947 and whose name is now associated with his invention, the "Holter Monitor." It originally weighed 83 pounds and was hardly very portable to be used in an ambulatory settring, but modern updated versions with two electrodes on the chest attached to a small box worn around the waist now weigh under a pound and newer subtypes, being mere small patches two to three inches in length and one to two inches wide at most, weighing but a few ounces and adhering to the chest wall, are widely used. These are made by several companies and can be worn for up to two weeks at a time, allowing intermittent abnormalities of the rhythm often to be detected when only 24-48 hours of most Holter monitor machines may miss them. These new versions allow all activities of daily life not to interfere with the recording, and the machine weighs only a few ounces and does not interfere with exercise. Occasionally a very small recording chip is buried under the skin, allowing monitoring and analysis for up to a year with external interrogation from time to time, determined by the physician. Pacemakers and internal defibrillators were only possible after the conduction system was discovered and explained. These are often placed by EP specialists and sometimes surgeons.

The modern way of monitoring a patient's heart rhythm is the use of a small patch, which can be worn regardless of activity. The one prohibition is that patients cannot swim or take a bath with it on but can shower as long as they turn away from the water source or the adhesive will weaken, preventing good electrical recordings. My patients knew my personality and my tendency to joke with them, so as a reminder not to get the monitor patch very wet and to keep their back to the shower, I would often say in jest, "Don't forget to turn away from the showerhead when taking a shower. I still feel guilty, as I lost three patients last year who were electrocuted in the shower because I forgot to tell them this." Then I quickly explain that they cannot be electrocuted with the patch getting wet but that the adhesive may no longer work. Hopefully my little prank helped them to remember.

GROUNDBREAKING WORK FOR UPPER HEART ARRHYTHMIAS, KNOWN AS ATRIAL ARRHYTHMIAS

The man considered the Father of Modern Electrophysiology is Dirk Durrer (1918-1984, born Schiedam, Netherlands, and died Amsterdam, Netherlands), who performed the groundwork for modern EP. First studying dogs' and goats' hearts' activation using an oscilloscope and stimulator built by a physicist college, Henk van der Tweel, he then began a project to study the normal human heart electrical activation. He noted that braindead patients had a pulse for one to seven hours after ventilation was stopped. But his most important contribution was being first, with his colleague Hein Wellens, to develop the technique known as programmed electrical stimulation (PES). In PES extra beats are delivered at the right time in the cardiac cycle by stimulating the right atrium by attaching a metal-tipped catheter placed in the heart to an electrical stimulator externally. Using this technique, they were able to initiate and terminate the rapid heart rate originating in the right atrium known as supraventricular tachycardia. Durrer and his college Hein Wellens (1935-2000, born the Hague, Netherlands, and died Maastricht, Netherlands) both Disruptors reported their results in 1967 on a patient with a rapid heart rate from the right atrium (supraventricular tachycardia) who had Wolf-Parkinson-White syndrome (WPW for short), named after the three cardiologists, Drs. Louis Wolf (whom I knew when I was a medical student and intern at the Beth Israel Hospital in Boston), John Parkinson, and Paul Dudley White, in which there is an abnormal anatomic electrical bypass tract from atrium to ventricle, circumventing the AV node, causing some patients to develop a rapid heart rhythm, 180-240 beats a minute.

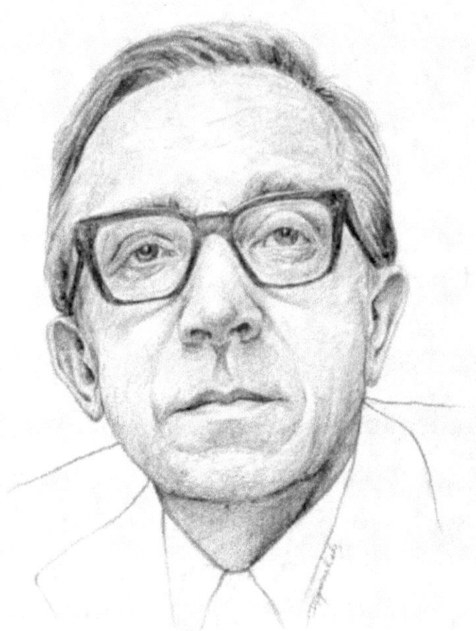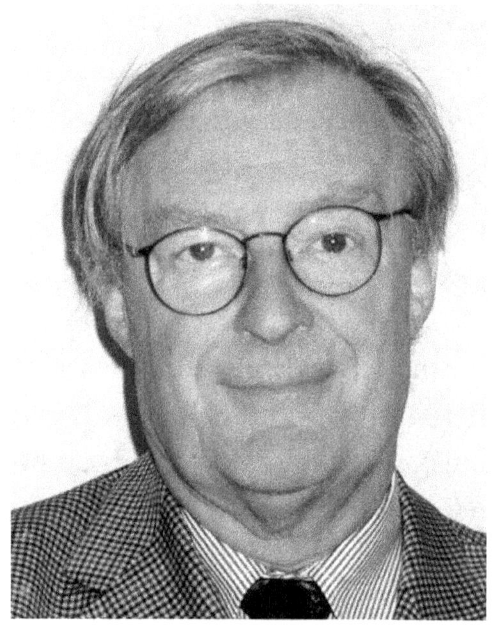

DIRK DURRER, permission of Lasker Foundation and redrawn by David Gavasheli

HEIN WELLENS, permission of Heart Rhythm Society

Almost simultaneously but after Durrer and Wellens performed programmed electrical stimulation and also in 1967, a French team led by Philippe Coumel (1935-2004, born Lyon, France, and died Paris, France) reported the same finding in a patient with a similar rapid atrial heart rhythm (being abnormal it is referred to as an arrhythmia). Coumel contributed hundreds of research papers during his career.

Dirk Durrer eventually used tiny needles as electrodes placed directly into the heart muscle to better understand the mechanism of the arrhythmia and recorded the sequence of electrical activation when the rhythm started and mapped its spread by recording multiple sites as the heart sent out electrical signals.

In the U.S., the mentor and teacher who trained many U.S. EP leaders was Anthony N. Damato, who headed the EP lab at Staten Island U.S. Public Health Hospital. Many future contributors and groundbreakers spent two years or more under his tutelage and leadership.

When Benjamin Scherlag (1932-, born Brooklyn, NY, U.S.) and Anthony N. Damato for in 1969 developed a method for recording the HIS bundle with a catheter inside the heart near the tricuspid valve, which separates the right atrium above from the right ventricle below, this was groundbreaking by two

Disruptors. It allowed cardiologists to better diagnose difficult to diagnose arrhythmias, especially those with abnormally wide QRS complexes, to help separate life-threatening ventricular tachycardias from more benign arrhythmias with wide QRS complexes. HIS bundle recordings not only helped to localize the site and cause of many arrhythmias but also served to map the path of their movement.

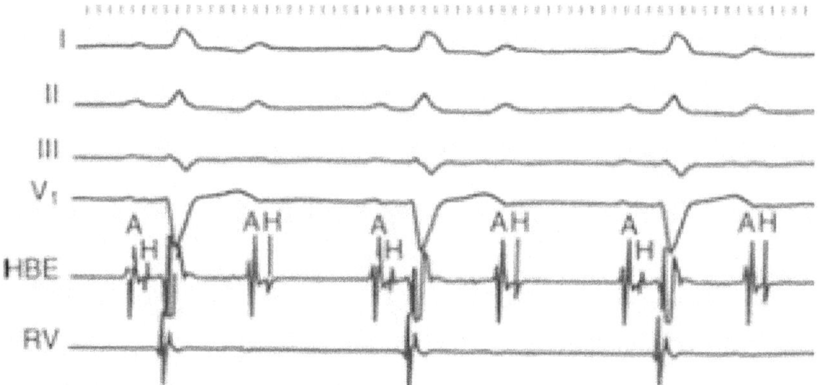

HIS bundle tracing (HBE) with a catheter in the right atrial floor, the first electrical recording is the atrium (A), then HIS bundle (H), and then the electricity from the ventricle (RV).
Note that there are two A and H for every V, indicating 2:1 block below the HIS bundle. From Atlantic Health EP lab

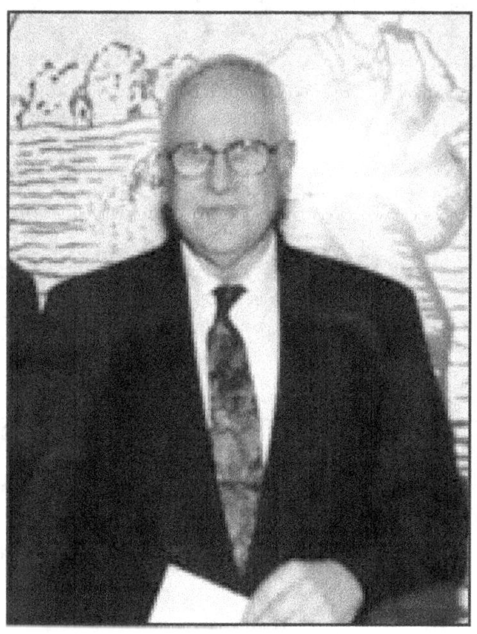

BENJAMIN SCHERLAG
courtesy Dr. Ronald Scherlag's personal collection

The Wolf-Parkinson-White syndrome (also known as preexcitation because the ventricles become electrically stimulated earlier than via the normal conduction system through the AV node due to an accessory or alternate
pathway around the AV node) was a gift to electrophysiologists, as it provided a more direct way to study electrical mapping as W-P-W had an anatomic alternate bypass tract from atrium to ventricle by bypassing the AV
node and HIS bundle fibers. Although Dirk Durrer first mapped the Wolf-
Parkinson-White accessory pathway, it took a Duke surgeon, Dr. Will Sealy
(1912-2001, born Roberta, Georgia, U.S. and died Greenville, North Carolina, U.S.) in 1968 to perform the first surgical interruption of this bypass
tract to cure the atrial arrhythmia associated with W-P-W operating on the
epicardium (outside surface of the heart). He then improved and reported
again on the improved procedure in 1974 and subsequently worked on techniques to rid the arrhythmia from the endocardial surface (i.e. inside the
heart where the heart muscle meets the blood pool). He is known as the
Father of Arrhythmia Surgery, a Disruptor.

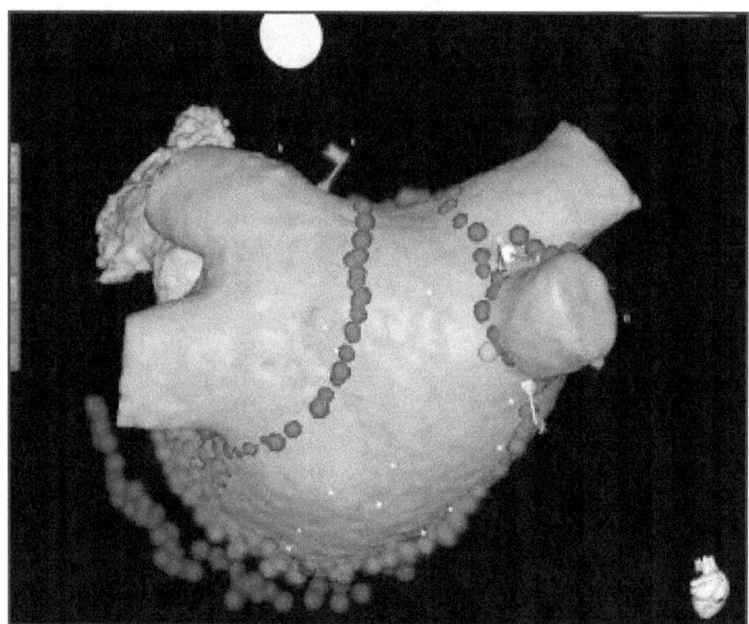

Carto electroanatomical map inside the heart, with red dots showing ablation
points in left atrium and green in coronary sinus
permission of EP Department, Morristown Memorial Hospital

John J. Gallagher (1943-2020, born Brooklyn, NY, U.S., and died Spartan-burg, South Carolina, U.S.), who was one of the students of Anthony Damato and Benjamin Scherlag at Staten Island in the EP laboratory, then went on to the faculty of Duke University Medical School as head of EP. While working with the surgeon Dr. Will Sealy, they pioneered intraoperative mapping of arrhythmias, especially Wolf-Parkinson-White syndrome and its bypass tracts, bypassing the AV node and HIS bundle to take the electrical impulse from atrium to ventricle. Their multi-sensing electrode array mapping device was like a sock placed on the heart and known as epicardial mapping (the outside surface of the heart is the epicardium), pioneered by two Disruptors.

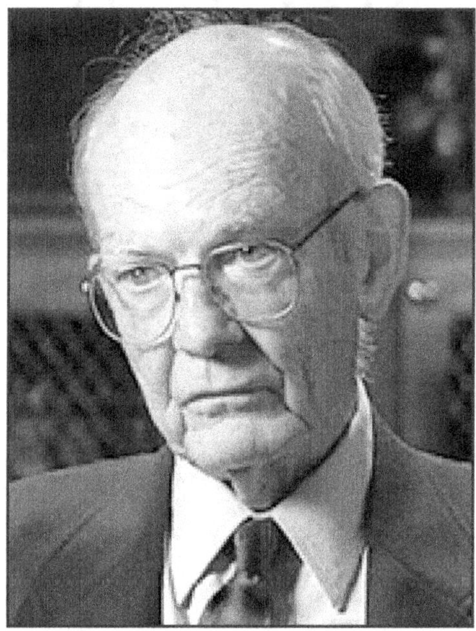

WILL SEALY,
permission of Heart Rhythm Society

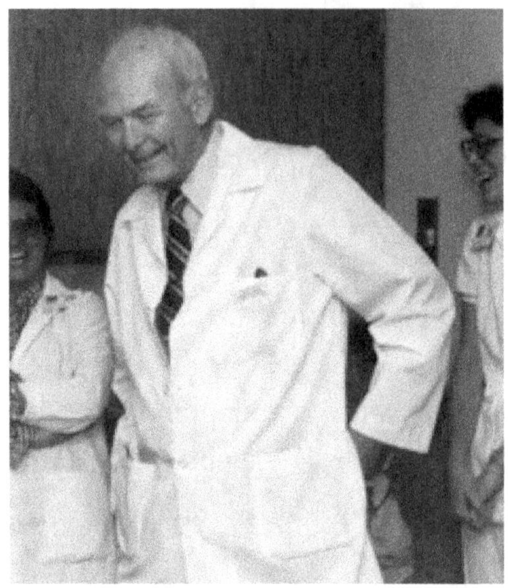
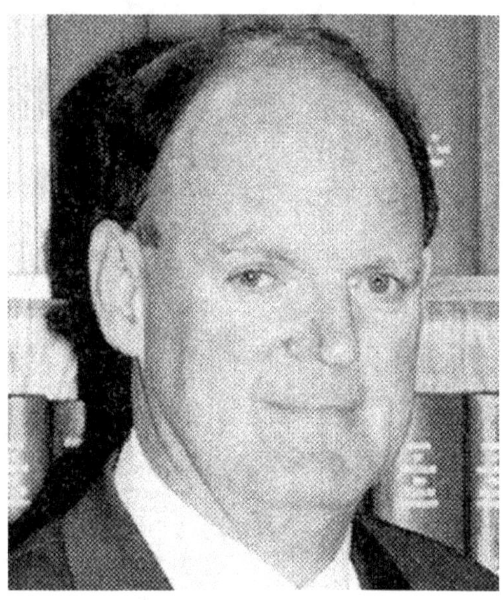

WILL SEALY
permission of Duke U Archives

JOHN GALLAGHER
permission of Heart Rhythm Society

Gallagher subsequently became involved with catheter ablation to replace the surgical approach and pioneered ablation, first starting with direct current and one of the earlier explorers of alternative ablation sources using cold cryoablation, which is now increasing in popularity by EP doctors.

Once arrhythmias were correctly localized and identified, the era of curing them was at hand. Although many medications have been used with varying degrees of success for arrhythmias, be they atrial or ventricular in origin, there has been a need to get patients off medications and permanently stop the arrhythmia. The entry of cardiac ablation into electrophysiology has been the answer. Although originally performed by a direct current ablation by Dr. Melvin Scheinman, the use of a radiofrequency ablation allowed the procedure to be performed without general anesthesia, limited surrounding tissue destruction, and did not cause subsequent arrhythmias. The 3D electricoanatomical mapping technique has revolutionized the ablation procedure by giving a visual picture to the proceduralist of where the arrhythmia begins and where its electrical path runs.

HEART BLOCK

A ventricular premature beat is a premature heart contraction that occurs early in the cycle, from one of the ventricles below, and usually interrupts the normal heart pattern, causing a feeling to the patient as if their heart temporarily stopped or fell into their abdomen (it does neither but, after a short lag, resets the normal cardiac cycle timing). To even the trained physician, such a pause while taking the pulse before diagnosing the abnormality with an EKG machine could be an atrial premature beat, ventricular premature beat, or even a type of heart block known as second degree, where most beats get through from the upper to the lower heart but some are blocked. These can all seem the same merely by feeling the pulse.

AV block can be first degree (seen in the EKG and is caused by slowing of the electricity in the AV node, second degree AV block, and third or complete AV block. In one type of second-degree block, every other beat is blocked with the alternate beat having no transmission of electricity into the ventricles below (sometimes known as Mobitz II). Another pattern is one type described by Dr. Karel Wenckebach (1864-1940, born the Hague, Netherlands, and died Vienna, Austria), with his name attached to this diagnosis. Supposedly he could take a patient's pulse and differentiate second-degree block from an atrial or ventricular premature beat (often called "skipped beats" by patients), even without an EKG (most cardiologists cannot).

Walter Gaskell, before the invention of the EKG, probably was describing complete or third-degree heart block rather than Wenckebach.

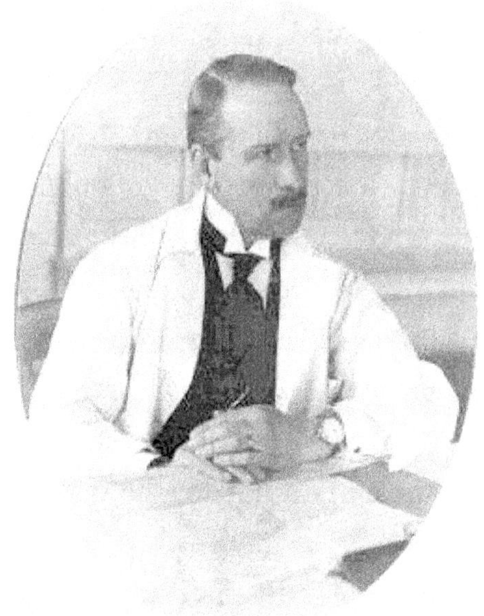

KAREL WENCKEBACH,
public domain

VENTRICULAR ARRHYTHMIAS

While at the Hospital of the University of Pennsylvania undergoing my cardiology residency training, I had the opportunity of performing EPS research with the rising star of the field, Dr. Mark Josephson, who had just finished two years at the famous Dr. Anthony Damato's electrophysiology lab in Staten Island, NY, and was now a year behind me in training at HUP. Our job was to place ventricular premature beats with a catheter placed in the right ventricle apex and gradually move the timing of these extra beats (one at a time) closer to the native EKG QRS complex to find the refractory period (when the electrical activity is blocked) to determine if this extra beat would suppress ventricular tachycardia using this technique. When two patients actually developed ventricular tachycardia during our research (both were quickly shocked and lived to tell the tale), we terminated the project after about a dozen patients in order to "reassess." I thought the subject was now taboo and finished and left the next year for a year's training in heart catheterization in Boston, leaving the field of electrophysiology forever and thinking that our research was a total bust, only to find out in a few years that it actually opened the door to amazing discoveries leading to lifesaving procedures, often pioneered by my friend Mark Josephson, who became chief of cardiology at HUP at age 38 before being recruited to the Beth Israel Hospital in Boston to lead the EP program. He unfortunately died much too early from bladder cancer.

VPCs can be benign or fatal if grouped into many successive beats for a period of time. VPC means "ventricular premature beat" or an early beat from the ventricle that resets the cardiac electrical cycle. But too many in succession can cause fainting or even lead to ventricular fibrillation and sudden death. After a heart attack, if over ten VPCs occur per hour on monitoring and the ejection fraction is under 40% (the percent of blood pumped out of the left ventricle with each heartbeat (normal is 55% or more), there is a marked increase of sudden death, as the VPC may degenerate into sustained ventricular tachycardia or even a totally disorganized rhythm from the ventricle known as ventricular fibrillation. This leads to death, as there is no output by the heart under this circumstance unless the rhythm is restored rapidly to normal by medication, electrical shock cardioversion externally or internally via an automatic defibrillator. Because of this, cardiologists since the 1970s have focused on VPCs and have tried to separate dangerous forms from benign types. Any VPC may arise from anxiety, overuse of alcohol, heart damage from heart attacks or viruses or various toxins known as cardiomyopathy or from genetically determined causes, severe valve disease, or poor sleep. They can be benign or lead to death. Three to five VPCs in a row (depending upon an arbitrary definition) is known as non-sustained ventricular tachycardia and sustained ventricular tachycardia as VPCs for thirty seconds or more, which is ominous. The problem is that cardiologists for years have tried to identify, with minimal success, who will be subject to a dangerous ventricular arrhythmia before it occurs.

Studies have found that low ejection fractions (i.e. 35% or less) are associated with more VPCs per hour. One study found 52% of the VPCs originating from the right ventricle and 48% from the left ventricle. Holter monitors of patients for 48 hours have demonstrated that 75% of normal subjects will have some VPCs but only 4% have more than 60/hour. Even a normally pumping heart with very frequent VPCs can become weakened and develop a very reduced ejection fraction if over 24% of heartbeats (i.e. about a quarter) are VPCs. This is called VPC-induced cardiomyopathy. Not all VPCs require treatment. Doctors reserve treatment for when the patient is severely bothered by them or at risk of dying suddenly, especially if an underlying cause is suggested.

Two of the pioneers of the field of electrophysiology were either a friend or teacher of mine when I was a cardiology resident (known as fellow) in 1972-1974 at the Hospital of the University of Pennsylvania in Philadelphia. Dr. Bruce Goldreyer was new to the institution and had already made a name for himself while at the Staten Island VA Hospital working with Dr. Anthony Damato. I had the privilege of performing early electrophysiologic research with Dr. Goldreyer and was lucky enough to even be first author on one of his publications. The other was a friend and a year behind me at HUP, Dr. Mark Josephson. He was short and had a low, gruff voice but was exceedingly friendly and understatedly brilliant with his sense of humor always shining through. He not only discovered many of the early findings in electrophysiology, EP as it is now known, but became known as a master teacher and mentor to many in the field who followed him. I went another direction as an interventional cardiologist in angioplasty and coronary artery stenting. One of my co-fellows, a friend and future cardiac partner in practice for over 47 years, Dr. Arthur Fisch, came into the EP lab one day during one of our studies on patients and somewhat jokingly said we were there to kill as many patients as possible with our research study. Fortunately no one died, but when two transiently required defibrillation I began to wonder. Several years after I left Penn for practice in NJ, I learned that the work I was helping on (it was really the research of Dr. Goldreyer and Josephson) led to many of the future discoveries on how to treat the life-threatening heart irregularity known as ventricular tachycardia. Of course, this allowed me to joke with my partner, Art Fisch, that what he called "killing our experiments" (none died) actually led to saving countless lives.

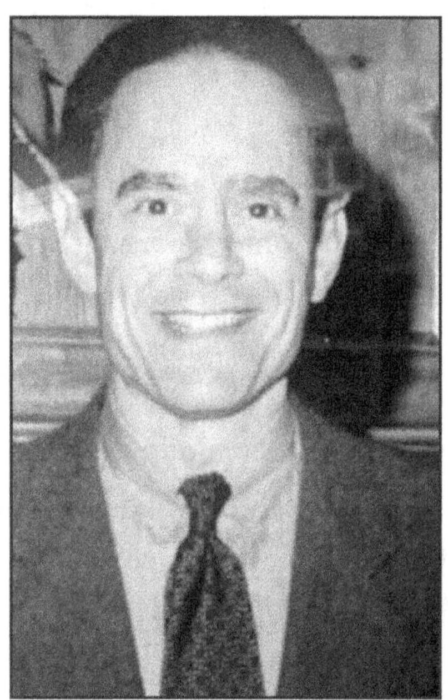

ARTHUR FISCH
Author's personal collection

One of the most important researchers to investigate ventricular arrhythmias was Dr. Mark Josephson. Dr. Mark Josephson (1943-2017, born NYC, NY, U.S., and died Boston, Massachusetts, U.S.) was a year behind me in cardiology residency at the Hospital of the University of Pennsylvania, and I considered him a friend. Short in stature but a giant intellectually and with a wry and sometimes biting sense of humor, any lack of height was more than made up for by his sharp intelligence, insight, creative scientific thinking, and friendliness. He had spent two years with Dr. Anthony Damato in his Staten Island, U.S., Public

Health Service Hospital lab as many of the pioneers of EP had previously done before Dr. Josephson came to the Hospital of the University of Pennsylvania.

He made his mark in cardiology and EP with ventricular premature beat mapping and stimulation that allowed cardiologists to identify where the dangerous ventricular arrhythmia was arising and how much of the damaged heart muscle was causing it, usually due to a heart attack. The ventricular tachycardia comes from barely alive tissue adjacent to the actual dead heart attack tissue. This led to a technique published in 1979 to cure the arrhythmia surgically by removing the inciting area. This is the research for which Josephson is best remembered. It became known as the "Pennsylvania Peel" (developed at the Hospital of the University of Pennsylvania), where the dead tissue along the inner lining of the left ventricle was mapped and removed. Technically it was called subendocardial resection. Dr. Josephson was the mapping physician and Dr. Alden Harken (1941-, born Boston, Mass., U.S.), son of the famous Dr. Dwight Harken, was the surgeon. Before his death Josephson wrote numerous papers and was known for his clinical teaching at seminars around the world. I am sure his wry humor kept everyone guessing but attentive. It can be said that Dr. Josephson helped transform "electrophysiology from a research tool to a powerful clinical tool." These scientists were important Disruptors.

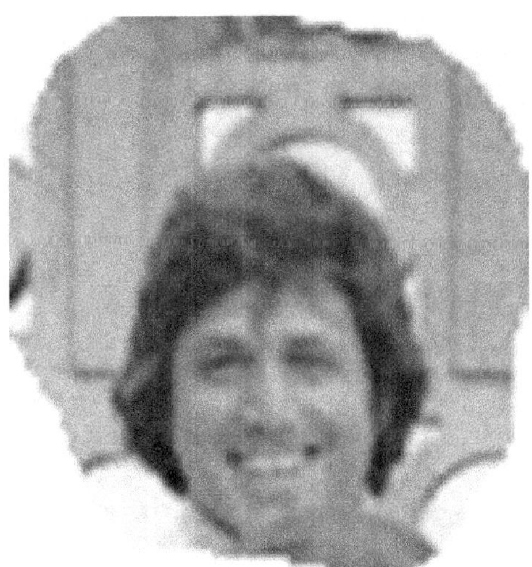

MARK JOSEPHSON,
as a fellow from author's personal
collection

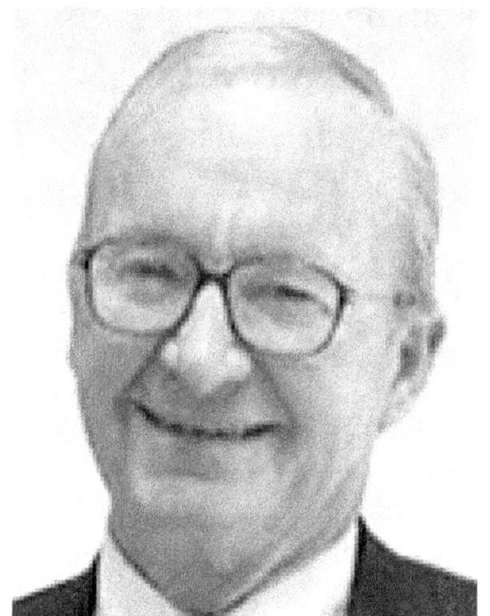

ALDEN HARKEN,
with his permission from Dr.
Harken's personal collection

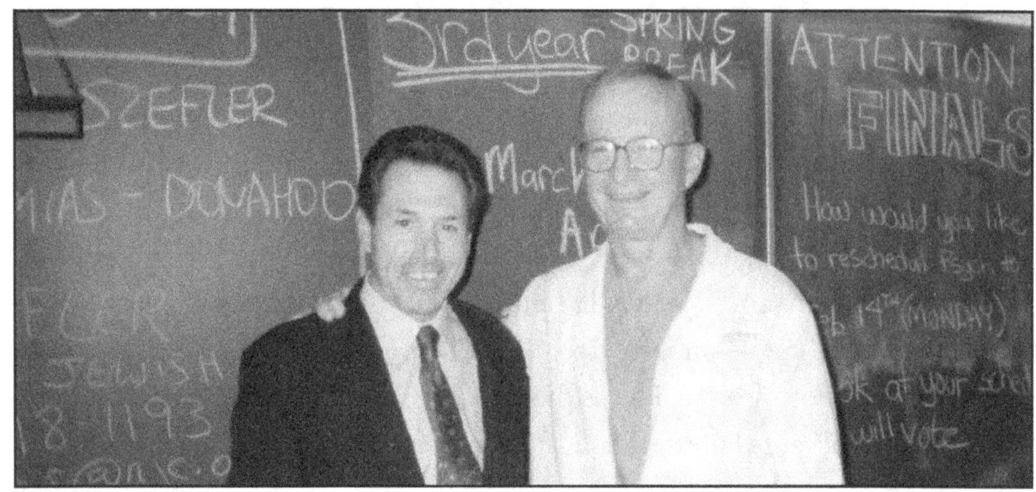

MARK JOSEPHSON AND ALDEN HARKEN, given with permission by Dr. Alden Harken, from his personal collection, photo taken by a friend

Hein Wellens, after his work with Dirk Durrer on atrial arrhythmia, reported triggering ventricular tachycardia in the laboratory with one appropriately placed and timed VPC in the right ventricle in five patients with previous attacks of ventricular tachycardia. He could then terminate the ventricular tachycardia (VT) with an appropriately timed single extra beat from his external stimulator. At the time he was criticized by the EP community as performing unethical and dangerous experiments, and the paper took one and one half years 'til it was finally accepted for publication and finally published in 1972. Once again we see the scenario of the Disruptor versus the Restrainers.

Over the years a multitude of anti-arrhythmic drugs for ventricular tachycardia have been abandoned except for beta blockers and a more potentially toxic amiodarone, as some studies showed excess mortality trying to suppress pharmacologically the ventricular tachycardia, possibly as a side-effect of the intended suppressive medication. Internal defibrillators invented by Mirowski have been the mainstay with some patients benefitting from ablation of the ventricular tachycardia source. Although automatic internal cardiac defibrillators (AICD) can treat ventricular tachycardia, the internal shock can be painful and produce future fear and anxiety. They are not a cure but a therapy.

Some attempts have been made to eliminate the substrate source of ventricular tachycardia (VT) by ablation. There has been limited success with this goal, but the recent data show improved and promising results. Remember that automatic implantable defibrillators discussed in Chapter 8 are to treat VT, not prevent it. Physicians sought to prevent VT by mapping the myocardial source and then eliminating it completely with radiofrequency ablation.

Originally there was some hope that bypassing blocked coronary arteries and excising the heart attack scar known as an aneurysm might prevent further ventricular tachycardia, and some of the earliest cases were reported by Charles Bailey in Philadelphia in 1955 and O. A. Couch in 1959, who reported successful excisions of aneurysms (dead ballooned-out left ventricular tissue) before the era of coronary artery bypass surgery. Subsequently, reports of combined aneurysm resections and coronary artery bypass for VT were published in the literature, but the results were unpredictable in prevention of subsequent sudden death. The Pennsylvania Peel was mentioned above in the discussion of Dr. Mark Josephson. Although mapping and then cutting out the inner-layer source of the VT was often successful and groundbreaking, in follow-up a relatively high mortality of 5-15% was obtained, especially if there was a previous heart attack.

However, ablation either from the outside of the heart (epicardial, which requires surgery) or from the inside via catheter is possible but has a limited patient referral source and is usually limited to patients who have failed or are intolerant of other therapies. They tend to be referred to this as a last resort. As a result, data on success of this technique for a wider group of patients who are early in their courses is quite limited. The patients are usually divided into two major groups with VT, those who have blocked coronary arteries usually with previous myocardial infarction (ischemic VT) and those who have VT from other causes, often genetically determined (nonischemic VT). However, knowing that the source of VT by EP mapping was from the endocardial layer of the ventricle (i.e. the layer close to the blood pool), the next logical step was to try ablation by cardiologists using catheters. The source of VT is not from the dead tissue but from live tissue adjacent to the heart attack scar, and often barely surviving in between the scarred and normal heart muscle. Francis Marchlinski (1951-, born Nanticoke, Pennsylvania, U.S.) of the Hospital of the University of Pennsylvania first performed catheter ablation for VT with radiofrequency and without detailed mapping in his early cases and reported his results in 2000. It mimicked surgical resection.

Moreover, non-ischemic (not due to coronary artery disease-produced scarring) can be more challenging and less effective for an ablation response, as the midportion of the heart muscle may be the source rather than the sub-endocardial (next to the blood pool) origin of VT as caused after a heart attack. One of the other pioneers in VT ablation is William G. Stevenson, who was at the Peter Bent Brigham Hospital in Boston and then moved to Vanderbilt Medical School in Nashville, Tennessee, in 2017. He is known for his work developing novel methods of mapping and innovative ablation techniques for VT. In 2007 a multigroup trial from the Massachusetts General Hospital and Beth Israel Hospital in Boston and Prague, Czech Republic, reported in the prestigious *New England Journal of Medicine* on a group of patients who had implantable AICD (defibrillators) after previous heart attacks, which caused a previous episode of VT. The group was evenly divided with 64 patients in the "AICD-only" group and 64 patients with an AICD but also mapped and ablated by a catheter to eliminate the VT focus in the heart. Both groups were at risk since in the follow-up of almost two years 33% of the AICD-only group had an appropriate shock for VT and would have died without their defibrillator vs. only 12% of the group that had both AICD and ablation required a shock after the ablation procedure. So there was some help with ablation, reducing recurrent VT, but it is not perfect.

Although the trend for a lower mortality in the ablation group was found (9% vs. 17%), the difference between the two groups did not reach statistical significance. Mortality may not have been the best measured outcome since the control group's lives were often saved since they had AICDs to shock a dangerous arrhythmia if it occurred.

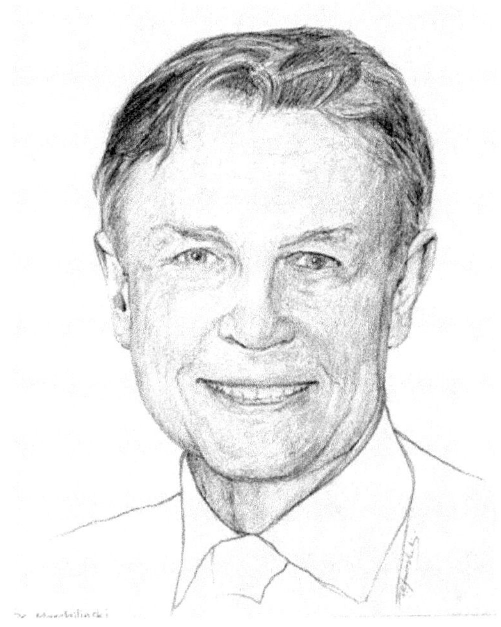 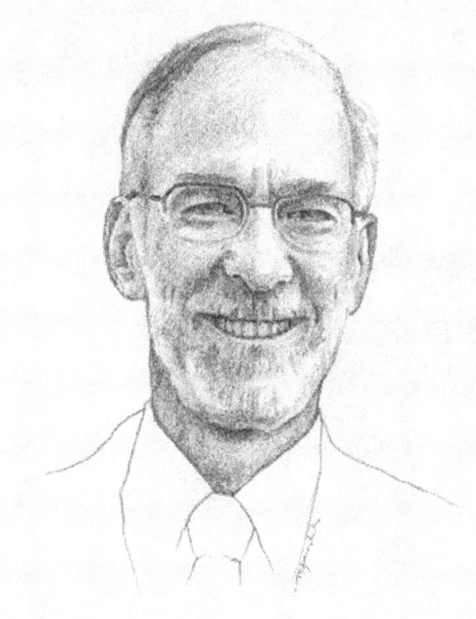

FRANCIS MARCHLINSKI, by D. Gavasheli   WILLIAM STEVENSON by D. Gavasheli

from photos permitted by Dr. Stevenson and Dr. Marchilinski

GLOSSARY CHAPTER 14

Ablation – burning out of a focus starting in heart muscle, usually with radio-frequency waves

Arrhythmia – any abnormal rhythm of the heart

Ventricular tachycardia – rapid and often fatal arrhythmia from the lower part of the heart, either from the right or left ventricle

CHAPTER 15

THE GOOD AND THE BAD AND? "THE UGLY" – CHOLESTEROL – THE RESEARCH THAT MADE STATINS POSSIBLE

Although cholesterol is thought of as bad, and too much can lead to vascular disease, including heart attacks, it is actually essential for life and is incorporated into the membrane of every living cell as a requirement for cell function and protection including, serving as a wall and gate to decide what to let into the cell and what to keep out. Ninety percent of the body's cholesterol is contained in these cell membranes (envelope surrounding cells). But cholesterol is also needed to make certain hormones such as testosterone (male hormone), estrogens (female hormone) and cortisol (anti-inflammation hormones). It is a balance between TOO much and TOO little that determines good and bad effects. So despite a public debate, cholesterol is not to be avoided but something we need to survive, although in moderation and, depending upon one's genetic makeup, occasionally avoided. Cholesterol is manufactured (synthesized) in the liver but also obtained exogenously from food in the diet, which is absorbed from the GI tract, packaged into particles and transported in the blood as small packets called lipoproteins (combination of fat and protein). As a rule of thumb, too high a level of LDL cholesterol is bad and a high level of HDL cholesterol is good, although the issue is much more complex and out of the realm of a discussion in a history book. People may have a condition known as familial hypercholesterolemia, with five times the level of cholesterol in the blood as normal if they inherit this gene from both parents (i.e. they have a double copy) or if only one parent's gene is inherited (i.e. one copy), and these people will have two to three times the level of cholesterol compared to normal people with neither genotype. Those with two copies of the gene develop atherosclerotic heart disease early in life, including in adolescence, and are known as homozygous hypercholesterolemia patients. With one copy the atherosclerosis, including heart attacks, occurs a bit later, usually age 35-50, but much more common than in a normal person and at a younger age than normal people. This type with one gene received is called heterozygous hypercholesterolemia. Twenty-five percent of the adult deaths in the western industrialized world are from blockages in the coronary arteries with atherosclerotic plaques.

Cholesterol was isolated from gallstones by the French physician and chemist Francois Poulletier (1719-1789, born Lyon, France, and died Paris, France), possibly in 1758 (his work was never published but his attribution is from contemporaries). Assuming this to be correct, he was the first to isolate pure cholesterol as crystals. Thirty years later Michel E. Chevreul (1786-1889, born Angers, France, and died Paris, France) named this substance "cholesterine" for bile (chole) and stereos (solid). He lived during the time of the French Revolution of 1789-1799. His main work revolutionized soaps. In addition he was the first to demonstrate that diabetics excreted glucose in the urine. He is among 72 scientists whose names are inscribed on the Eiffel Tower. In 1888 the Austrian botanist Friedrich Reinitzer (1857-1927, born Prague, Czechoslovakia, and died Graz, Austria) established the molecular formula for cholesterol. But the actual structure for cholesterol was discovered by Heinrich O. Wieland (1877-1957, born Pforzheim, Germany, and died Starnberg, Germany) and Adolf Windaus (1876-1959, born Berlin, Germany, and died Gottingen, Germany), who both received Nobel Prizes for their efforts in 1927 (Wieland) and 1928 (Windaus). Their Nobel Prizes were given between WWI and WWII, just before the great worldwide depression of 1929-1939, which led to the dictatorial takeover of Germany by Adolf Hitler from 1933 to 1945. Windaus also discovered in 1910 that the cheesy substance in plaques (atherosclerosis) contained cholesterol.

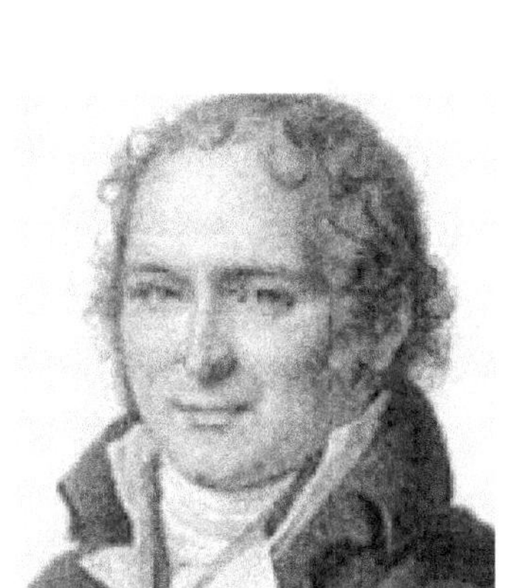

FRANÇOIS POULLETIER,
public domain

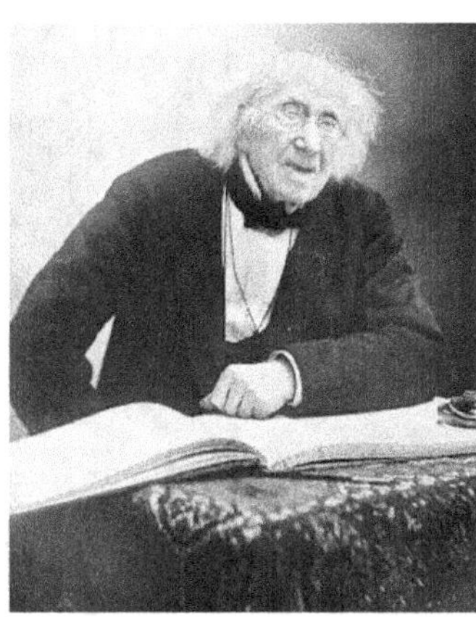

EUGENE CHEVREUL,
public domain

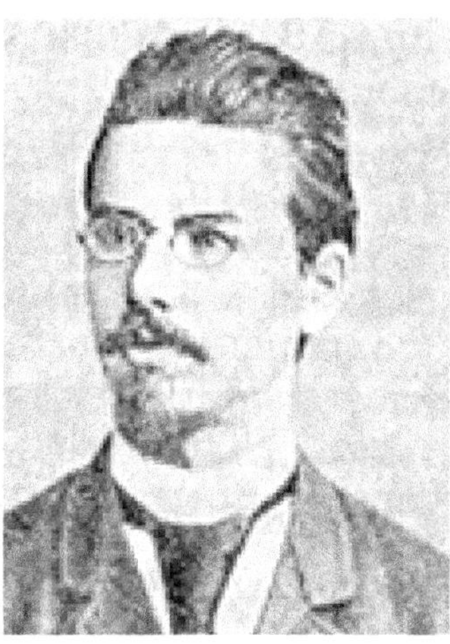

FRIEDRICH REINITZER,
public domain

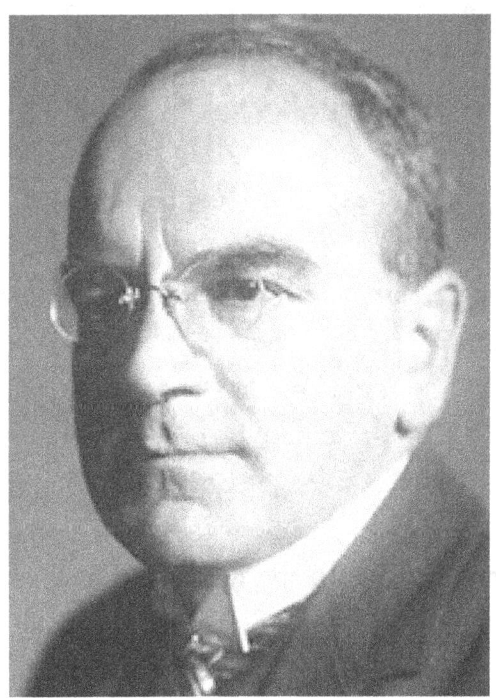

HEINRICH OTTO WIELAND
public domain

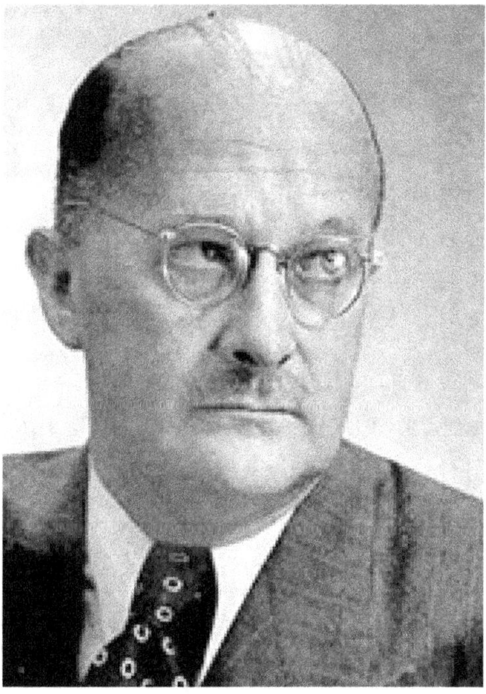

ADOLF WINDAUS
public domain

Windaus was the first to hint at the cardiovascular effects of cholesterol accumulation when he reported in 1910 that plaques (accumulations of fatty substances) in the aorta (the main artery exiting the heart) contained twenty times the amount of cholesterol as normal aortas. Three years later the Russian scientist Nikolay Anichkov (1885-1964, born and died St. Petersburg, Russia) in 1913 fed pure cholesterol to his experimental rabbits and produced high blood cholesterol levels in the animals and atherosclerotic plaques in their aortas. Thus, he is the first scientist to link dietary cholesterol intake to atherosclerosis.

Anichkov lived from the time of the last czars of Russia through much of the Communist regime of the Soviet Union, including during the leadership of Nikita Khrushchev, who famously hammered his shoe at the United Nations in 1960 but withdrew his guided missiles aimed at the U.S. from Cuba during the infamous Cuban Missile Crisis of 1962, averting a world war. Khrushchev also introduced some liberalization in the Soviet Union, known as "The Thaw," after Joseph Stalin died in 1953, including reducing the number of political prisoners in the Gulag camps. In 1956 he denounced Stalin and the "cult of personality." A 1957 coup against Khruschev failed, and he expelled his enemies from the Communist Party. His policy of "Peaceful Coexistence" with the U.S. led to the Geneva Summit and traveling to Camp David in 1959 to meet with President Eisenhower. But the thaw was damaged by the downing of a U.S. spy plane over the Soviet Union, flown by Francis Gary Powers, in 1960, the construction of the Berlin Wall in 1961 and, of course, the Cuban Missile Crisis in 1962. At the UN in 1960, when Khrushchev may have hammered his shoe on the podium during his speech against colonialism (there is debate whether he actually used it as a gavel or only removed his shoe and pretended to bang the table with it, setting himself up as a hotheaded buffoon), a representative of the government of the Philippines charged that he was a hypocrite since the Soviet Union dominated over much of Eastern Europe.

Two findings gave inspiration to Michael S. Brown and Joseph L. Goldstein, the discoverers of the LDL receptor. In 1933 Rudolph Schoenheimer (1898-1941, born Berlin, Germany, and died New York, NY, U.S.), a German-American working in Germany, placed mice in a sealed bottle and fed them a cholesterol-free diet. Despite this, he found that the cholesterol content of the bottle increased, showing mice were capable of synthesizing cholesterol even without dietary intake of this fat. When fed a diet high in cholesterol, the mice no longer produced cholesterol in the bottle, demonstrating a negative feedback or inhibition of cholesterol synthesis when given in large amounts to animals. This, according to Brown and

Goldstein (see below), "laid the groundwork for the discovery of LDL receptors in the 1970s." Schoenheimer also helped establish that cholesterol was a risk factor in atherosclerosis. He unfortunately committed suicide using cyanide in 1941, having suffered manic depression all of his life.

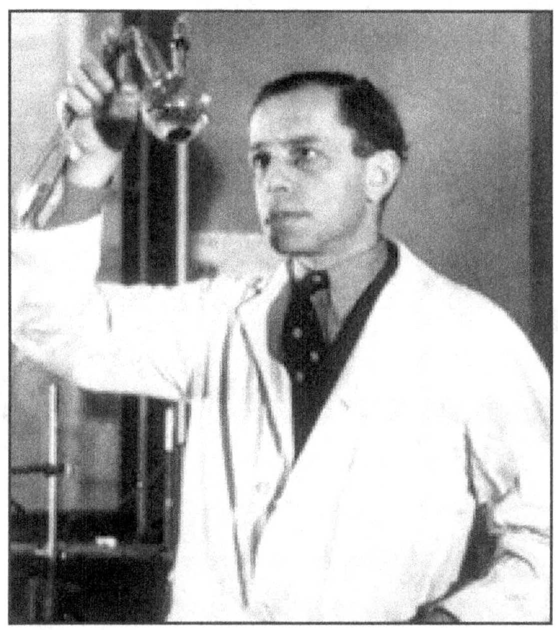

ADOLF SCHOENHEIMER,
public domain

Konrad E. Bloch (1912-2000, born Neisse, Poland (Silesia), and died Burlington, Massachusetts, U.S.) and Feodor Lynen (1911-1979, born and died Munich, Germany) worked out the thirty crucial enzymatic steps in the synthesis of cholesterol. Bloch fled the Nazi persecution of Jews and came to the U.S. in 1936, receiving his Ph.D. from Columbia University and finally becoming a Harvard professor of biochemistry. Bloch and Lynen shared the Nobel Prize for Physiology or Medicine in 1964. The third reaction in the first of four stages in cholesterol synthesis is due to HMG-CoA conversion to mevalonate, and its enzyme (enzymes allow chemical reactions to occur) when blocked by statin drugs inhibits the production of cholesterol in the liver, leading to a reduction of blood cholesterol and LDL cholesterol levels.

They both received the Nobel Prize in 1964.

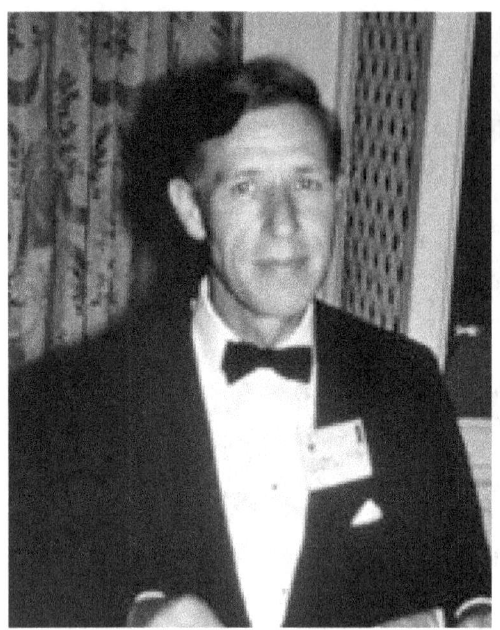
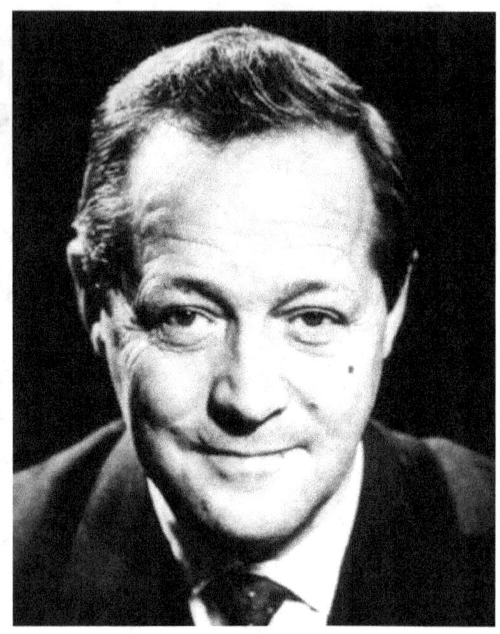

KONRAD E. BLOCH
by Peter Geymeyer, released license
to public domain

FEODOR LYNEN
National Library of
Medicine/Science photo library

In 1938 a Norwegian physician, Carl Muller (1886-1983), described families with high plasma cholesterol levels (serum is the liquid removed from clotted blood, but plasma is the light yellow liquid portion of unclotted blood) transmitted as an autosomal dominant (i.e. a person with only one gene from either the mother or from the father will have the disease), known as familial heterozygous hypercholesterolemia, with a twentyfold increased risk of heart attacks compared to the general population. Despite little data, he correctly advised his patient to adhere to a low-cholesterol diet. Muller was the first to recognize the association between high blood cholesterol and nodules of cholesterol over tendons called xanthomata.

In 1964 Avedis K. Khachadurian (1926-2022, born Beirut, Lebanon, and died New Brunswick, NJ, U.S.A.) discovered an even rarer form of hypercholesterolemia in Lebanon with 52 patients having a genetic disease where patients have a gene from each parent (homozygous whereas Muller's patients with one gene only were heterozygous) have an even higher blood cholesterol level and even more heart disease at an extremely young ages 5-25 years vs. 35-60 years of age in Muller's patients. Fortunately, the homozygous form affects only one in one million people vs. about one in 1500 people with the Muller heterozygous form.

In 1951 Dr. Paul Dudley White (1886-1973, born Roxbury, Mass., and died Boston, Mass., U.S.) and coworkers, including Menard M. Gertler (1920-2015, born Saskatoon, Canada, and died NY, NY, U.S. – no photo available) at the Massachusetts General Hospital in Boston (Harvard), recognized a group of characteristics that increased a person's chances of a heart attack—male sex, high blood cholesterol, high blood pressure, smoking cigarettes, a family history of premature coronary disease, and obesity. These factors continue to be relevant today.

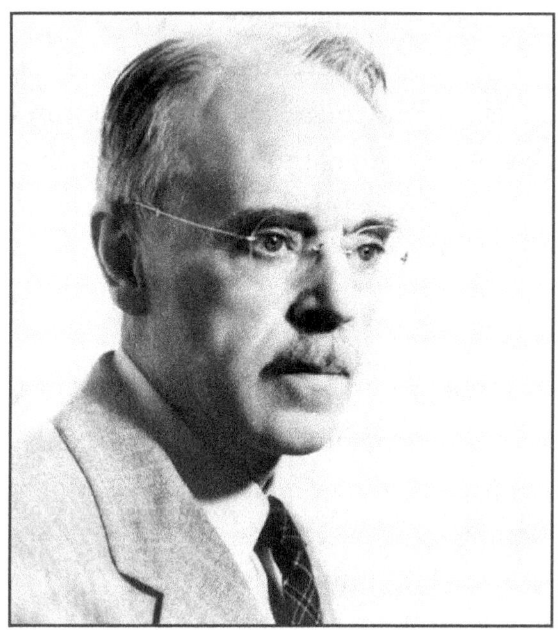

PAUL DUDLEY WHITE
permission: Lasker Foundation

In 1953 Ancel Keys (1904-2004, born Colorado Springs, Colorado, U.S., and died Minneapolis, Minnesota, U.S.) from the University of Minnesota started a large international study of heart attack patients in sixteen different countries. A group of men ages 40-60 were followed for ten years, recording fatal and nonfatal heart attacks and blood levels of cholesterol. The two extremes of baseline cholesterol measurements were as low as 165mg/dl (milligrams per deciliter of blood) in Japanese fishermen primarily on a diet of fish and vegetables vs. 270mg/dl in Finnish lumbermen who ate a large amount of red meat. The Finns had a thirteenfold increase in heart attacks compared to their Japanese counterparts. He concluded that a diet rich in fat and cholesterol not only raised the blood cholesterol (serum) but the incidence of heart attacks. Keys also noted that Japanese populations in Japan, Hawaii and California had a greater dietary fat intake as they moved eastward toward the U.S. mainland. Similarly blood cholesterols levels also increased with this migration pattern. This was the first epidemiologic study of diet and cholesterol intake. The mechanism of a heart attack is a plaque that enlarges until it splits in one area (ruptures), leading to formation of a blood clot and a heart attack. Where in-flammation enters in this process is uncertain but probably is a component and possibly the initiating factor. Keys developed a complex formula but found that saturated fats increased total cholesterol and LDL cholesterol twice as much as polyunsaturated fats, which tended to lower cholesterol and LDL choles-terol. Keys had his critics, including those who pointed out that France, which has a high-fat diet, also has a low coronary heart disease incidence but was left out of his study. Such "picking and choosing" or "cherry picking" may have biased his overall results. Nor did he consider whether sugar played a part in heart disease.

Around the same time the FRAMINGHAM HEART STUDY was launched in 1948 with government money by the U.S. Public Health Service in over five thousand male and female people in Framingham, Massachusetts, ages 30-61 years old. The goal was to identify risk factors that contribute to coronary artery disease. Currently the population followed has increased to fourteen thousand people over three generations. The results of this longitudi-nal study helped to identify high blood cholesterol and high blood pressure as two major contributors to developing coronary artery disease. Phase II started in 1971, enrolling 5124 people of the second generation, and in 2002 Phase III enrolled the third generation. A score was developed, and if one's score was 16% chance of heart disease development or more over five years, it was considered a high risk of having a heart attack or stroke or other blood vessel disease. The calculator is still used but is not perfect and sometimes inaccurate, so a new test known as the Coronary Artery Calcium Score, which is more precise (see chap-ter on new technologies) in detecting current and predicting future disease, came along. Thomas Royle Dawber (1913-2005, born Duncan, British Columbia, Canada, and died Naples, Florida, U.S.) was the first Framingham Heart Study director from 1949 to 1966. He left due to budget cuts and moved from Framingham to Boston and continued to raise money to keep the study going.

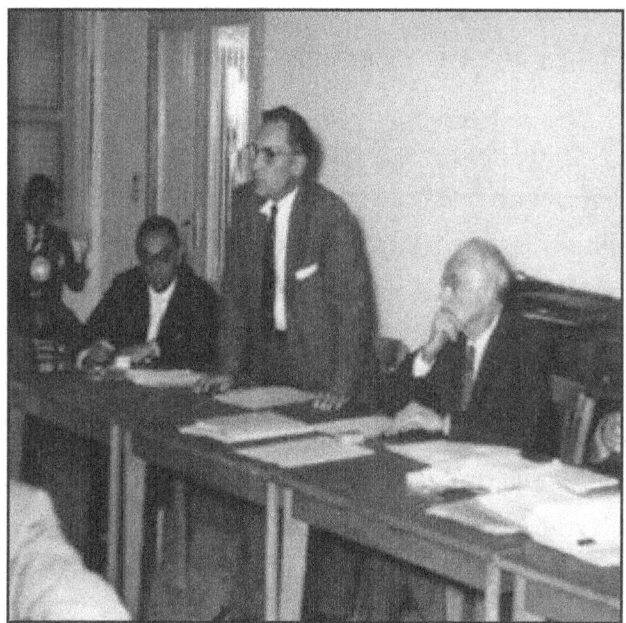

ANCEL CANCEL KEYS
standing and Paul D. White sitting Alamy License

John Gofman (1918-2007, born Cleveland, Ohio, U.S., and died San Francisco, California, U.S.) is considered the "Father of Clinical Lipidology. " Interestingly Gofman went to work on the Manhattan Project as his first career, as he was in nuclear physics and chemistry. He co-discovered Uranium-233 and recognized its fission ability. At J. Robert Oppenheimer's request, he isolated milligram quantities of plutonium. Using one of the few world's ultracentrifuges he discovered "protein X," later found to be the LDL cholesterol component. This extremely important discovery by John Gofman was made in 1955. However, the start of his career on the Manhattan Project would not predict the end of his career as a cholesterol researcher who separated cholesterol components by the density of their carrier proteins using similar ultracentrifuges. He discovered LDL and HDL and, at the time, made the correlation between patients with heart attacks and high levels of LDL cholesterol as well as low levels of HDL cholesterol (although this second observation was ignored for two decades). His lipid research was actually aided by his experience on the Manhattan

Project using sophisticated centrifuges. The relationship between heart attacks and LDL levels even applies to other mammals (so take care of your dogs and cats). The LDL particle contains molecules of cholesterol in the center surrounded by a phospholipid (another kind of fat with a phosphorus group called phosphate) coat and a single large protein known as apolipoprotein B, or apoB for short.

The apoB is recognized by white blood cells known as macrophages, which swallow up the apoB with its cholesterol, creating foam cells that incite inflammation by releasing certain irritating chemicals called cytokines. In response to this inflammation, the lining of arteries produces substances leading to growth of plaque formation. These plaques eventually form splits and cause clots to form on and/or within the splits, which block the artery blood flow, causing a heart attack or stroke. As Brown and Goldstein wrote, "all in all, the higher the LDL, the faster the plaque evolves." The risk factors described by Paul D. White and M. Gertler accelerate this process also.

Two investigators and Disruptors who spent their professional careers studying cholesterol were Michael S. Brown (1941-, born Brooklyn, NY, U.S.) and Joseph L. Goldstein (1940-, born Sumter, South Carolina, U.S.). Both shared the Nobel Prize for medicine for their work in 1985 on the regulation of cholesterol. In 1973 they discovered the receptor in cells that takes up and incorporates cholesterol into the cell. Brown graduated from the U of Pennsylvania School of Medicine in 1966 and met Joseph Goldstein at the Massachusetts General Hospital, where they were both interns and residents in internal medicine and became friends. Brown went to the NIH (National Institutes of Health in Bethesda, Maryland) for research in 1966-1971, where he learned enzymology under Earl R. Stadtman, a pioneer in the field. After leaving the NIH in 1971 to join the staff of Southwestern Medical School in Dallas, Brown joined forces with his friend who was already there, Joseph Goldstein. There Brown synthesized 3-hydroxy-3-methylglutaryl coenzymes A reductase, found to be the controlling enzyme for cholesterol biosynthesis in the liver. He collaborated with Dr. Joseph Goldstein in 1972 and combined their labs in 1974. Although both also served as attending physicians teaching medical students and medical residents, they were extremely productive in the lab as well. Goldstein had also gone to the NIH where he worked for Marshall W. Nirenberg (Nobel Laureate in Physiology or Medicine in 1968) and also worked with Donald S. Fredrickson, a world's expert in lipid disorders. He convinced Brown to come to the University of Texas Health Science Center in Dallas to collaborate on genetic cholesterol metabolism. Together Brown and Goldstein discovered the LDL receptor, which takes up cholesterol into liver cells as the LDL receptor binds the LDL-cholesterol in the blood. When taken up into the cell, the LDL inhibits HMG-CoA reductase, which would normally help the cell make its own cholesterol. There are no functional receptors in the homozygous familial hyper-cholesterol patients (ala Khachadurian) with two copies of the gene (having either none or all nonfunctional LDL receptors) and fewer than the normal amount of receptors if only one copy of the gene was present (heterozygous hypercholesterolemia ala Muller). Furthermore, they discovered the LDL receptor not only binds the LDL cholesterol, but it regulates the passage into the cell of cholesterol. This in turn inhibits the cell not only from making more LDL receptors but also from manufacturing more cholesterol by inhibiting the enzyme HMG-CoA reductase, which initiates cholesterol pathway of synthesis within the cell. With no receptors, there is no inhibition of this process, a bad prognosis for that person. With fewer than normal receptors (one gene), only half the normal inhibition occurs, also bad but not as bad. With not enough functional LDL receptors, the turned away LDL-cholesterol may end up invading arteries and creating a process to block arteries, known as atherosclerosis. Brown and Goldstein chemically characterized the LDL receptor as well as describing its function. For their work Brown and Goldstein were awarded the 1985 Nobel Prize for Physiology or Medicine. Their discoveries have helped shape treatment today and in the future, including leading to the discovery of statin drugs to lower blood cholesterol and reduce cardiovascular disease. At the Nobel ceremony presentation to Brown and Goldstein in 1985, the presenter said, "Brown and Goldstein's discoveries have lead to new principles for treatment and prevention of atherosclerosis." He added, "It may one day be possible for people to have their steak and live to enjoy it, too." The importance of cholesterol in disease is highlighted by the fact that thirteen Nobel Prizes have been awarded to scientists studying the chemical cholesterol.

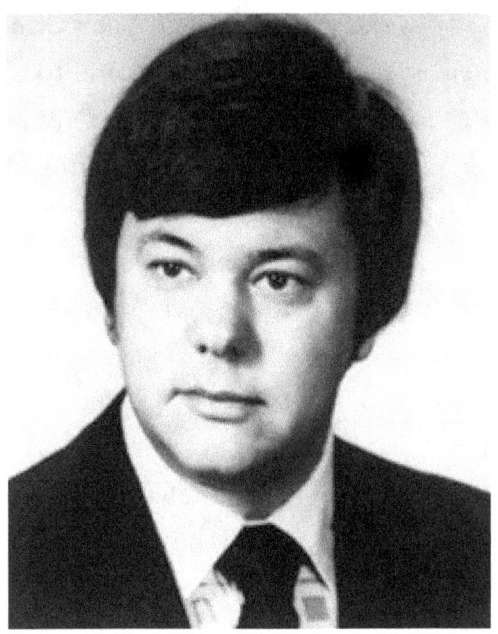

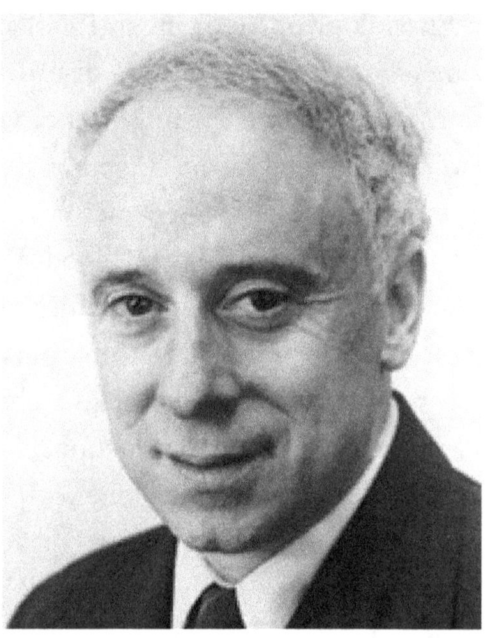

MICHAEL S. BROWN
permission of the Lasker Foundation

JOSEPH L. GOLDSTEIN permission of the Lasker Foundation

FINALLY A TREATMENT TO LOWER CHOLESTEROL LEVELS AND REDUCE THE OCCURRENCE OF HEART DISEASE

Although Brown and Goldstein discovered that LDL-receptors take up LDL cholesterol and inhibit HMG-CoA reductase from allowing cellular synthesis of cholesterol, it took a Japanese scientist working at Sankyo Laboratories to find the way to medically lower cholesterol leading to clinical treatments. Akiro Endo (1933-, born Higashiyuri, Akita, Japan) pioneered the efforts to produce the statins that have been manufactured and taken by millions of patients to lower blood cholesterol.

Cholestyramine was developed by Dow Chemical in 1957. Cholestyramine, which is not a statin, is not absorbed but prevents cholesterol absorption in the gut by binding to it similar to charcoal binding chemicals. This was the first treatment to lower cholesterol. The treatment, although still used today as an adjunct, was not very efficient in lowering cholesterol and caused side-effects such as constipation. Hence its use is more prevalent now to treat diarrhea than to lower cholesterol. In 1954 clofibrate (brand name Atromid) came onto the market, although it mainly lowered triglycerides. However, it was found to lower coronary events in a Finnish study.

In 1976 Akira Endo isolated a substance he called "compactin" from a mold. It blocked HMG-CoA reductase, the important chemical step in the body to make cholesterol. Compactin was found to lower blood cholesterol, but its development by Sankyo was stopped when dogs given it developed lymphomas. However, these dogs were given two hundred times the amount later given to patients. In 1979 Merck isolated mevinolin (very similar to compactin) from another mold, which led to the eventual marketing of the first statin drug, Mevacor (lovastatin is the generic name), approved by the FDA for use in 1987. The FDA then approved Zocor (simvastatin) in 1989, Pravachol (pravastatin) 1991, Lescol (Fluvastatin) 1994, Lipitor (atorvastatin) 1997, Baycol (cerivastatin) 1998 (Baycol was withdrawn from market by Bayer due to severe muscle destruction), Crestor (rosuvastatin) 2003, and Livalo (pitavastatin) 2009. All are similar in action and effects, with some patients tolerating one and not another of this class of drugs and some patients responding better to one than to another of the drugs. As a class of drugs (with individual patient success), they lower LDL cholesterol and total serum cholesterol. The data on whether cardiac events are reduced is robust and impressive. The well-publicized 4S Study from Scandinavia, published in Lancet 1994, demonstrated LDL lowering in 2222 patients in the simvastatin treatment group compared to the 2222 patients in the non-treatment group (the Scandinavian Simvastatin Survival Study). All 4444 subjects had known coronary artery disease (angina pectoris or previous heart attack) with baseline high-serum cholesterol in both groups even on a low-fat diet. They were followed on average for 5.4 years, with some patients even longer so that a six-year result could be tracked. At the end of that time, those on simvastatin lowered their total serum cholesterol 25% and LDL cholesterol 35% compared to the control group. Twelve percent died in the control (no simvastatin) group compared to 8% in the treatment group on simvastatin over six years, a 33% relative risk reduction but only 0.66% absolute percentage reduction per year (about a half-percent plus). The 33% is known as a relative reduction rate and seems much more impressive than the absolute number of 0.66%/yr. It is important to realize that not everyone in the control group died, and the six-year probability of surviving in the control group was pretty high, at 87.6%, vs. 91.3% in the treated group. This is statistically significant, but the absolute numbers of reduction in deaths are not as impressive as the relative percent reduction in deaths, as there were 267 deaths in the control group and 178 in the simvastatin group over six years, 89 fewer deaths in the simvastatin group's 2222 enrollees. Nevertheless, this study with two other important studies has dictated how most cardiologists have treated people for the last thirty-plus years, as we recommend statin to everyone with known coronary heart (coronary artery) disease and even those with no previous disease who have high blood cholesterol levels, especially with other risk factors such as family history of coronary artery disease at a young age, diabetes, smoking, high blood pressure or obesity. Everyone must decide for themselves if fewer deaths per year is worth an entire group of 2222 people taking a daily drug, just in case.. As for prevention of heart attacks, the control group had 528 heart attacks vs. the simvastatin group's 367, a 30% reduction (the heart attacks included the 189 in the placebo and 111 in the treatment group who died).

Furthermore, when other studies looked at treatment vs. control groups on other statin drugs, if both groups never had a previous coronary problem the results were even less impressive with the death rate reduction being only a quarter percent per year (that is right—one person saved for four hundred treated) rather than the 0.66% per year if you entered treatment after having a known coronary event. I am only presenting the numbers and not advocating a recommendation FOR statin use or not. These are discussions to be had with one's physician. Clearly, it depends on an individual's risk tolerance and fear of a coronary event.

Subsequently ezetimibe, whether by itself or in combination with a statin, was developed and lowers LDL cholesterol about 10% over just using a statin. It works by preventing absorption of dietary cholesterol in the gut. Subsequently two new medications given by subcutaneous needle (just under the skin) have been developed and are known as PCSK-9 inhibitors, which interfere with LDL cholesterol uptake through interfering with messenger RNA. They also have been shown not only to lower LDL but to reduce heart attacks. They have been expensive and until recently difficult for physicians to convince insurance companies to reimburse patients. The two drugs developed so far are Praluent (generic alirocumab) and Repatha (generic evolocumab). Finally, recently another medication, bempoic acid (brand Nexletal), which inhibits cholesterol production in one of the enzymatic steps before HMG-CoA required for cholesterol synthesis, is now on the market. It effectively lowers cholesterol but is also quite expensive, difficult to get reimbursement as of this writing from insurance companies, and has no studies yet completed to show reduction in adverse cardiac events, i.e. heart attacks.

Much to most cardiologists' surprise, an omega-3 pill, which uses only one of the two components of fish oil, has been found to not only lower triglycerides but to reduce cardiac events 25% as well, although it has no significant effect on cholesterol reduction. It is called Vascepa (generic icosapent ethyl) and sold only by prescription.

The future suggests that other ways to treat high cholesterol that reduce heart attacks will be discovered.

Patients often said to me when I placed them on strict low-cholesterol and low-fat diets, "Doc, even if I don't live longer on this diet you gave me, it sure will seems like longer."

On the other hand, I was known on more than one occasion to write on a prescription pad for a coronary bypass patient after surgery who was having trouble adjusting to a low-cholesterol diet, "ONE FILET MIGNON." Hopefully they understood what I was doing and did not present the prescription to Walgreens or CVS or for daily use.

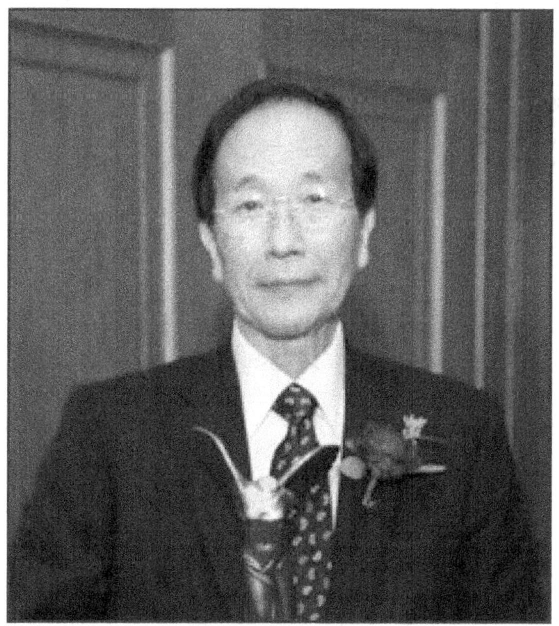

AKIRA ENDO
with permission for use by Lasker Foundation

Cholesterol – a fat component required for cells to survive and contained in the protective envelopes, called membranes of cells. It is made in the liver.

Lipoprotein – small packets of fat and a protein transported in the blood

HDL cholesterol – high-density lipoprotein cholesterol thought to be protective against coronary artery disease

LDL cholesterol – low-density lipoprotein cholesterol thought to be the "culprit" in producing heart attacks and strokes

Phospholipid – a phosphorus component attached to a cholesterol component, and both are surrounded by a protein envelope known as apolipoprotein B, or apoB for short

Serum cholesterol – cholesterol measured in the liquid after blood clots in a test tube. Plasma cholesterol is the measured cholesterol in a test tube not allowed to clot due to a chemical inside the tube.

Heterozygous – receiving only one gene for a disease, i.e. from only one parent

Homozygous – receiving a gene for a genetically transmitted disease from each parent, i.e. having two copies of the gene

CHAPTER 16
LEST WE FORGET – IMPORTANT SCIENTISTS

This chapter is devoted to a series of scientists not yet mentioned in this book but who are equally important. They are listed separately since together they do not fit together as a single related chapter topic.

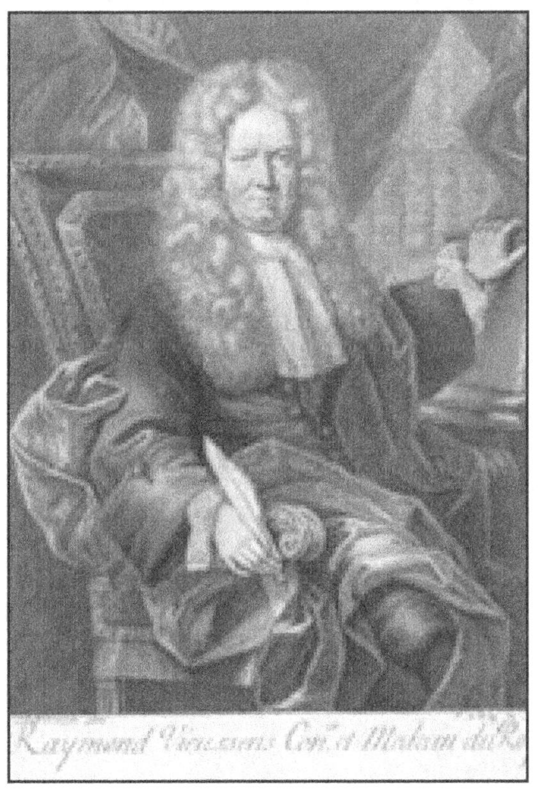

RAYMOND VIEUSSENS, Alamy License

In 1708 Raymond Vieussens (1641-1715, born Vigan City, Philippines, and died Montpellier, France) wrote a book describing the anatomy of coronary arteries (which bring oxygenated blood to the heart muscle) and also described the first anatomic findings in the thickening and reduced opening of the valve dividing the left heart's upper chamber (left atrium) from the lower chamber (left ventricle), a condition known as mitral stenosis. He was also the first to describe the anatomic findings of aortic insufficiency (also known as aortic regurgitation), the leakiness of the valve that controls blood flow out of the heart from the left ventricle to the main artery the aorta.

Albrecht Von Haller (1708-1777, born Bern, Switzerland, and died Bern, Switzerland) was the first to describe calcification of the covering of the heart, the pericardium. In his age many if not nearly all of the hearts with this finding were due to tuberculosis, a common disease at the time and cause of death. It is rare today, but cardiologists occasionally see patients with calcium in the pericardium. When the calcium encircles or partially encircles the heart, one is taught to think of tuberculosis involving the pericardium.

Switzerland at this time was not all cows and yodeling. Multiple peasant wars occurred between 1653 and 1755, including revolts against the leadership in Bern and Basel. Swiss scholars calling for reform founded the Helvetic Society in 1761. A Swiss revolution in 1798 occurred with farmers becoming free citizens, supported by the French in the western part of Switzerland. Between 1798 and 1802, the Helvetic Republic was formed with a centralized parliament based on the French model. Parts of Switzerland, however, became occupied by Napoleon and the French Army until the end of the Napoleonic Wars.

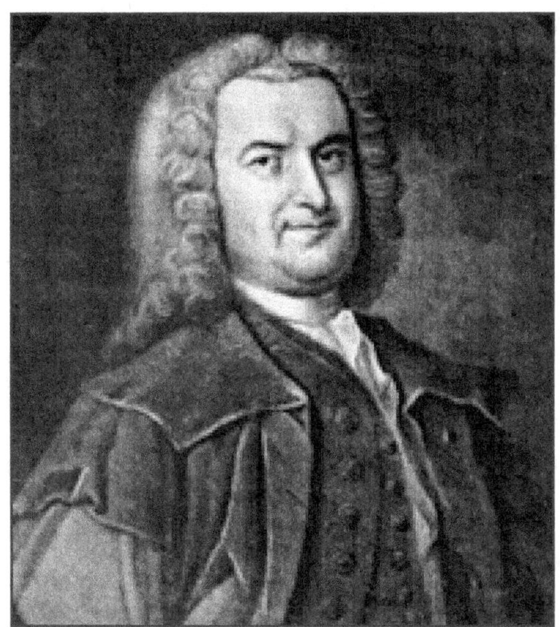

ALBRECT VON HALLER, public domain

Jean-Baptiste Bouillaud's (1796-1881, born Garta, France, and died Paris, France) contribution to cardiology was being the first to recognize the stages of inflammation of the heart associated with rheumatism (joint and tendon pain), including the lining at the blood interface of the left ventricle in his papers of 1824 and 1826 (most probably acute rheumatic fever). He called this endocarditis, although Bouillaud's term has subsequently been associated not with the condition described by Bouillaud but with bacterial infection of heart valves. During Bouillaud's lifetime the discovery of bacteria was made, but the association of rheumatism and heart involvement with the streptococcus bacterium would come much later. Bouillaud was not the first to write about the association of the heart with episodes of rheumatism. So did William C. Wells (1757-1817, born Charlestown, SC, U.S., and died London, UK), who wrote an excellent paper on the subject in 1812 describing patients, many with autopsies, but Wells did not go into the details of inflammation that Bouillaud did. Bouillaud described the symptoms of joint pains, fevers, chest pain and rapid heart rates in his patients.

Bouillaud's contributions to cardiology also included studies on heart sounds and the differentiation of normal heart rhythms from abnormal heart rhythms (without an EKG, still to be invented in 1906).

RUDOLPH VIRCHOW'S (1821-1902, born Spidwin, Poland, and died Munich, Germany) importance to cardiology lies in his magnificent studies of thrombosis and embolism (clot starting at point A and travelling to point B) in 1856. They were simple, well-proved, and convincing experiments, important for heart and blood vessel disease.

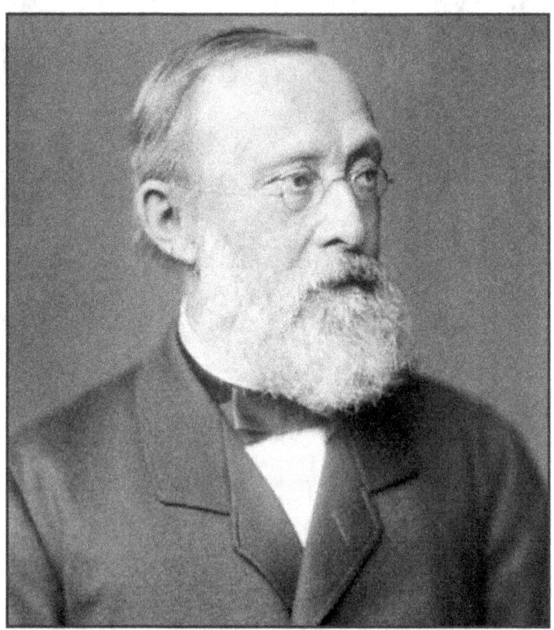

RUDOLPH VIRCHOW, public domain

Previous scientists left the field in a confusing state, so he decided to perform a systematic study. He soon understood that inflammation played a major part in formation of blood clots and that the inflammation arose in the blood vessel wall rather than in the clot itself. In a postmortem study of a patient with a clot in the lung (pulmonary embolus), he noted that the clot stopped when it reached a blood vessel smaller than the head of the clot. He also noted that the tail in the lung perfectly fit the head of the clot in the leg like a jigsaw puzzle. Therefore, he reasoned that it had to embolize (after splitting into two portions) via the veins from the leg and into the lung artery. He very elegantly but simply showed the source of the clot and its destination in the lung. He also showed that arterial clots could travel via the arteries into the spleen, arm, kidney or brain. This obstruction of the blood vessel demonstrated that blood vessels could produce serious mechanical consequences. His findings have not only endured but have served as a basis for even newer findings by others. He is also known for launching the field of cellular pathology, and he is known for his famous expression, "Every cell stems from another cell." However, his theory on coronary artery disease and heart attacks held back the field for a number of years, as he was certain that heart attacks were primarily the result of local or systemic inflammation directly within the heart muscle and not due to blocked coronary arteries arising from inflammation and clots of the coronary arteries.

He lived during the unification and commercial, industrial, cultural, and military growth of Germany under Kaiser Wilhelm I.

LOUIS PASTEUR (1822-1895, born Dole, France, and died Marne-la-Coquette, France) was the father of bacteriology and without his discoveries, infections of the heart would continue to be an enigma. He started his career studying fermentation in the alcohol industry of France and, in so doing, literally saved the French beer, wine, and silk industries. In addition he is known for developing vaccines against anthrax and rabies. Although an excellent artist and a decorated sergeant major in the Napoleonic Wars, receiving from Napoleon the Legion of Honor, fortunately for the world he became a chemist and microbiologist and not a professional soldier. His research of crystals made him conclude that asymmetry was a fundamental characteristic of living matter.

By studying fermentation in the alcohol industry, he also was led to finding that lactic acid was responsible for souring of milk. In 1857, having moved back to Paris from Lille, he presented his research and evidence for living organisms being responsible for fermentation, giving rise to the germ theory of fermentation. He also discovered that some bacteria could live only in the presence of oxygen while some could not live in an oxygen environment (aerobic and anaerobic bacteria), which led him to conclude that he could stop fermentation by passing air (contains oxygen) through the fermenting fluid (the Pasteur effect). Wine in the 19th century was having contamination issues. Simply heating the wine to 120-140 degrees, he discovered that he could kill the bacteria causing the problem, a process now known as pasteurization. (Wines that benefit from aging no longer are pasteurized, but milk, cheese, and many foods are.) Next he studied beer and developed a process to prevent deterioration during shipping.

He is often quoted, "Chance only favors the prepared mind." He noted by chance that cultures of chicken cholera (now called Pasteurella) lost their virulence over generations, leading him to studying immunization and developing vaccines. After Robert Koch announced the isolation of the anthrax bacillus, Pasteur and Koch independently announced that the organism responsible for the killing sheep and some people was anthrax. This established the germ theory as the basis of microbiology. Pasteur then performed experiments of inoculating sheep with the bacteria after immunizing them with low virulent anthrax cultures. A second control group with no inoculation all died but not the vaccinated group. The ones given weakened bacteria as vaccines when later injected with live virulent organisms did not develop anthrax. This experiment was carried out in 1881. He went on to develop a rabies vaccine also in 1882. Subsequently, it was found that rabies was a virus and not seen under the microscope, but his studies also led to a class of inactivated vaccines, neutralizing viruses by desiccation (drying them out). Although not directly studying heart disease, the diagnosis and treatment of infectious endocarditis, an infection of a heart valve, depends upon the principles he laid down and discovered. Furthermore, some scientists think coronary artery disease is a process starting with an infection from the mouth, leading to inflammation of the artery, which causes plaque and thrombus (clot) formation.

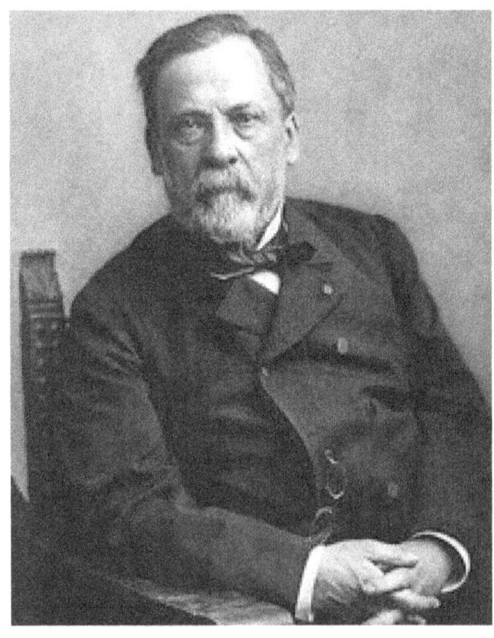

LOUIS PASTEUR,
public domain

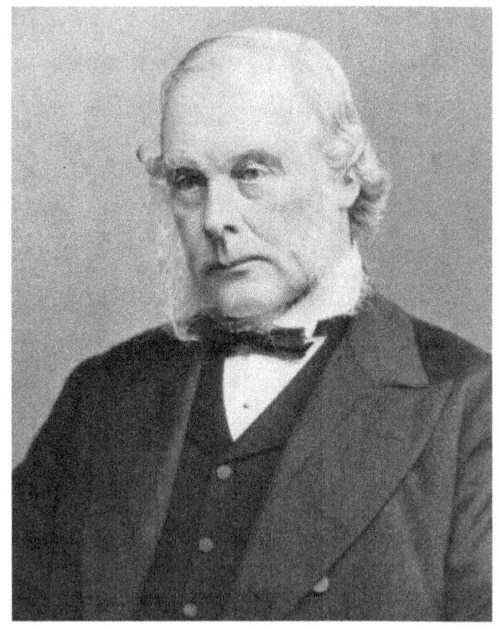

JOSEPH LISTER,
public domain

Joseph Lister (1827-1912, born West Ham, England, and died Kent, England) was not able to attend Oxford or Cambridge, as he was barred for his religious beliefs, being a Quaker, and attended the University College London Medical School. He worked with the famous surgeon John Erichsen (see Chapter 2). As a surgeon seeing his mentor, John Erichsen, he noted that debriding and cleaning wounds sometimes allowed healing, indicating that the problem was not from bad air as some, including Erichsen, believed but within the area wound (i.e. bacteria). A little boy who died of hospital gangrene, as it was called, had his arm amputated. Lister noted that the young boy's arm showed pus coming out of the bone at the elbow. Lister's first operation was on a woman stabbed in the abdomen by her husband, who was convicted and sent to Australia for fifteen years' punishment. She healed after Lister operated on her.

In 1853 Lister went to Edinburgh to apply his skills and began studying inflammation, which he observed led to post-operative problems (heat, redness, swelling, and pain). He read Pasteur's papers and was influenced by Pasteur's findings and in 1871 performed experiments showing that air could carry organisms that could be killed by heating. He became convinced that the organisms causing surgical wound infection could be eliminated. He began experimenting with carbolic acid derived from coal tar, but this was a failure, and his treated patient died. He obtained a purer form of phenol (from his carbolic acid application) in crystals that could be dissolved in water heated to 80 degrees F and used as a lotion for an antiseptic. His success came in 1865, when he applied a pad with carbolic acid to a young boy with a compound bone fracture after a cart ran over his leg. Not only did he not develop an infection and pus, but his bones healed. His second patient, in 1866, had a crane chain break holding a metal mold, which landed on his leg. He also was treated with an improved phenol (carbolic acid) by Lister. He healed without infection. Lister published the case in 1867. Subsequently he had surgeons wash their hands before and after surgery with 5% carbolic acid and wear gloves at surgery. Surgical instruments were also cleaned in the same solution. He started using gauze and sprays successfully. The age of aseptic surgery was born. However, when he lectured in London, he was met with indifference, apathy, and even hostility (Disruptor vs. Restrainer). Once again the words of Sir William Osler reverberate, "How eminent soever a man may become in science, he is apt to carry with him errors which were in vogue when he was young—errors that darken his understanding, and make him incapable of accepting the most obvious truths" (see Osler, Chapter 1). However in Leipzig, Germany, and Copenhagen, Denmark, his technique was adopted but for some reason neglected at its most crucially needed time, during the Franco-Prussian War of 1870-1871, when war wounds were aplenty. Finally, by 1874 Germany widely used his technique, his findings having spread much faster in Germany than any other country.

Robert Koch (1843-1910, born Clausthal-Zellerfeld, Germany, and died Baden-Baden, Germany) received the Nobel Prize in Physiology or Medicine in 1905 for his discovery and research into the tuberculosis bacterium, the scourge of Europe, which he discovered in 1882. Before Koch, tuberculosis was thought to be an inherited disease because so many people in families suffered from it. Like Pasteur, he is one of the main founders of microbiology, with his discovery of the anthrax bacillus in 1876, and he is considered the Father of Medical Bacteriology. He used new techniques to make the microscope an even more important tool, allowing smaller objects to be seen, and he invented the use of agar as a culture method for growing bacteria on glass plates. Subsequently he developed the Petri dish, named after his assistant, Julius Richard Petri. For those interested in trivia, he first tried to grow bacteria on potato slices but this was not satisfactory. To determine the cause of a disease with its pathogen, his development of Koch's postulates became known worldwide. Originally his development of tuberculin, which he thought might become a cure for tuberculosis, was not successful, but it has been used for over one hundred years diagnostically for tuberculosis. He died of a heart attack at age 66, much too young. His cardiac death was ironic, as it was the illness that his own and Pasteur's research served to divert many otherwise cardiac researchers away from coronary artery study and toward bacteriology, which seemed more interesting and important at the time. Nevertheless, Pasteur, Koch, and Lister are three extremely important Disruptors of cardiology and science.

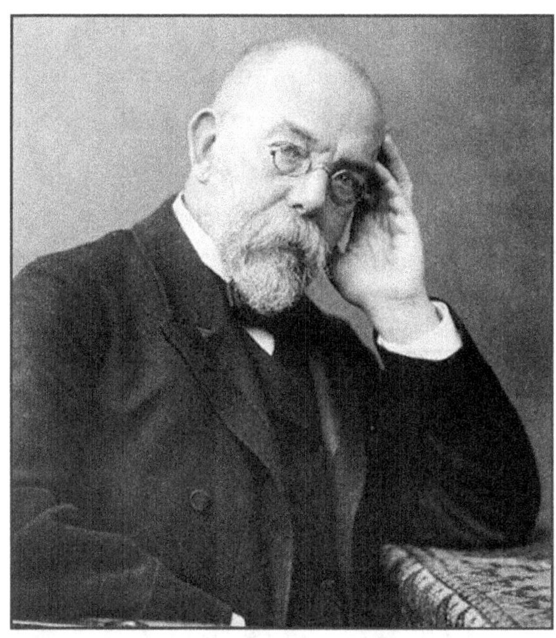

ROBERT KOCH, public domain

EMANUEL FREDRICK HAGBARTH WINGE (1827-1894, born Stvern, Norway, and died Oslo, Norway) made only one contribution to cardiology, but it was very important. Winge's contribution to cardiology is a single-case report in 1869 of a man paring his foot bunion with an unclean knife. The area became red, painful, swollen, and abscessed with puss. He then developed fever and chills and died from his illness. The autopsy showed a cauliflower-like mass with pus on a heart valve, as well in the kidney and spleen. In the pus he found micro-organisms but mistook these for parasites, as germ theory was just being promulgated by Louis Pasteur (1822-1895, born Dole, France, and died Marnes-la-Coquette, France), and Robert Koch (1843-1910, born Clausthal-Zellerfeld, Germany, and died Baden-Baden, Germany). Pasteur was learning about bacteria for wine and beer fermentation at the time, and Koch did not perform his famous anthrax experiments on mice from infected cow blood until the 1880s, proving that the bacteria caused the disease (fulfilling what was later called "Koch's Postulates"). So Winge came very close to not only making a good description of bacterial endocarditis with septic emboli and knowing for the first time that it was an infection that caused endocarditis, but he just missed the actual bacterial cause due to limited knowledge and techniques at the time. He recognized the entrance of germs into the body could cause heart damage even if the actual organism cause awaited bacterial identification.

Thanks to Winge's report, an explosion in the medical literature on endocarditis subsequently occurred. Infectious endocarditis became divided into two entities, acute and subacute. Even the great physician Sir William Osler (1849-1919, born Bradford, West Gwillimbury, Canada, and died Oxford, UK), who at the time was professor of medicine at the University of Pennsylvania, delivered a lecture in London in 1885 on malignant endocarditis (now called acute bacterial endocarditis). But at that time, bacterial identification still was not a lab test accessible to physicians.

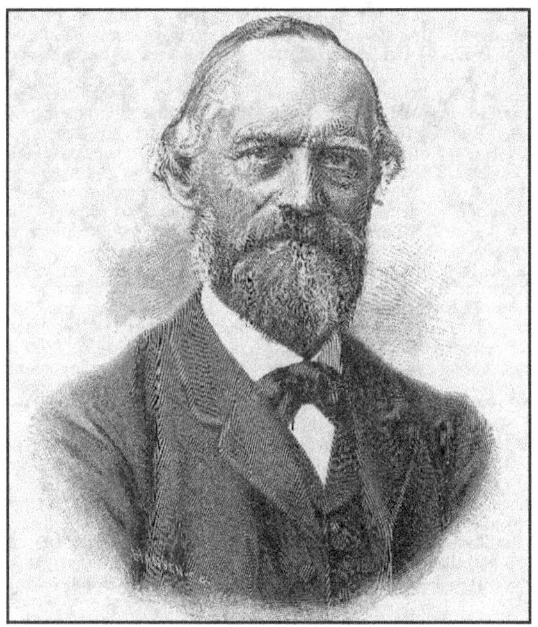

EMANUEL WINGE, public domain

In 1903 Hermann Lenhartz (1854-1910, born Ladbergen, Germany, and died Hamburg, Germany) wrote a book detailing the bacteriology known at the time and also detailed in his book the known bacterial types causing endocarditis and the clinical manifestations. He advocated for the use of blood cultures for isolating and identifying the endocarditis-causing bacterium. Today this is the standard for identifying and diagnosing endocarditis.

It was not until 1910 that Hugo Schotmueller (1867-1936, born Trebbin, Germany, and died Hamburg, Germany) identified streptococcus viridans as the cause of most indolent (now called subacute bacterial endocarditis) infections of the heart valve.

WILLIAM RASHKIND (1922-1986, born Paterson, NJ, and died Marion, PA, U.S.) was one of my own personal heroes and great Disruptors in cardiology. I met him in July of 1972, when I was sent over to Children's Hospital in Philadelphia on a rotation in pediatric cardiology that lasted six months and almost made me change from adult to children's heart disease. Dr. Rashkind was brilliant and due to him, many a child with congenital heart disease are now alive today who would have died in early years. His optimistic and cheerful personality filled the room when he entered. He was funny and always nice to his cardiology residents, including me. He was always willing to teach and answer any questions the residents had. He was world renowned but never outwardly impressed with himself. He was a giant in pediatric cardiology research and skillful in the cardiac catheterization laboratory, where I assisted him on numerous cases.

His genius led him to devise the balloon atrial septostomy procedure in 1966, only six years before I arrived, creating with a balloon on the tip of a catheter in a locally anesthetized patient a larger hole between the upper-right and upper-left atrium so that red oxygenated blood could pass through to provide adequate oxygen to the body of the blue baby or young child. Usually the procedure was done on a patient with a reversal of circulation, a condition known as Transposition of the Great Vessels. His procedure became known worldwide as the "Rashkind Procedure," and he became legitimately known as the "Father of Pediatric Interventional Cardiology."

I can vividly recall helping him in another procedure for which he devised a new system to close an open connection between the main artery going to the body's organs, the aorta, and the main artery traveling to the lungs, the pulmonary artery. Normally this connection, which is a fetal blood vessel, aids in utero transfer of a mother's bright red blood to enter the left side of the body for a baby to survive in utero. But when it does not close at birth and is no longer needed, the consequences can send the baby into heart failure and growth failure. The defect is known as a patent ductus arteriosus, or PDA for short. Originally, the solution was open heart surgery, but Dr. Rashkind's invention allowed many children to have this repair without surgery. Although Werner Porstmann in Berlin, Germany, in 1966 first placed a catheter delivered plug for the patent ductus, it was a system that could not be used for small children and babies. By 1976 Michael A. Heymann demonstrated medical closure of the PDA using anti-inflammatory medications such as indomethacin in premature patients. Dr. Rashkind reported his results in 1979 using a double-disc system on a 3.5kg baby (7.7 pounds) without surgery but using his system through the skin (percutaneous) using the procedure he developed. This remains today the most commonly used system and device.

I can still picture assisting Dr. Rashkind in his development of a PDA plug in the summer of 1972, when I was sent to Children's Hospital in Philadelphia from the Hospital of the University of Pennsylvania on a long rotation in pediatric cardiology. Although at first disappointed that I could not start my training in heart disease on adults, this rotation became my favorite of my three years in training.. The system Dr. Rashkind devised was to deliver a double-disc closure device into the patent ductus of a small infant. Ingeniously Dr. Rashkind devised a method placing one catheter in the vein of the groin and one catheter in the artery on the opposite groin and eventually hooking each to the other with his "plug" in between. Then we would pull or release each side until he positioned the closure device exactly where he wanted it to lie. This closed the small and short open tubelike tissue between the aorta and pulmonary artery, which did not close normally at birth. I would tighten or relax the venous side for him as he would pull the arterial side. He published his results in 1979. That day I understood why the pediatric cardiology residents sometimes called him "Wild Bill" Rashkind. Wild, perhaps, but amazingly smart and always worried about his small patient and the waiting parents.

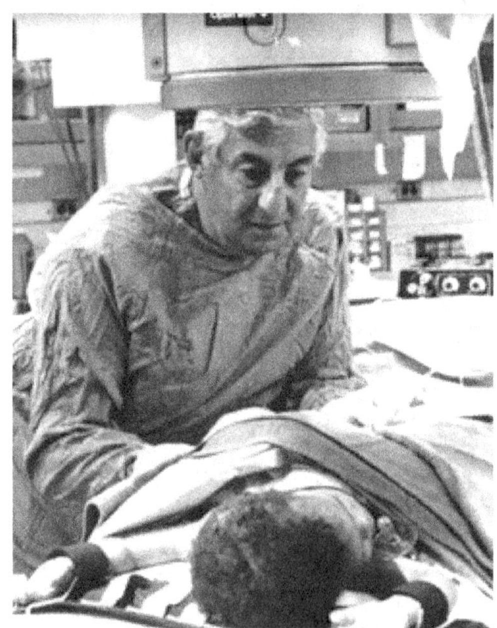

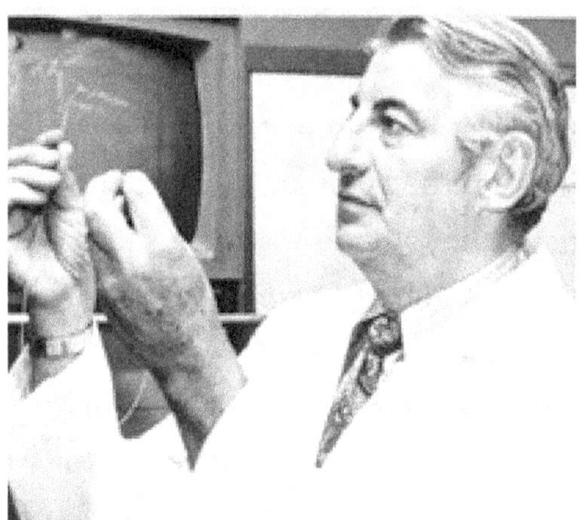

WILLIAM RASHKIND   WILLIAM RASHKIND
both photos by permission: Children's Hospital of Philadelphia

Eugene Braunwald (1929-, born Vienna, Austria) is hard to characterize for this book, although clearly he is one of the giants of cardiology of the 20th and 21st centuries and another personal hero of mine. He came to the U.S. as a child with his parents who fled Hitler's takeover of Vienna and Austria.. In his 90s he continued to be a researcher, clinical trials investigator, administrator, cardiology classic textbook editor, author of over one thousand research articles, and lecturer, including one I personally heard in 2019, given at age ninety. While chief of cardiology at the National Institutes of Health, he made great contributions to our understanding of an important disease, hypertrophic cardiomyopathy, where the heart muscle between the two ventricles is disproportionately thickened compared to the outside wall and can lead to chest pain, shortness of breath, dizziness, fainting, and even sudden death. Young athletes with sudden death often have this genetic problem. Occasionally but rarely, heart transplantation is required. Eventually, becoming chairman of Cardiology at the Brigham and Women's Hospital in Boston, Dr. Braunwald brought and fostered famous or soon-to-become famous cardiologists to his staff. One of his great contributions was starting the study group to assess the utility of clot-busting agents known as thrombolytics. At the time of this writing, he continues to be the Hersey Distinguished Professor of the Theory and Practice of Physics at Harvard Medical School. When I interviewed him by phone in June of 2023, I asked him what his cardiology achievements were of which he was most proud. His response was "My research on hypertrophic cardiomyopathy and my research limiting the size of heart attacks." Then he thought for a few seconds and amended his response: "I think the order should be 1) my research showing how heart attack size can be limited with medications, 2) my research on hypertrophic cardiomyopathy." He explained that a single patient led him to consider a way to study how to reduce the size of a heart attack at least a decade before clot-busting agents to dissolve the clot of a heart attack came to be used. This patient had an electrical wire attached to the nerve bundle in the neck surrounding the carotid artery (known as the carotid body), with its external sleeve connected to an electrical stimulator, which would control the heart rate through the autonomic nervous system, which the carotid body influences. He found that when his patient had severe chest pain over and over again, known as "status anginosis" or preinfarction angina" (often leading to a heart attack), turning on the electrical stimulator slowed his heart rate and lowered the systolic blood pressure (both reduce the heart's demand for oxygen and readjusts the supply/demand balancer when narrowed coronary arteries are present) with a corresponding normalization of the EKG and resolution of his patient's pain. It would not be an exaggeration to say that Dr. Braunwald "is a giant on whose shoulders the cardiology profession stands" and an important Disruptor.

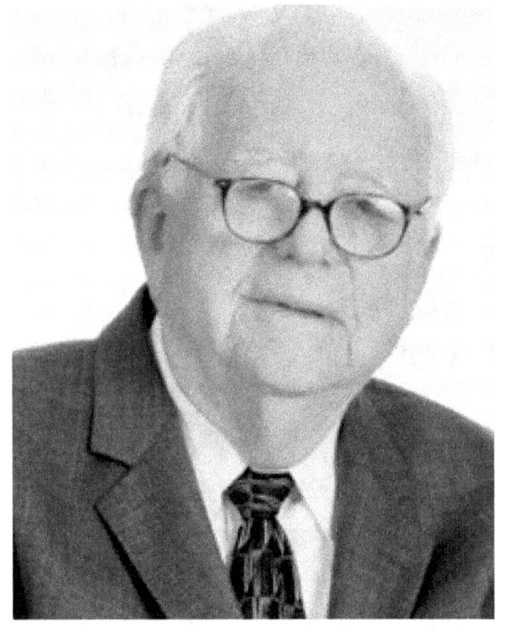

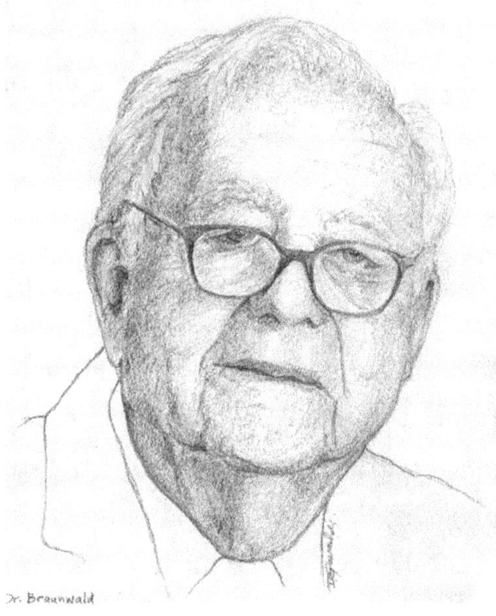

Left: EUGENE BRAUNWALD, by permission: American College of Cardiology

Right: drawn by David Gavasheli from a photo, author's personal collection

I was a clinical associate at the National Institutes of Health not long after Dr. Braunwald left as the chief of cardiology. His research on hypertrophic cardiomyopathy is still remembered by us who were around at that time, and it has determined the treatment for this fairly common disease. Later, I treated many patients with intravenous clot busters for heart attacks because of his collecting thousands of patients in trials, which convinced the medical procession to use these drugs for heart attack treatment. It would not be an exaggeration to say that he is already a "legend in his own time."

Pericardium – double-layer tissue surrounding the heart

Mitral stenosis – thickening of the mitral valve separating the upper- and lower-left chambers, which then limits the flow of blood crossing so that blood backs up into the lungs

Endocarditis – infection of a heart valve and sometimes the inner lining of the heart with a bacterium

Pulmonary embolism – clot travelling usually from the leg to the pulmonary artery

Aseptic technique – performing a procedure sterilely

Transposition of the great vessels – a congenital heart defect where the normal left-sided blood vessels now exit the right side of the heart and bring deoxygenated blood to the "blue" baby

Hypertrophic cardiomyopathy – thickening of the muscle separating the right and left ventricles disproportionately to the outside-left ventricular wall

CHAPTER 17
NEW MEDICAL TREATMENTS AND DEVICES

The end of the twentieth and beginning of the twenty-first centuries has seen an explosion in medications to treat cardiac diseases, especially coronary artery disease, heart failure, high blood cholesterol, hypertension, and clotting. Arrhythmia treatment started in the 1960s with a plethora of medications, but these have nearly stopped development in favor of radiofrequency ablative treatment for arrhythmias.

The main technological developments of the last one hundred and twenty-five years are the x-ray machine, cardiac catheterization, EKG (ECG) machine, Holter monitor, echocardiogram machine, cardiac CTA, cardiac MRI, nuclear stress testing, and biventricular pacing known as CRT.

I have written in Chapter 2 about the development of the x-ray machine (which was the forerunner of coronary angiography (Chapter 5)) and the EKG machine (Chapter 2). The Holter monitor was discussed in Chapter 13. It became a necessary extension of the Coronary Care Units (CCU), which came into being in the 1960s for monitoring patients at a central station. But early CCUs used a hard wire tethered to the patient and limited the patient's mobility and range to three to four feet, whereas today patients can often walk the hospital hallways while their EKG rhythm is still monitored by technicians at a central station.

ECHOCARDIOGRAPHY

The echocardiogram was the next major device to come along, "the next big thing." Its origins go back to Lazzaro Spallanzani (1729-1799, born Scandiano, Italy, and died Pavia, Italy), who recognized that bats used inaudible sounds to navigate their way (i.e. ultrasound or sonar). This was the inspirational starting point in a long series of discoveries leading to the development of clinical echocardiography about seventy years ago. Ironically, it is the only major cardiac imaging modality for which no one has received a Nobel Prize, possibly because there were so many historical points and a gradual evolution in its development rather than a single "ah-ha" moment. However, the modern start for echocardiography probably can be attributed to the invention by Paul Langevin (1972-1946, born and died Paris, France), who was a physicist. He studied under Pierre Curie, and during World War I he invented sonar to detect submarines. Evidently, after Pierre Curie died in an auto accident in 1910, Langevin and Madame Marie Curie, 43 years old at the time and he being five years younger, had a love affair and rented an apartment near the Sorbonne, where they secretly rendezvoused.

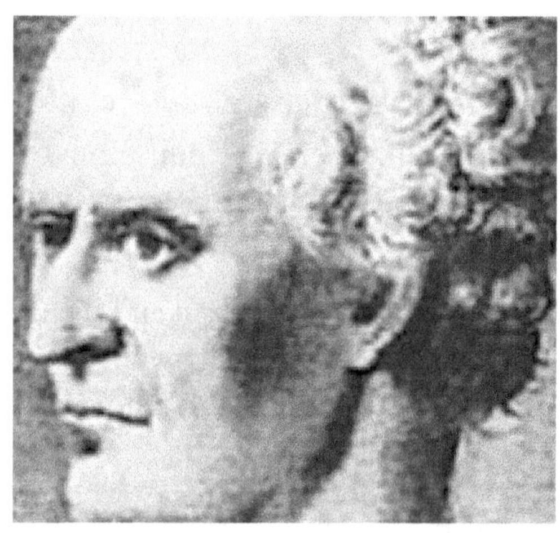

LAZZARO SPALLANZANI,
public domain

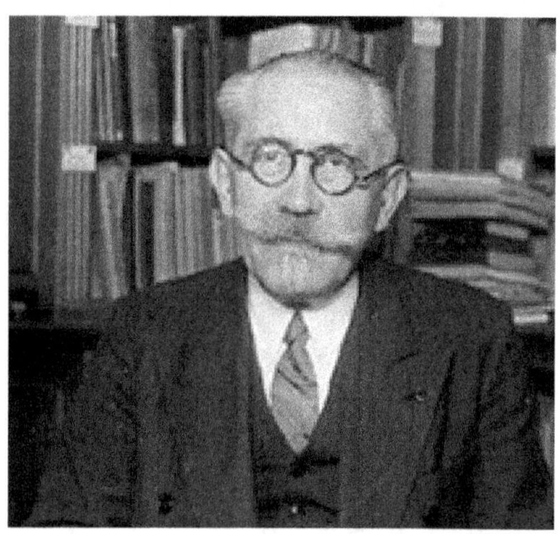

PAUL LANGEVIN,
public domain

Despite some early uses for the brain and breast masses, echocardiography for the heart owes its existence to the Swedish cardiologist Inge Edler (1911-2001, born Burlov, Sweden), a medical doctor, and Carl Hellmuth Hertz (1920-1990, born Berlin, German, and died Lund, Sweden), a physicist. In 1953 in Lund, Sweden, Edler wondered about using radar to detect heart disease, but Hertz suggested sonar and knew of its use in Sweden to detect flaws in the metal of ships. Edler was the head of cardiology at the University Hospital in Lund, Sweden. Carl Hertz was the son of the Nobel Laureate Gustav Hertz. Carl Hertz was a graduate student in nuclear physics at the University of Lund, where he met Edler. They borrowed the equipment from Tekniska Rontgencentralen, whose equipment was used in a shipyard in Malmo, Sweden, to detect structural flaws in ships.

First the two scientists tested the sonar on their own hearts in 1953. Although simple and primitive by today's standards, they became certain that ultrasound had a utility in detecting heart function and heart disease, especially of the mitral valve, which interested Edler. Edler used it primarily to diagnose mitral stenosis, a thickening of the mitral valve leaflets from rheumatic heart disease caused by streptococcus bacteria. They used M-mode echocardiography, which was used until the 1970s. M-mode echocardiogram beamed a narrow band of ultrasound at the heart and recorded the motion of whatever structure in the heart it struck as it was reflected back and as the beamed structure moved within the heart. Edler and Hertz called their technique ultrasound cardiography (UCG), which was later changed to echocardiography, not to confuse it with the ECG. Together they were awarded the prestigious Lasker Award in 1977 for their contributions. Many thought they both deserved a Nobel Prize, although this was not to occur.

Subsequently in 1972, using a single beam not recorded over time like the M-mode echo but as a single point in time (A-mode) and gradually moving the beam very slowly, a better picture of the heart called Compound B imaging briefly was tested. Because this required acquiring many images with each adjacent to the previous one to create a two-dimensional still picture of the heart, it was cumbersome and slow.

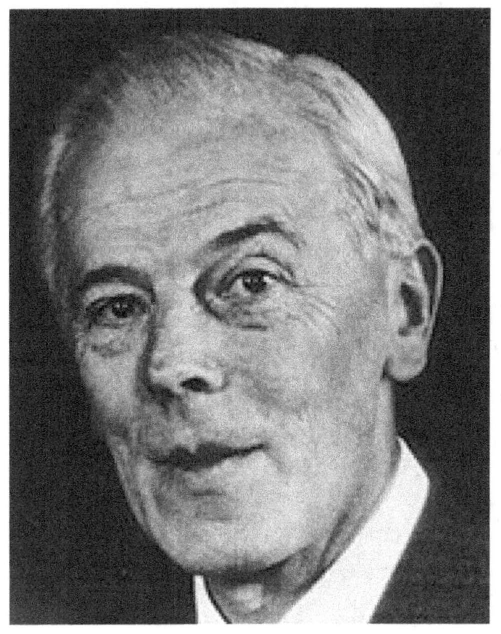

INGE EDLER,
public domain

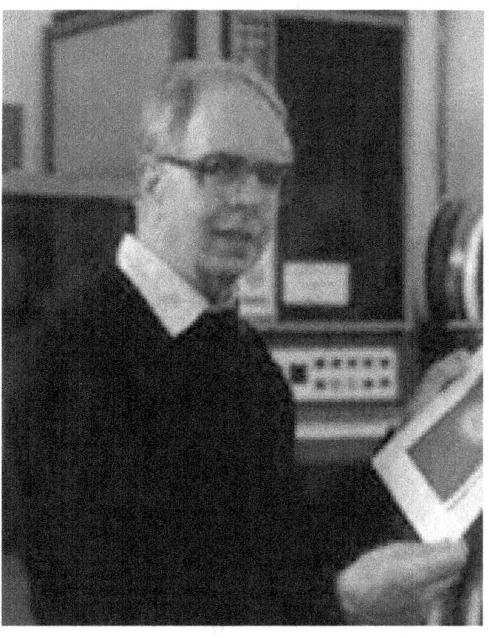

CARL H. HERTZ,
public domain

This process was not just slow but painstakingly slow. I was involved in its early use at the Hospital of the University of Pennsylvania, where I published a paper using this technique with Dr. Morris Kotler, a staff cardiologist, brilliant teacher and an early pioneer in the field of echocardiography. Not long after my paper's publication, this time-consuming, impractical technique was replaced with the 2D echocardiography of today, which not only obtains 2D pictures of the heart in various planes but allows visualization of real-time cardiac motion very quickly. Most cardiac patients have had such an echo taken of their hearts. The historical development of 2D echo is complicated, quite technical, and would require thirty pages, which is more than the scope of this book, as its developers include many physicians and engineers and many theoretical issues. But the person who pushed clinical research in the U.S. using echocardiography was Dr. Harvey Feigenbaum (born 1933-, East Chicago, Indiana) in Indianapolis, Indiana, U.S., and he is called the Father of Echocardiography (no public domain photo available).

The echocardiogram today also has other modes, including a three-dimensional mode, color doppler to determine blood flow direction for valve leakage, and a transesophageal probe to look at the heart without air and bones intervening to give a better picture. There are also intravascular probes and a technique to determine "strain" to assess subtleties of abnormal heart pumping. In short, it remains the most useful and most cost-effective clinical tool in cardiology today. It is portable and even comes in a miniaturized form for the pocket. The echocardiogram's main purpose is to identify 1) how the heart muscle is pumping in systole and in the relaxing diastolic phase, 2) whether there is fluid in the bag around the heart (pericardium), 3) how the valves are functioning (opening properly or less than perfectly, called stenosis, or not closing properly, known at insufficiency or regurgitation), 4) tumors in the heart's muscles or on the valves, 5) if infections of the valves with masses called vegetations are present, and 6) if an abnormal protein called amyloid is infiltrating the heart muscle. The echo is rarely helpful in identifying narrowed coronary arteries but with exercise echocardiography, looking for reduction in regional wall area motion after exercise and not present at rest before the treadmill walking will suggest blocked coronary arteries supplying these areas.

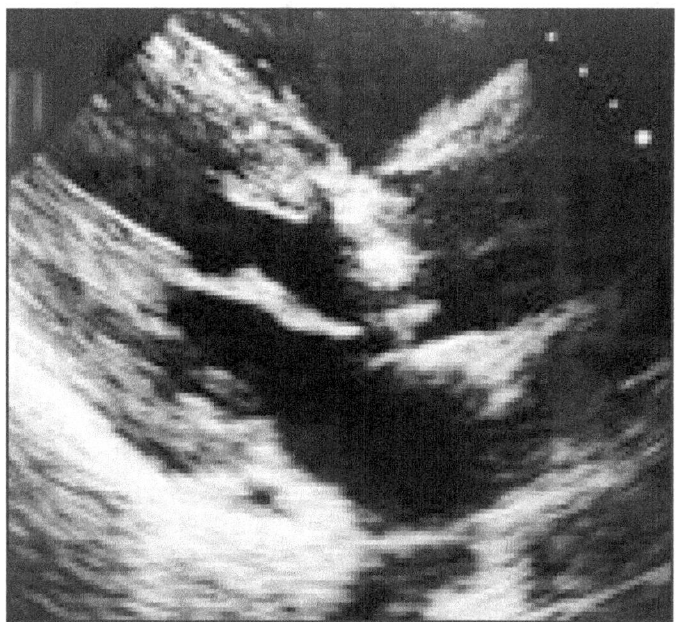

Long-axis echocardiogram showing left ventricle to the left and calcified aortic valve upper center From author's files

CORONARY ARTERY CALCIUM SCORING

Coronary artery calcium scores and CTA (computerized tomographic angiography) is a special ultrafast CT of the chest with no contrast that makes multiple thin (5mm) sections through the heart from up to bottom or vice versa, looking for calcium in the coronary arteries that can be seen. With a light pen, all areas of white calcium within the coronary arteries are circled, producing a score. Although very unusual, having plaque buildup within the coronary artery rarely gives a score of zero, and one study demonstrated a ten-year event rate with a calcium score of zero of only 1% in nearly twenty thousand patients followed. The higher the score, the more likely a patient will suffer a cardiac event over the next five to ten years. The score is a noninvasive technique to estimate plaque burden and future risk. The score, known as the Agatston Score, was first researched and pioneered by Dr. Arthur Agatston (of South Beach Diet fame), a cardiologist, with his radiologist colleague, Warren Janowitz, in Miami, Florida. It is better as a predictor for future events than serum cholesterol or LDL cholesterol levels or the Framingham risk score. Dr. Matthew Budoff of Los Angeles, California, has extensively studied its utility and value in large number of patients and has taught many cardiologists this test over the years. Zero scores often allow physicians to stop statin drugs, and very high scores over 300 (I have seen some over 3000!!) require further cardiac testing for significant blockage by nuclear stress testing or cardiac catheterization. Although there is an association between future cardiac events and the level of the score, the degree of narrowing within a coronary artery or a single coronary artery lesion cannot be determined from this test. Rather, the test gives a range of total coronary artery plaque burden.

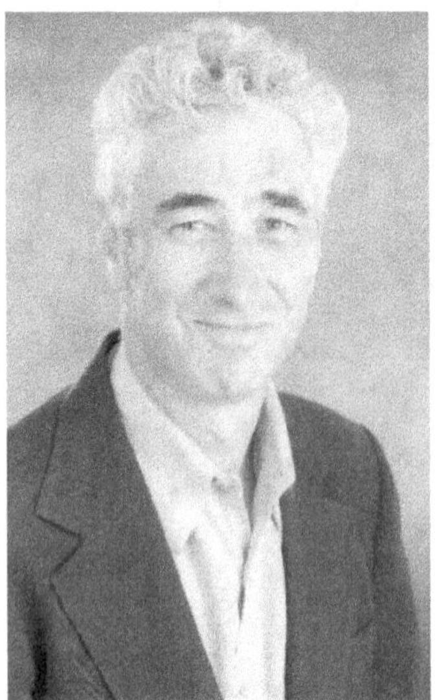

Dr. Matthew Budoff permission to use from his personal collection

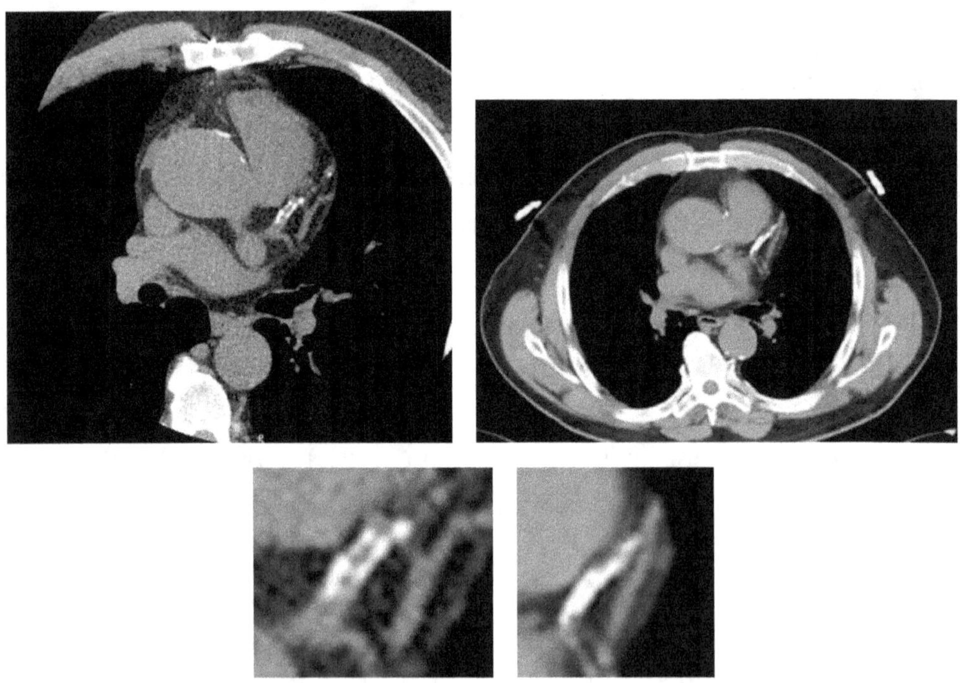

Coronary artery calcium score, 2014, and same patient, 2023
Note how linear white calcium in the left anterior descending has become worse over time as more plaque has built up and calcified – from author's files

CTA (COMPUTERIZED TOMOGRAPHIC ANGIOGRAPHY) is a step beyond the coronary artery calcium score. The procedure uses rapid thin CT images that, due to computer software, can be manipulated and viewed either in a 2D or 3D mode. The patient enters the CT scan and has x-ray contract injected into a vein. The information can be obtained by breath holding for only thirty seconds and, in some cases, can replace an invasive heart catheterization and coronary angiography. Very high coronary calcium scores and previous metal coronary stenting may make interpretation less accurate. Although more expensive than various stress tests, many studies have found the CTA very predictive of future events so it may become more extensively used as costs come down.

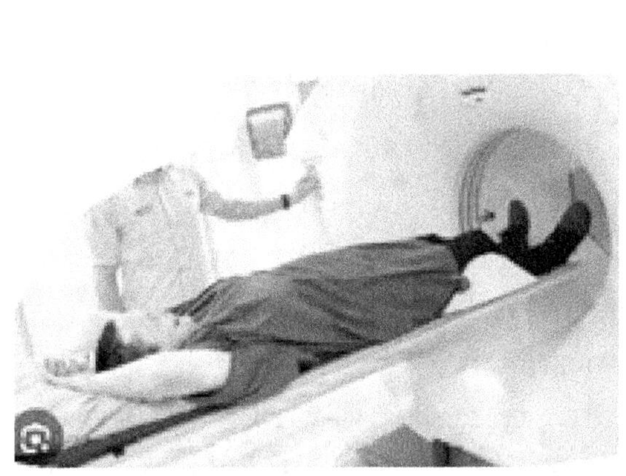

CT machine for CTA
from author's personal collection

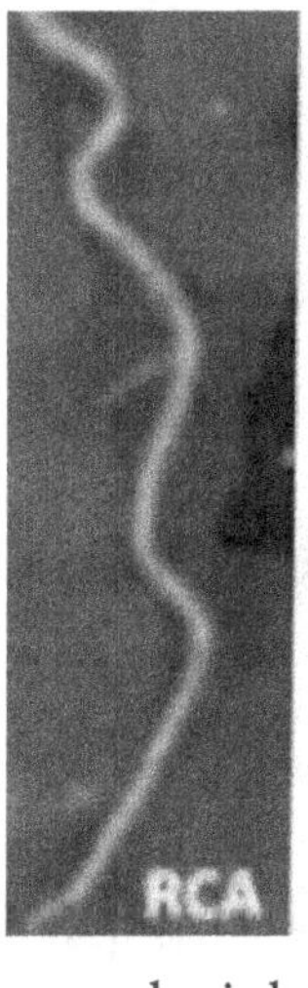

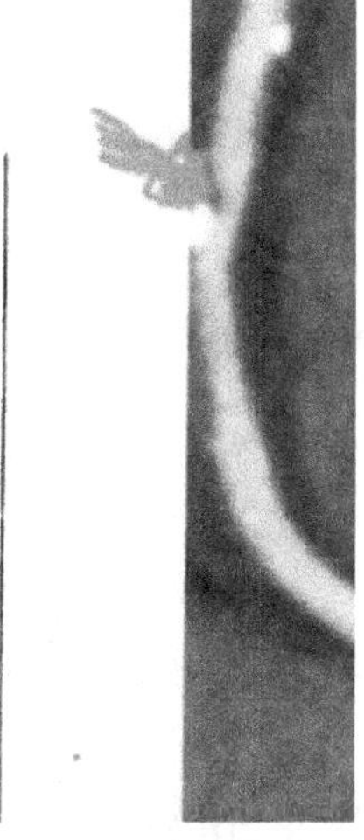

normal, right coronary artcry CTA (both pictures)

CT machine for CTA right coronary with arrow pointing to plaque-narrowing channel and calcium From author's collection

CARDIAC MRI (MAGNETIC RESONANCE IMAGING) (KNOWN AS C-MRI) is one of the newest cardiac imaging techniques to help cardiologists diagnose disease and effects of therapy. Using large magnets, pictures of the heart can be obtained. Beginning first in the 1970s as a tool to measure heart muscle metabolism, in the 1980s it was found useful for imaging the heart structure and function. By the 1990s ways to determine blood supply, heart muscle death, and location of scarring became possible. All of these studies were able to be performed with no radiation exposure and with high-resolution images. First described in examining liquid and solid crystals in 1946, Felix Bloch at Stanford and Edwin Purcell at Harvard independently reported their results at the same time. Because of their research, both received the Nobel Prize for Physics in 1952. The basis for C-MRI is complicated mathematics and physics and beyond the scope of this book, but the bottom line is that these scientists (five received Nobel Prizes in this field) found a way to take the field from the chemistry lab to the radiology suite with images that would help cardiologists diagnose heart disease.

Richard Ernst, Ph.D., in 1966 figured out the physics equations that led to a more efficient use of NMR (it was first called nuclear magnetic resonance and changed to MRI (magnetic resonance imaging)) so that patients would not fear that they were receiving nuclear material (which they were not). In 1991 Dr. Ernst received a Nobel Prize for his research.

In 1970 Drs. Paul Lauterbur and Peter Mansfield, both Ph.Ds., discovered the basis for NMR imaging when they added an additional small magnet. They received a Nobel Prize for their work in 2003. The earliest imaging occurred at the University of Nottingham in the United Kingdom.

The first clinical laboratory using medical NMR was the University of California in San Francisco under Dr. Alexander Margulis.

In 1980 one of the earliest research centers for C-MRI was started at the Massachusetts General Hospital in Boston, headed by Dr. Gerald Pohost, working with Joanne S. Ingewall, Ph.D., and Mark Goldman, MD, who brought the field into the clinical practical sphere for diagnosing heart disease. By the 1990s myocardial scar detection was possible. Johnson & Johnson and Technicare were the two early companies in producing machines.

Today C-MRI can diagnose heart function, valve leakages and failure to open properly (regurgitation and stenosis), cardiac tumors, holes in the heart, heart attack scars, abnormal proteins in the heart such as amyloidosis, thickening of heart muscle in a condition known as hypertrophic cardiomyopathy, reduced coronary artery blood flow, and narrowing upstream in the largest part of the coronary artery. The C-MRI is more accurate in detecting the left ventricular ejection fraction (percent of blood pumped out of the heart with each heartbeat, normal 55-60%) than an echocardiogram. One of the complaints patients have during C-MRI is being claustrophobic in a small tunnel for 45 minutes and the banging sound of the magnets. The C-MRI often has an injection of gadolinium to make images more visible.

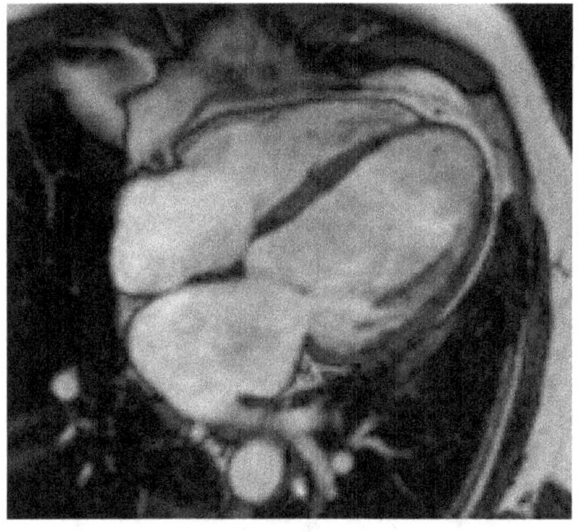

Normal long axis view of all four
heart chambers
From author's collection

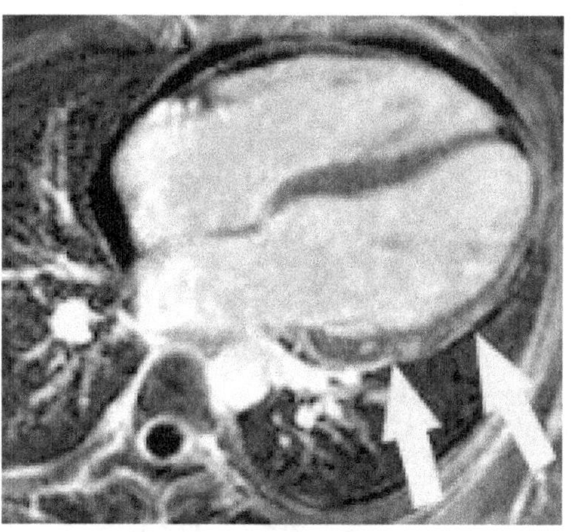

arrows point to a white white scar in
lv muscle (normal black)
from author's personal collection

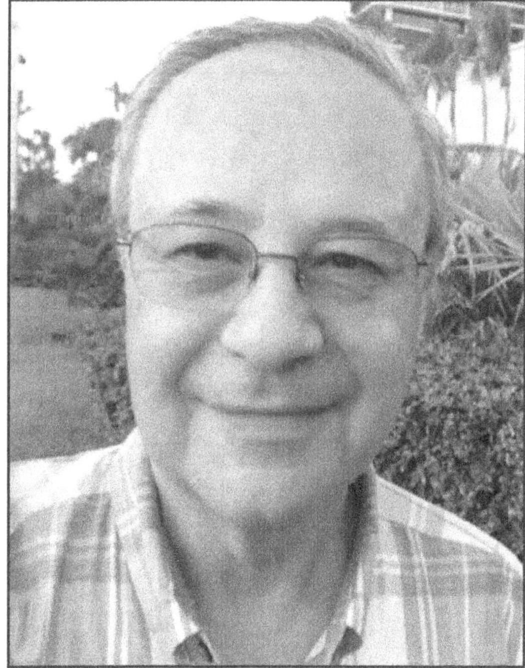

DR MARK GOLDMAN,
from his personal collection with permission for use

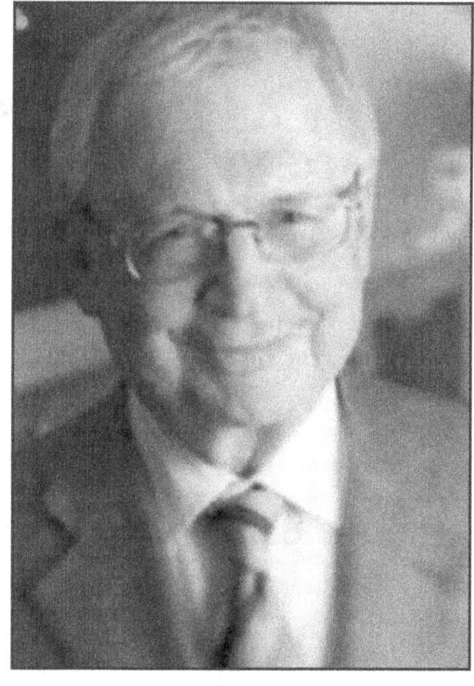

DR GERALD POHOST
From Dr Pohost's personal collection with permission to use

CARDIC PET SCANNING

PET stands for "proton emission tomography" to look at cellular level function in organs. It can more accurately diagnose reduced blood flow to heart muscle than other stress tests can.

PET scans are painless but require an injection of a specially prepared isotope radioactive tracer, given intravenously. Although also used to detect certain cancers, it is useful to measure blood flow to the areas of the heart muscle similar to nuclear stress testing but without exercising and more accurate, although more costly. In cardiology it has been used primarily to assess live vs. dead heart muscle and to diagnose a disease known as sarcoidosis, which can affect the heart or lung, or both.

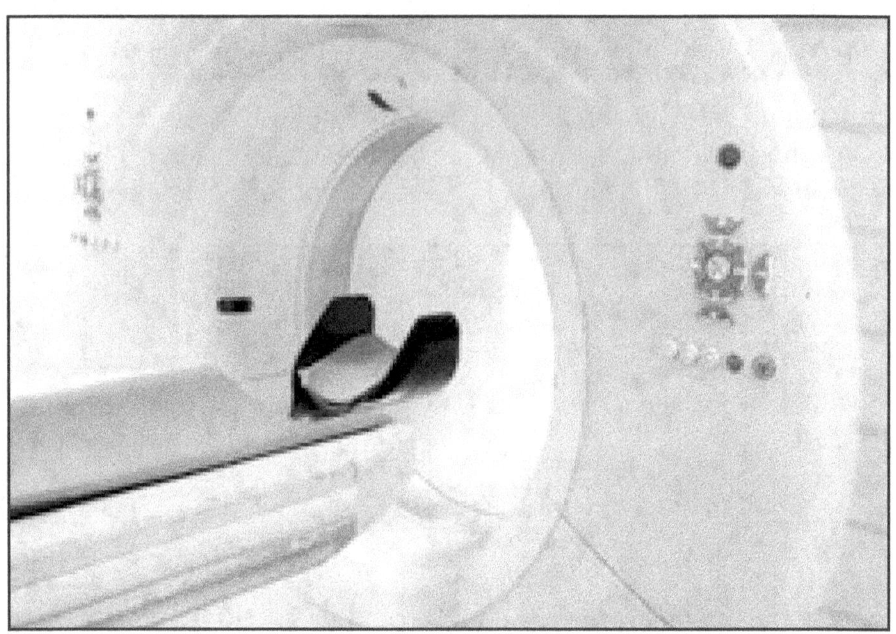

PET SCANNING MACHINE
From author's collection

CARDIAC RESYNCHRONIZATION THERAPY (CRT)

CRT is a type of pacing for weakened hearts causing congestive heart failure. Many times people have a left ventricle that is out of phase with the outside wall not pumping inwardly to meet the inside wall (as a rubber ball would when compressed with one's hand), called the interventricular septum. We cardiologists call this "asynchrony." This is usually associated with an EKG abnormality known as a left bundle branch block (LBBB for short). People with heart failure, even mild, but with an abnormally wide EKG complex and a very low ejection fraction of the left ventricle under 35% (the percent of blood pumped out of the heart with each heartbeat—normal 55-65%), may benefit from CRT. CRT in some patients allows the heart to shrink in size and pump more effectively. This in turn can improve a patient's symptoms.

Basically, CRT is a pacemaker procedure where instead of only a single pacing electrode wire at the tip of the right ventricle and often a second in the right atrium, a third wire to pace the left ventricle is also used. Although early attempts to place this wire through the skin and directly into the left ventricle were tried, these wires tended to clot with the risk of travelling to other parts of the body (embolization). The problem has been solved by placing this wire into a large vein, which empties the coronary artery flow into the floor of the right atrium, known as the coronary sinus. The wire is then fished upstream through the coronary sinus and into a connecting vein, which runs along the outside of the left ventricle on the far-left side of the heart. When timed to pace with the right ventricular wire, many patients will benefit with improved heart pumping. This is known as CRT and sometimes as biventricular pacing since both ventricles are nearly simultaneously paced. When an appropriate patient with heart failure responds to this technique, the heart may shrink in size, pump more efficiently, and have symptomatic relief of heart failure and shortness of breath. Data also shows that life may be prolonged and hospitalizations for heart failure reduced with CRT. When the heart shrinks in size (more toward normal size), the medical term for this favorable outcome is "reverse remodeling" (remodeling is not good, as the heart enlarges abnormally). The first trial of CRT was the MUSTIC TRIAL in 2001, but too few patients were enrolled to show a survival benefit. In 2002 the MIRACLE TRIAL randomized 53 patients with a normal rhythm but a low ejection fraction of under 35% and a wide EKG complex, usually with a left bundle branch block pattern. These patients were short of breath with minimal effort or at rest. At one year the group given CRT had a statistically significant survival improvement over the control non-CRT group. No defibrillator was given to either group (see Chapter 8: Pacemakers and Defibrillators). Several other trials were published, including the DASH CRT trial, which was published in 2009 with 1820 patients. Although patients felt better, no proof of living longer was found. However, since mild heart failure patients were the bulk of this trial, there was now proof of concept that even mildly affected patients would feel better with CRT.

INTRA-AORTIC BALLOON PUMP

The intra-aortic balloon pump, or IABP, is a hollow catheter or tube inserted in one of the two femoral arteries at the groin through the skin (percutaneously), which has a long deflated sausage-shaped balloon on the far end, which varies in length from 180mm to 270mm and, when inflated with helium or carbon dioxide, has a volume of 25 to 50cc and inflated diameter of 13 to 18mm. The balloon is connected to a console and inflated and deflated with each heartbeat if the rate is not too fast or 1:2 or even 1:3 when required. The timing of inflation is in the relaxing phase of the heart, known as diastole, and deflation in the active pumping phase, or systole.

This allows blood to be pushed through the body and into the coronary arteries in diastole while producing a negative pressure in the abdominal aorta in systole, creating less work for the heart. Cardiologists call this reducing "afterload." The IABP can be left in the body for up to ten days and requires a blood thinner to prevent clotting known as heparin. The balloon is usually advanced up the aorta under fluoroscope x-ray guidance and is used for people in non-blood loss shock, usually from a heart attack or a severe infection and other causes of a weakened heart muscle. The normal heart pumping output of four to five liters a minute is much less than required, and IABP only increases the flow out of the heart by only an additional 0.5 to 1.0 liters (about a quart) per minute. It is a form of treatment known as counter-pulsation.

Earliest studies using early primitive models were performed at Western Reserve in 1951 by Adrial Kantrowitz, and preliminary animal studies were performed in 1961 by S. Moulopoulos, working with Wilhelm Kolff and published in 1962. The first human clinical use was in 1966 by Adrian Kantrowitz in two patients, one who died after 24 hours and one after eleven days. But he was impressed by the blood pressure support provided. In 1970 Mortimer Buckley, Robert Leinbach, and John Kastor at the Massachusetts General Hospital in Boston reported its use after cardiac surgery in a weakened heart patient. By 1975 the technique was used in many institutions, including ours for a young woman with toxic shock syndrome. And by 1980 over 50,000 IABP pumps were implanted.

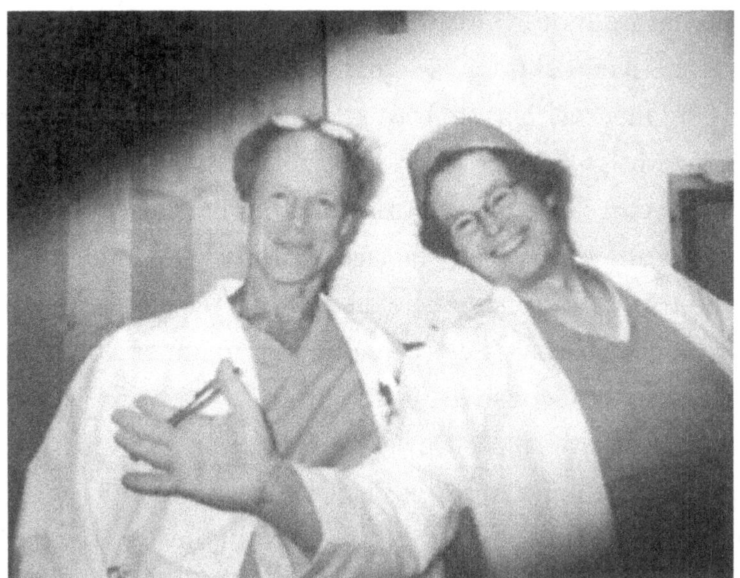

Drs Robert Leinbach and Dr Herman"Chip"Gold
permission to use from Dr Palacios' personal collection

THE IMPELLA HEART PUMP

A competitor to the IABP was developed and FDA approved in 2008. Its invention is owed to a physician, Dr. Richard Wampler, who visited Egypt in 1976 and became interested in irrigation pumps for wells and recognized that the ancient Egyptian Archimedes Screw might be useful for the weakened heart. The Archimedes Screw is a helical metal device attached around the outside of a central metal pole and then set inside a cylindrical shaft (i.e.a hollow tube). It is used to remove water from a pool by trapping the water in air pockets when the helical shaft is turned or cranked to lift the water out. It must be at an incline angle to work and will not work when vertical. It has been used for centuries to scoop up water from a lake or well. Wampler recognized that the principle might be used to empty blood from the left ventricle into the aorta when the left ventricle was weak.

In 1985 Wampler developed the first Hemopump (Medtronic, Minneapolis), which was the precursor to the Impella Heart Pump. Dr. O. H. Frazier, in 1988 at the Texas Heart Institute made headlines when he placed the first Hemopump in a patient's heart. Despite its initial clinical success, it did not become a commercial success and was discontinued. In 1991 a group of Germans led by Seiss in Aachen, Germany, redesigned the system using a much shorter rotating impeller rather than a long screw, which the Hemopump had. He also attached a miniature motor to turn the pump. Although Seiss is given credit for its design, the eventual Impella actually owes its birth to Dr Helmuth Ruel, a biomedical engineer with a PhD from the University of Houston. Ruel had conversations with Dr Frazier when Dr Ruel was still in Houston after they met at a social event. He went to work when he returned to Achen, Germany on what later became the Impella Device and shortened the pump and miniaturized the motor. Unfortunately, he died of lung cancer before he could see his device brought to market. Seiss actually worked under Ruel. A hollow catheter is inserted percutaneously from the groin over a wire, which is then removed with the catheter placed into the tip of the left ventricle, stabilized because the catheter tip is shaped like a curved pig's tail. It has a series of holes from the curled tip up the catheter shaft to draw in the blood with the impeller motorized rotator inside the left ventricle itself. Meynes and colleagues in 2000 and 2003 evaluated the newer device in Leuven, Belgium. Europe approved its use in 2005 and the U.S. F.D.A. approved its use in 2008.

Despite the ability to pump two and a half or five liters of blood per minute and decompress the left ventricle and its ability to perfuse tissues better than the IABP, the survival in studies was no different between these two devices in early studies. A recent study in 2022, however, showed a survival advantage for the Impella. The price of the Impella device is much greater than the IABP. Both devices continue to be used in cardiogenic shock and high-risk coronary stenting procedures and improve blood pressure, coronary artery blood flow, and reduce the work of the heart's left ventricle.

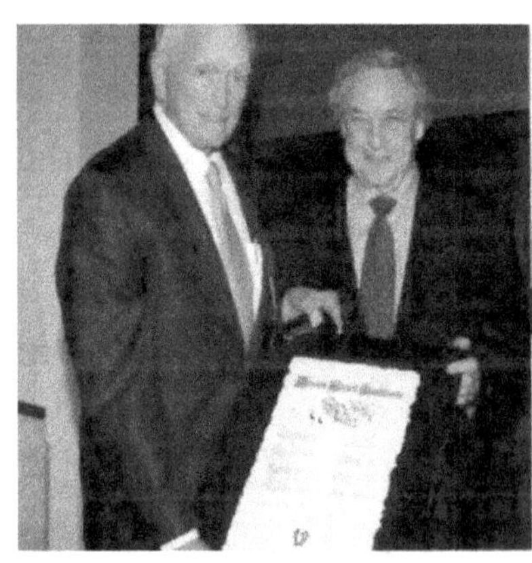

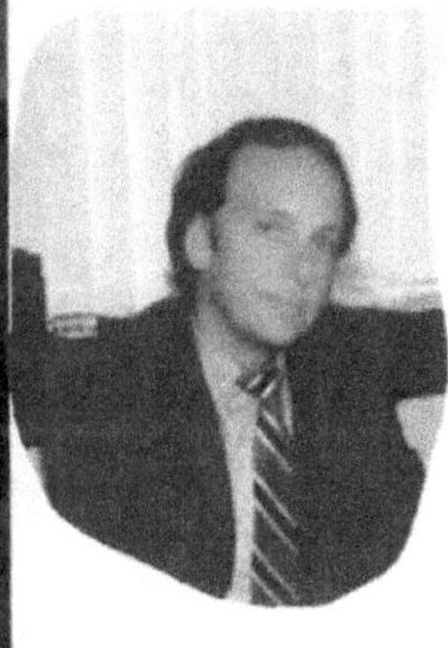

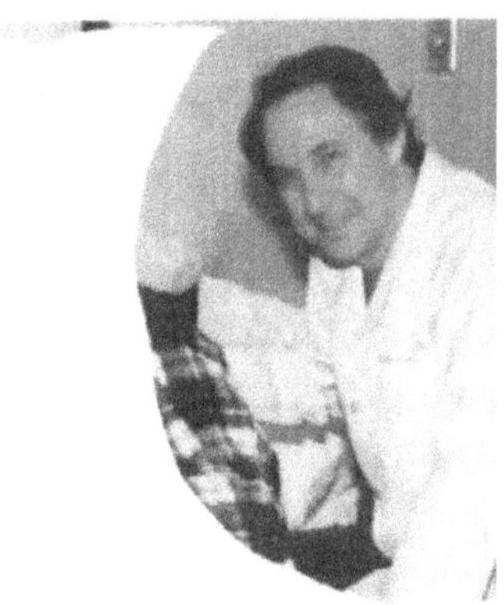

Dr Denton Cooley   Dr Richard Wampler   Dr O. H. "Bud" Frazier
and Dr O.H. Frazier

permission to use from Dr Frazier's personal collection

ECMO (EXTRACORPOREAL MEMBRANE OXYGENATION)

ECMO is the third "bailout" device for cardiogenic shock. It is called "an artificial life support" system, to help a patient with lung and heart failure. The system pumps blood out of the body to a machine, which oxygenates the blood and rids it of the carbon dioxide. It then pumps the oxygenated blood back into the body. This allows the body to function while the heart and lungs are resting. Although not as frequently used as IABP and the IMPELLA. In 2021 twenty thousand patients worldwide received its benefits. Dr. Robert Bartlett first used ECMO in a baby in 1971 after performing research on sheep. He is considered the Father of ECMO and led the program at the University of Michigan Hospital.

ROBOTIC ANGIOPLASTY

Angioplasty historically has been performed with the operator standing at the right side of the recumbent patient on an x-ray table and pushing and twisting catheters to the appropriate position. I worked for five years on a robotic angioplasty device to perform it, sitting away from the x-ray machine to reduce stress on the neck and back from heavy leaded aprons, which protect from x-ray scatter and even to theoretically perform the procedure at a great distance away from the patient. My two partners and I dropped the project (although we developed a prototype) for want of funding and when an Israeli company beat us to a European patent. The Corpath is one such system today, but for some reason only a few hospitals have at the time of this writing accepted the need for robotic angioplasty.

MEDICAL THERAPEUTICS

1. Heart failure, along with diuretics and beta blockers such as metoprolol and carvedilol, the newest medications in the cardiologist's armamentarium, includes the use of aldosterone (a mild diuretic acting differently from most other diuretics and helping symptoms of heart failure), Farxiga and Jardiance, which were meant originally as diabetic drugs but reduce death and hospitalizations from heart failure even in nondiabetics, and Entresto (sacubitril in combination with valsartan), a drug that improves cardiac function by unloading the heart and reducing its resistance to pumping blood out so the heart need not work as hard. Heart

failure is either systolic (the pumping phase) or diastolic (the resting phase) or a combination of both. In systolic heart failure, the left ventricle pumps poorly with a reduced amount of blood pumped out with each heartbeat (ejection fraction). This is also known as HFrEF (heart failure with reduced ejection fraction (pronounced "hef ref")). In diastolic heart failure, the heart is stiff and cannot accept the normal filling from the left atrium and often backs up the blood into the lung, which the left ventricle cannot adequately accommodate, although the pumping fraction of blood remains normal. This is known as HFpEF (heart failure with preserved ejection fraction and is pronounced "hef pef").

2. Cholesterol treatment – see Chapter 15

3. Amyloidosis treatment – Vyndaqel and Vindamax are related oral drugs to treat cardiac amyloidosis by preventing further deposition in the left ventricle. Amyloid is an abnormal protein produced by the liver or the bone marrow, which prevents normal sliding of heart muscle fibers to shorten as the heart pumps blood out. A new drug to remove amyloid from the heart is now in therapeutic trials as well.

GLOSSARY CHAPTER 17

Echocardiogram – ultrasound obtaining pictures of the heart's motion, size and valves

C-MRI (Cardiac MRI) – Cardiac Magnetic Resonance Imaging, test to obtain pictures of the heart using high-powered magnets. The patient is in a tunnel, sometimes preventing claustrophobic patients from completing the test.

Cardiac PET – an imaging test using radioactive sugar to see if a disease known as sarcoidosis is affecting the heart

CRT (cardiac resynchronization therapy – a second pacer wire is inserted in the base of the right atrium and fished up the coronary sinus to the outer-left side of the heart to allow simultaneous pacing the right ventricular wire to improve heart performance.

REFERENCES

CHAPTER 1

Cardiac Classics. A Collection of Classic Works on the Heart and Circulation with Comprehensive Biographic Accounts of the Authors. By Fredrick A. Willius and Thomas E. Keys. C. V. Mosby Co. 1941, pp. 191-216, pp. 323-382, pp. 80-811.

A Short History of Cardiology. By James B. Herrick. Charles C. Thomas, Publisher, 1942,

History of Cardiology. By H. A. Snellen Donker Academic Publications, the Netherlands, 1984, p. 243.

The Collected Essays of Sir William Osler. Edited by John P. McGovern and Charles G. Roland. The Classics of Medicine Library, 1985.

Profiles in Cardiology. Edited by J. Willis Hurst, C. Richard Conti, and W. Bruce Fye, 2003.

Medical History, 1989, 33:42-71. The Cardiology of R.T.H. Laennec, Jacalyn M. Duffin.

CHAPTER 2

A Short History of Cardiology, 1942. By James B. Herrick. Charles C. Thomas, Publisher, Chicago.

DE HUMANI CORPORIS FABRICA (1543). Vesalius.

MOTU CORDIS ET SANGUINIS (Movement of the Heart and Blood), William Harvey, 1728. De Motu Cordis et Aneurysmatibus (Motion of the Heart and on Aneurysms), Lancisi Cardiac Classics, 1941. Willius, F. A.; and Keys, T. E.

1733 HAEMASTATICKS, Stephen Hales.

1691, Tractus de Corde, Richard Lower.

1802, "Commentaries on the History and Cure of Disease," (Willius) Heberden.

Profiles in Cardiology. Edited by J. Wilis Hurst, C. Richard Conti and W. Bruce Fye, 2003.

Texas Heart Journal, 2002, 29(3), pp. 164-171, Mehta, N.; and Khan, I.

Coronary Thrombosis and Myocardial Infarction, Classic Papers. Edited by W. Bruce Fye. Gryphon Editions, 2008.

History of Cardiology – A Brief Outline of the 350 Years' Prelude to an Explosive Growth, 1984. Snellen, H. A., Donker Academic Publications, Rotterdam.

Cardiac Classics, 1941. A Collection of Classic Works on the Heart and Circulation with Comprehensive Biographic Accounts of the Authors. Willius, F. A.; Keya, T. E.; C. V. Mosby, St. Louis.

CHAPTER 3

Cardiac Classics: A Collection of Classic Works on the Heart and Circulation with Comprehensive Biographic Accounts of the Authors. By Fredrick A. Willius and Thomas E. Keys. C. V. Mosby Co., 1941.

The Lancet, Jan. 18, 1879. Murrell, W. Nitro-Glycerin as a Remedy for Angina Pectoris.

CHAPTER 4

Kidney Blood Press Res (2005) 28 (4) 259-3 Paskalevm, Dm; Kiurcheva, A.; Krivoshiev, S. A. Century of Auscultatory Blood Pressure Measurement: A Tribute to Nikolai Korotkoff.

Profiles in Cardiology. Edited by J. Willis Hurst, C. Richard Conti and W. Bruce Fye, 2003.

CHAPTER 5

Profiles in Cardiology. Edited by J. Willis Hurst, C. Richard Conti and W. Bruce Fye, 2003.

Circulation, 70 no. 5, 1984, pp. 781-787. Coronary arteriography – It took a long time?

American Heart Journal, Mar. 1950, pp. 357-359. Zimmerman, H.; Scott, R.; Becker, N. Catheterization of the Left Side of the Heart in Man.

Nobel Lecture, Dec. 12, 1956. Forssmann, W. The Role of Heart Catheterization and Angiocardiography in the Development of Modern Medicine.

Circulation 2992, 106: pp. 752-756. Ryan, T. J. The Coronary Angiogram and its Seminal Contributions to Cardiovascular Medicine over Five Decades.

European Heart Journal, 10 December 2007. Letter to the Editor: Otto Klein – the forgotten founder of diagnostic cardiac catheterization.

Journal American College of Cardiology, 45, 3, 2004. Stern, S. A Note on the History of Cardiology: Dr. Otto Klein, 1881-1968.

Journal Clinical Investigation, 1945, 24 (1), pp. 106-116. Cournand, A.; Riley, R. L.; Breed, E. S.; Richards, D. W.; Lester, M. S.; Jones, M. Measurement of Cardiac Output in Man Using the Technique of Catheterization of the Right Auricle or Ventricle.

Acta Radiology, 1953, 39: pp. 368-376. Seldinger, S. I. Catheter Replacement of the Needle in Percutaneous Arteriography.

Radiology, 1967, 89, pp. 815-824. Judkins, M. P. Selective Coronary Arteriography: I: A Percutaneous Transfemoral Technique.

American Heart Journal, 1960: 60, pp. 762-776. Dodge, H. T.; Sandler, J.; Ballew, D. W., et al. The Use of Biplane Angiocardiography for the Measurement of Left Ventricular Volume in Man.

Texas Heart Institute Journal, 2000, 27 (3) pp. 234-235. Cooley, D. A. In Memoriam: Tribute to Ake Senning, Pioneering Cardiovascular Surgeon.

CHAPTER 6

Rentrop (Clinical Cardiology, vol. 2, pp. 354-63, 1979).

New England Journal of Medicine, 1980, 303: pp. 897-902. DeWood, M. A.; Spores, J.; Notske, R.; Mouser, L.; Burroughs, M. D.; Golden, M. S.; and Lang, H. T. Prevalence of Total Coronary Occlusion during the Early Hours of Transmural Myocardial Infarction.

Texas Heart Institute Journal, 1984, Mar. 11 (1), pp. 44-51. Selinger, S. L.; Berg, R.; Leonard, J. J.; Coleman, W. S.; DeWood, M. A. Surgical Intervention in Acute Myocardial Infarction.

New England Journal of Medicine, 1984, No. 23, vol. 311, pp. 1457-1463. Rentrop, K. P., et al. Effects of Intracoronary streptokinase and Intracoronary Nitroglycerin Infusion on Coronary Angiographic Patterns and Mortality in Patients with Acute Myocardial Infarction.

Clinical Cardiology, 1978. 1, pp. 101-106. Rentrop, P.; DeVivie, R.; Karsch, K. R.; Kreuzer, H. Acute Coronary Occlusion with Impending Infarction as an Angiographic Complication Relieved by Guide Wire Recanalization.

National Academy of Sciences, 1993. Lawrence, H. S. William Smith Tillett: 1892-1974: A Biographical Memoir.

CHAPTER 7

Texas Heart Institute Journal, 2001:28 (1), pp. 28-38. Payne, M. M. Charles Theodore Dotter: Father of Intervention.

Profiles in Cardiology. Edited by J. Willis Hurst, C. Richard Conti and W. Bruce Fye, 2003.

New England Journal of Medicine, 1979; 301: pp. 61-68. Gruentzig, A. R.; Seining, A.; Siegenthaler, W. E. Non-Operative Dilation of Coronary Artery Stenosis in Percutaneous Transluminal Coronary Angioplasty.

New England Journal of Medicine, 316 (12): pp. 701-706. Sigwart, U.; Puel, J., et al. Intravascular Stents to Prevent Occlusion and Restenosis after Transluminal Angioplasty.

Roubin, Gary S. The First Balloon Expandable Coronary Stent – An Expedition That Changed Cardiovascular Medicine, A Memoir, University of Queensland Press.

CHAPTER 8

Circ. 71:1985, pp. 858-865. Fye, W. B. Ventricular fibrillation and defibrillation: historical perspectives with emphasis on the contributions of John MacWilliam, Carl Wiggers, and William Kouwenhoven.

Circulation, 1998, 97, 1978-1991. Jeffrey, K.; Parsonnet, V.

Cardiac Pacing, 1960-1985. A Quarter Century of Medical and Industrial Innovation.

Physiology 8:296, 1887, MacWilliam, J. A.), Fibrillar Contraction of the Heart.

CHAPTER 9

Circ. 2003:107:2168-2170. Cohn, L. Fifty Years of Open-Heart Surgery.

Circulation, 28 Sept., 1999. 217, 1364. Cooley, D. A. C. Walton Lillehei, the Father of Open Heart Surgery Anesthesia, 61, 10, pp. 984-995. Lim, M. W. The History of Extracorporeal Oxygenators.

CHAPTER 10

Circulation, 1998; 98; pp. 466-478. Favaloro, R. Landmarks in the Development of Coronary Artery Bypass Surgery.

CHAPTER 11

Cardiovascular Medicine, 29 September 2021. Andersen, H. R. How Transcatheter Aortic Valve Implantation (TAVI) Was Born: The Struggle for a New Invention.

American Journal of Cardiology , Feb 17 , 2024 In Memoriam: Alain Cribier

American Journal of Cardiology , July 20, 2017 Harold, J.G., Harold on History:The Evolution of Transcatheter Aortic Valve Replacement

Interv Cardiology 2014, April 9(2) 121-125 Noorani, A and Bapat, V, Differences in Outcomes and Indications between Sapien and Core Valve Transcatheter Aortic Valve Implantation

Journal of Thoracic Surgery, Vol. 36, No. 6, pp. 839-856. Glover, R. P.; Gadboys, H. L. Seven Years' Experience with Transventricular Aortic Commissurotomy.

CHAPTER 12

Published in 1965, Lower, R. R.; Dong, E.; Shumway, N. E. Long-term survival of cardiac homografts. Surgery 1965:58: pp. 110-119.

CHAPTER 13

At the Smithsonian, April 2019. Swartz, M. The Rivalry Between Two Doctors to Implant the First Artificial Heart.

Profiles in Cardiology. Edited by J. Willis Hurst, C. Richard Conti and W. Bruce Fye, 2003.

CHAPTER 14

Scherlag, B. J.; Lau, S. H.; Helfant, R. H.; Berkowitz, W. D.; Stein, E.; and

Damato, A. N. Circ. 1969, 39, pp. 13-18. Catheter Technique for Recording HIS Bundle Recordings in Man.

New England Journal of Medicine, 1998. Haissaguerre, M.; Jais, P.; Shah, D. C., et al. NEJM

(Petra Kuijpers, History in Medicine. The Road to Clinical Electrophysiology. European Society of Cardiology, 21: pp. 13-15, 2021).

Durrer, D.; Schoo, L.; Schullenburg, R. M.; and Wellens, H. J. Circ. 1967:36, pp. 544-662. The role of premature beats in the initiation and termination of supraventricular in the Wolf-Parkinson-White syndrome.

Circulation, 57, no. 5, May 1978, pp. 854-866. Gallaher, J. J.; Kassel, J.; Sealy, W., et al. Epicardial Mapping in the Wolff-Parkinson-White Syndrome.

Heart Rhythm Disorders History, Mechanisms, and Management Perspectives. Springer, Gomes, J. A. Springer, 2020.

Journal of the American College of Cardiology, 44; 6; 2004, pp. 1155-1163. Wellens, H. J. J. Cardiac Arrhythmias: The Quest for a Cure; a Historical Perspective.

Josephson, M. E.; Harken, A. H.; Hurwitz, L.; Ann Thorac Surg, 1979: 60: pp. 1430-39.

Endocardial excision: A new surgical technique for the treatment of recurrent ventricular tachycardia.

Journal of Cardiology, Practice 21 (13), 15 December 2021. Kuijpers, M. J. C. History in Medicine: The Road to Clinical Electrophysiology.

CHAPTER 15

Lancet (1994, pp. 1383-1389. Randomized trial of cholesterol lowering in 4444 patients – the 4-S Trial.

Nobel Prize Press Release, 1985. Michael Brown and Joseph Goldstein, Nobel Prize in Physiology or Medicine, 1985.

Circulation, Jan. 7, 2014, pp. 77-86. Martin, S., et al. Dyslipidemia, Coronary Artery Calcium, and Incident Atherosclerotic Cardiovascular Disease, Implications for Statin Therapy from the Multi-Ethnic Study of Atherosclerosis Cell, 2015. Mar. 26; 161(1), pp. 161-172. Goldstein, J.; Brown, M. S. A Century of Cholesterol and Coronaries: From Plaque to Genes to Statins.

European Society of Cardiology Journal, vol. 19 (9), pp. 9-13, 2021. Kuljpers, P. M. J. C. History in Medicine: The Story of Cholesterol, Lipids and Cardiology.

CHAPTER 16

Cardiac Classics, 1941. Willius, F. A.; Keys, T. E; C. V. Mosby Co., St. Louis.

A Short History of Cardiology, 1942. Herrick, J. B.; Charles C. Thomas, Chicago.

History of Cardiology – A Brief Outline of the 350 Years' Prelude to an Explosive Growth, 1984. Snellen, H. A. Donker Academic Publications, Rotterdam.

Autopsy and Case Reports 2013: 3(4):5-12 Geller, S , Infective Endocarditis: A History of the Development of Its Understanding

CHAPTER 17

European Heart Journal, 2002, 23(9), pp. 1130-1143. Fraser, A. F.; Monaghan, M. J. A Concise History of Echocardiography: Timeline, Pioneers, and Landmark Publications.

New England Journal of Medicine, 2009; 361: pp. 1329-1338. Moss, A. J., et al. Cardiac Resynchronization Therapy for the Prevention of Heart Failure Events.

Journal of the American College of Cardiology, 1 (5) 2008, pp. 672-678. Pohost, G. M. The History of Cardiovascular Magnetic Resonance.

Int J Angiol, 2019, Jun;28 (2) : 118-123 Glazier, J and Kaki, A, The Impella Device: Historical Background, Clinical Applications and Future Directions

INDEX

Beck, Claude 164

Bernard, Claude 82,83

Bicuspid Aortic Valve 171

Blalock, Alfred 156

Bleichroeder, Fritz 84

Bloch, Felix 268

Bloch, Konrad 234

Blood pressure 75,76,77,78

Borel, Jean 192

Braunwald, Eugene 257,258

Braunwald, Nina 177

Brown, Michael 238, 240

Brunton, Thomas Lauder 68, 69

Buchner, Johann Andreas 71

Buchard, Henri 143

Budoff, Matthew 265,266

Bundle of HIS 205,215

Burns, Allan 50

CABG 161

Capillaries 31

Cappelin, Axel 152

Cardiac catheterization 81-98

Cardiac MRI 267, 268, 269

Cardiac PET scanning 270

Carrel, Alexis 163,187

Caves, Phillip 188, 190

Chardack, William 144, 145

Chauveau, Auguste 85

Chirac, Pierre 42

Cholesterol 229

Circumflex coronary artery 21

Cohnheim, Julius Friedrich 52,53

Cooley, Denton 191,196,197

Compactin 241

Diuretic 70

Dodge, Harold 96

Dotter, Charles 112,113

Durrer, Dirk 213,214

ECMO (extra corporeal membrane oxygenator) 275

Edler, Inge 262,263

ECG (EKG) 57, 58

Echocardiogram 261, 262, 263

Effler, Donald 165

Einthoven, Willem 57, 58

Emmanuelsson, Haakon

Endo, Akiro 241,242,243

Endocarditis 295

EP (electrophysiology) 201-227

Erichsen, John 51

Ernst, Richard 268

Ethacrynic acid 70

Farxiga and Jardiance 275

Favaloro, Rene 168

Flack, Martin 208

Fisch, Arthur 98, 222

Flint, Austin 173

Forssmann Werner 85-88

Fothergill, John 47

Framingham Heart Study 236

Frazier, O.H. 273. 274

Frank, Howard 145

Furman, Seymour 148

Galen 20

Gallagher, John 217, 218

Gangee, Arthur 69

Gaskell, Walter 206, 207

Ganz, William 95

Geng, Yong jian 127

Marey,Etienne-Jules 86

Marchlinski, Francis 25. 226. 227

MacWilliam, John Alexander 132, 133

Mann, Frank C 187

Master, Arthur 61

Matteucci, Carlo 204

Medtronic Hall valve 176

Mercuriale, Geronimo

Mevacor 241

Miracle Trial 271

Mirowski, Michel 148

Morgangni, Giovanni (Giambattista) 44

Mower, Martin 148

Muller, Carl 234

Murrell, William 69

Myler, Richard 119

Nitroglycerin 68

Nuclear powered pacemaker 146

Osler, William 10, 11, 12

Pacemaker 139, 140

Palacios, Igor 178

Palmaz, Julio 124,125

Pardee, Harold 61

Parr, Grant 151,152

Parry, Caleb Hillier 48, 49

Parsonnet, Victor 146

Pasteur, Louis 249, 250

Pennsylvania Peel 223

Pericardium 246

Perloff, Joseph 13, 14, 15

Physical diagnosis 1

POBA (plain old balloon angioplasty) 119

Pohost, Gerald 268, 269

Poulletier, Francois 230, 231